D0302012

Research and Development in Mental Health

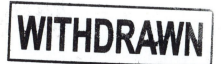

WITHDRAWN

Commissioning Editor: Susan Young
Development Editor: Catherine Jackson
Project Manager: Cheryl Brant
Designer: Judith Wright
Illustration Manager: John Marshall

WITHDRAWN

Research and Development in Mental Health

Theory, Frameworks and Models

Edited by

David Sallah PhD MSc RN

Director of Research, Ethics and Consultancy, School of Health,
University of Wolverhampton; Professor of Mental Health, UK

Michael Clark PhD MPhil BA(Hons)

National Portfolio Manager for Mental Health Research and Development,
Department of Health; Research and Development Manager
Wolverhampton City Primary Care Trust, UK

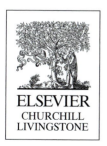

ELSEVIER
CHURCHILL
LIVINGSTONE

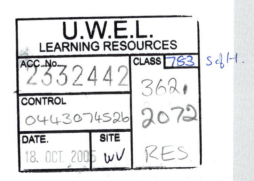

U.W.E.L.
LEARNING RESOURCES

ACC.No. 2332442

CONTROL 0443074526

DATE. 18. OCT. 2005 SITE wV

CLASS 753 sdH.

362.

2072

RES

EDINBURGH   LONDON   NEW YORK   OXFORD   PHILADELPHIA   ST LOUIS   SYDNEY   TORONTO   2005

ELSEVIER
CHURCHILL
LIVINGSTONE

An imprint of Elsevier Limited

© 2005, Elsevier Limited. All rights reserved.

The right of David Sallah and Michael Clark to be identified as editors of this work has been asserted by them in accordance with the Copyright, Designs and Patents Act 1988.

No part of this publication may be reproduced, stored in a retrieval system, or transmitted in any form or by any means, electronic, mechanical, photocopying, recording or otherwise, without either the prior permission of the publishers or a licence permitting restricted copying in the United Kingdom issued by the Copyright Licensing Agency, 90 Tottenham Court Road, London W1T 4LP. Permissions may be sought directly from Elsevier's Health Sciences Rights Department in Philadelphia, USA: phone: (+1) 215 238 7869, fax: (+1) 215 238 2239, e-mail: healthpermissions@elsevier.com. You may also complete your request on-line via the Elsevier homepage (http://www.elsevier.com), by selecting 'Customer Support' and then 'Obtaining Permissions'.

First published 2005

ISBN 0 4430 7452 6

British Library Cataloguing in Publication Data
A catalogue record for this book is available from the British Library

Library of Congress Cataloging in Publication Data
A catalog record for this book is available from the Library of Congress

Notice

Medical knowledge and best practice in this field are constantly changing. As new research and experience broaden our knowledge, changes in practice, treatment and drug therapy may become necessary or appropriate. Readers are advised to check the most current information provided (i) on procedures featured or (ii) by the manufacturer of each product to be administered, to verify the recommended dose or formula, the method and duration of administration, and contraindications. It is the responsibility of the practitioner, relying on their own experience and knowledge of the patient, to make diagnoses, to determine dosages and the best treatment for each individual patient, and to take all appropriate safety precautions. To the fullest extent of the law, neither the publisher nor the editors assumes any liability for any injury and/or damage.

The Publisher

your source for books,
journals and multimedia
in the health sciences
www.elsevierhealth.com

The
publisher's
policy is to use
**paper manufactured
from sustainable forests**

Printed in China

Contents

Part III – METHODS AND FRAMEWORKS

About the editors

Dr David Sallah is Professor of Mental Health and Director of Research, Ethics and Consultancy in the School of Health, University of Wolverhampton. Professor Sallah was a service practitioner (nurse, manager, service development consultant) before his academic appointment. He has worked in the Department of Health and also has experience as a member of national committees. He works with a plethora of national organizations helping to shape services for people with mental health problems.

Dr Mike Clark is the Research and Development Manager for Wolverhampton City Primary Care Trust and the National Manager for the Mental Health Research and Development Portfolio at the Department of Health. He has a PhD and is an Honorary Research Fellow with the University of Wolverhampton.

Contributors

Piers Allott DipSocStud CertAppSocStud CQSW
*NIMHE Fellow for Recovery, Senior Service Development Fellow,
University of Wolverhampton, UK*

Zaubia Alyas
Consultant Psychiatrist, East London & City Mental Health Trust

Susan Barnes BA
Senior Research Manager, Department of Health (retired August 2004)

Kamaldeep Bhui
*Professor of Cultural Psychiatry & Epidemiology, Barts & The London
School of Medicine, Queen Mary, London*

Max Birchwood DSc FBPsS
*Director, Birmingham Early Intervention Service; Professor of Mental
Health, University of Birmingham, UK*

Clair Chilvers DSc FFPH
*Director, NHS Research and Development Portfolio in Mental Health
Research Director, National Institute for Mental Health in England,
Nottingham, UK*

Michael Clark PhD MPhil BA(Hons)
*National Portfolio Manager for Mental Health Research and
Development, Department of Health; Research and Development
Manager, Wolverhampton City Primary Care Trust, UK*

John R. Cutcliffe RMN RGN BSc(Hons)Nrsg PhD
*Professor and Chair of Nursing, University of Northern British Columbia,
Canada*

Ann Davis
*Professor of Social Work and Deputy Dean of Arts and Social Sciences,
University of Birmingham, UK*

Tim Freeman BA MSc
Lecturer, Health Sciences Management Centre, University of Birmingham, UK

Kevin M. Hogan PhD
Associate Dean and Head of Psychology, School of Applied Sciences, University of Wolverhampton, UK

David Jolley BSc MSc FRCPsych
Director of Dementia Plus, University of Wolverhampton; Consultant Psychiatrist, Wolverhampton Primary Care Trust, UK

Frank Keating BSocSci(SW)Hons Doctor of Social Work (DSW)
Senior Research Fellow, The Sainsbury Centre for Mental Health, London, UK

Alison Longwill
Women's Programme Lead: National Institute for Mental Health in England West Midlands Regional Development Centre

Alistair McIntyre BSc(Hons) DMS
Deputy Director, National Institute for Mental Health in England West Midlands Mental Health Development Centre, UK

Elizabeth Newton BSc(Psych) DClinPsy
Birmingham Early Intervention Service, UK

Peter Nolan PhD MEd BEd(Hons) BA(Hons) RMN RGN DN RNT
Professor of Mental Health Nursing, School of Health, Staffordshire University, UK

Sarah Orme BSc(Hons)
Research Fellow, University of Wolverhampton, UK

Kate Read MA(Gerontology)
Executive Director, Dementia Plus, University of Wolverhampton, UK

David Rogers BA(Hons)
Assistant Chief Executive, Hyndburn and Ribble Valley Primary Care Trust, Accrington, Lancashire, UK

David Sallah PhD MSc RN
Director of Research, Ethics and Consultancy, School of Health;
Professor of Mental Health, University of Wolverhampton, UK

Antony Sheehan DSci MPhil BEd(Hons) RN DHSM CertEd(FE)
Director of Care Services, The Department of Health; Professor of Health
and Social Care Strategy, University of Central Lancashire, UK

Sue Spiers PhD
Assistant Programme Manager, The National Forensic Mental Health
Programme, University of Liverpool, UK

Ingrid Steele BA(Hons)
Director of Underpinning Strategies, National Institute for Mental Health
in England, Leeds, UK

Judy Whitmarsh MA PGCE RGN
Doctoral Student, University of Wolverhampton, UK

Introduction

David Sallah and Michael Clark

Mental health is one of the top three clinical health priorities, alongside coronary heart disease and cancer, for the United Kingdom. It is fair to say that the Government's approach to developing mental health services has presented the services with the best opportunity for improving the lives of people at a time when they are vulnerable. The publication of the *National service framework for mental health* (DoH 1999), the first National Service Framework (NSF), was a landmark event in mental health care in England. It was an important marker in the operationalisation of health policy, namely that of increased central direction of broad health policy. It also expressed a desire for greater use of the evidence base to guide central policy making and local service delivery. The *National service framework for mental health* (p. 4) contains a commitment to the established hierarchy of evidence, with the experience and views of professionals and users at the bottom, moving up through evidence from a range of research methods, to that from randomised controlled trials and then systematic reviews at the pinnacle. In other words, a commitment to the orthodoxy of research evidence. Yet, it is clear in the *National service framework for mental health*, and has become even more apparent since, that the evidence base for some of the service development proposed in both that and subsequent policy statements, such as the *NHS plan* (DoH 1999), did not always match up to the preferred forms in this hierarchy.

There have been continued efforts to identify research priorities for mental health. The Mental Health Topic Working Group (MHTWG) (1999) of the Clarke Review of NHS R&D reported priority areas that included evaluating service models relevant to achieving delivery of the standards of the *National service framework for mental health*. Thornicroft *et al.* (2002) similarly identified a set of research priorities and questions with regard to the *National service framework for mental health*. In essence, both publications are endeavouring to set a research agenda that the authors feel is seen to be more closely allied to current policy and service needs. They are seeking to contribute to closing the gap between research and development. As the MHTWG (1999, p. 4) said of its report:

The emphasis is heavily on the development side of R&D. We need to know a great deal more about the effectiveness, the costs, user satisfaction and engagement rates with interventions whose efficacy has already been established in small scale trials. We need to know whether existing services, and service models to be implemented with the National Service Framework, actually deliver what is intended in a range of circumstances.

Further developments in mental health care have some bearing on this relationship between research and development. The establishment of the National Institute for Mental Health in England (NIMHE) is an attempt to establish an organisation to provide leadership to mental health service development throughout England. Its Regional Development Centres (RDCs) provide a national network for disseminating mental health policy and good practice. Alongside the RDCs, we have a developing Mental Health Research Network (MHRN). The 'hubs' of this provide an interface between academic organisations and clinical settings with a view that they will provide both the ideas and participants for large-scale research projects ultimately aimed at improving care. It remains to be seen what the impact of these developments will be on R&D in mental health care, and especially on the relationship between research and development.

This espoused commitment to the use of research in practice is a key theme of this book. The complex issues in the interaction between Research (R) and Development (D) are at the heart of an R&D strategy. The R&D strategy for the NHS was a significant development.

Throughout its comparatively short history, though, the strategy has been the subject of marked changes, often reinforcing the extent of concern about the lack of stability in the environment within which it is to be implemented. From the standpoint of the summer of 2004, it seems very likely that further developments are coming soon. Two significant reports are being given high-level attention within the Department of Health. The first, the report from the Academy of Medical Sciences (2003) argues a case for the need to strengthen clinical research to close a perceived gap between new discoveries in basic science research and their application to innovations to improve health. The Academy argues that, factors such as an underdeveloped infrastructure, inadequate funding, and increasingly complex bureaucracy mean that there are not enough clinical trials and too little experimental medicine research in the UK. The Academy's report contains a number of recommendations intended to remedy its analysis of the problem. These include creating a national network for clinical research within the NHS; new funding, including increasing the proportion of the NHS budget dedicated to R&D to 1.5% of its turnover; better career structures and incentives for clinical researchers; improving the regulatory framework for clinical research; and promoting greater public involvement. Whilst not new recommendations, put together and articulated in this way they are presenting a powerful case.

The second report, *Bioscience 2015: improving national health, increasing national wealth* (Bioscience Innovation & Growth Team 2003) (BIG T), argues for a better environment in the UK to facilitate the development and testing of products from the biosciences. This includes proposing the creation of a National Clinical Trials Agency (NCTA) to support excellence in clinical trials and clinical research, having a regulatory environment supportive of innovation, ensuring appropriate funding, developing capacity amongst staff, and establishing a Bioscience Leadership Council (comprising industry representatives and six other strategic stakeholders) to make all this happen. The detail of the Government's response to these recommendations is yet to be explained; however, it is apparent that there is a clear drive for substantial support for clinical trials. What the implications of this will be, across the range of research, remains to be seen.

Both of these reports refer to the whole of NHS R&D across health issues. Whilst they are not specific to mental health, if their recommendations are acted upon, they will have implications for research in this field.

The close cousin of NHS R&D is the world of academic research. Here too, in Higher Education (HE) we see, at the time of writing, major debates that are likely to have significant impact on mental health R&D. Feverish debates are ongoing about the funding and structure of teaching and research in institutions of HE.

Given the prominence being placed on R&D in mental health service development and the policy shifts in NHS R&D and HE, it is particularly appropriate to review the current situation of research and development in mental health. Whilst this will have a predominantly English perspective, a great deal of the discussion in this book will be of interest in other countries.

This book is organised into three main parts, each on a separate, but related, theme. The first part is that of *Theory and methodology* in relation to mental health R&D. The discussions and debates presented here will be of interest beyond England. In Part II, we present discussions relating to policy. Whilst the policies reviewed are more specific to England, and to some extent the United Kingdom in general, again many of the issues that are being addressed are of wider concern. In the third part of the book, we present some models currently in operation that may be ways of bringing research and development closer together. The application of these approaches will be interesting for others beyond England.

The first chapter in Part I is a discussion of the relationship between research and development in terms of the emerging conceptual framework of a Health Research System (HRS). It includes an overview of the historical development of the NHS R&D strategy, with a discussion of its uncertain settlement that has led policy makers to tinker with it regularly to address, amongst other things, the perceived relevance and importance of the strategy and the links between research and development.

The next two chapters in Part I take up the discussions relating to methodological perspectives in mental health research; firstly by making the case for continuance of the quantitative method, and secondly by making the case for qualitative methods in terms of its popularity and relevance. The established hierarchy of research used in the *National service framework for mental health* places, as we have seen, quantitative methodologies towards the top. Clearly the dominance of the quantitative paradigm both in terms of funding (and consequently the preferred choice of method by researchers) has in a way relegated the qualitative approaches to the lower priority areas of research funding. In recent times, the Mental Health Topic Working Group (1999, p. 6), reported that those commissioning research to support mental health policy development should consider using methodologies and disciplines (such as social sciences and anthropology) that have not traditionally been widely used in mental health research. In these two chapters in Part I, the arguments for and against reliance on the one method at the expense of the other are discussed and the case is made that the choice of method should be dependent upon the nature of the topic and the population being researched. The emerging viewpoint is that scholars and researchers who recognise and espouse a pluralistic approach to research and knowledge generation should be encouraged as there is evidence that the value of qualitative studies is increasingly being recognised as these approaches are starting to receive major funding.

Chapter 4 in this part of the book addresses other approaches to developing a research and development framework in mental health. The author of this chapter develops an understanding by showing the range of research that has been carried out into mental health care, with a view to improving our knowledge of why research does or does not influence practice. In this chapter, the various descriptive and investigative approaches that have been used through the centuries are outlined. Reference is made to creative thinking and innovative treatments and to the impact they have had on mental health care, and to the analysis of the evolution of mental health research to facilitate a better understanding of how effective research could be undertaken today.

In Chapter 5 the author addresses the concept of race and ethnicity in the context of modern day mental health practice. It has been noted that ethnic minorities often receive poor quality mental health services and that this situation presents particular research priorities (Thornicroft *et al.* 2002; NSCStHA 2003). It is argued here that these constructs are shrouded in complexity, fraught with contradictions and tend to evoke a variety of emotional responses that could range from fear to denial and prejudice. Utilising these constructs in research therefore brings us to one of the most contentious spheres of knowledge construction as well as bringing us to policy and service development in mental health. It is suggested in this chapter that the epistemological and ontological considerations that inform research should be taken into account when researchers investigate 'race' and mental health, reflecting this complex area of need in the process.

In Chapter 6 a selective overview and critique of research relating to women is presented. Showalter (1987) provided a timely look at how cultural ideas about 'proper' feminine behaviour have shaped the definition and treatment of mental disorder in women. Chapter 6 builds on the argument for effective and appropriate services for women from the perspective that, although women make up over half of the general population and play a pivotal role in the development of society, the association of women and irrationality over the years has resulted in gender blindness in their diagnosis, treatment and care. It is argued in this chapter that because modern psychiatry has been characterised by the quest for a 'pill for all ills' philosophy it has created a paucity of high-quality evidence to support various assertions which play important roles in the design and development of services for women. The recent government strategy (DoH 2003) for improving the quality of care for women forms the backdrop to the focus of analysis in this chapter.

Part I is concluded by highlighting the need for mental health service users to be included, and even to lead mental health services research.

The author outlines why mental health service-user involvement has emerged as an important concern in the R&D field, what issues it raises for those involved in R&D and the implications of this development for the service user and the R&D communities. It is argued in this chapter that to understand and work productively with the current service-user involvement agenda in R&D, it is important to understand the context in which it has evolved. The point of view is that the focus on service-user involvement in this sphere has its roots in several approaches, not least government action over the years. In this chapter, it is revealed that the most dominant approach reflects the way in which public services in the UK have been increasingly viewed by government as key players in a market of health and welfare provision. As such they have been exhorted to place the interests of those on the receiving end at the heart of their endeavours mirroring the pronouncement in the *NHS plan* which states 'patients are the most important people in the health service'.

Part II of this book discusses what various policy pronouncements mean for mental health research and development. In the first of four chapters in this part, the higher education White Paper is discussed. This White Paper has created many opportunities and, to some extent, challenges for researchers in the university sector and the health economy, particularly in attempts to bridge the gap between research and practice. The locus of this chapter is that the NHS alone cannot address the issues that relate to improving the care and treatment of patients and deliver improved systems of care provision to foster partnership and collaborative working. In calling for this approach, the authors draw attention to the fact that some of the policies shaping the continuing modernisation of the NHS could stymie progress and innovation in the development of a programme of clinical or any other type of research in the health and social care sector.

Next, we address the research and development policy and its context. In Chapter 9 the authors discuss the fact that mental health as a ministerial priority reflects not only the burden of mental ill health and its devastating social consequences, but also the low priority that has been given to improving health and social care services for people suffering from mental distress. They argue that the stigma associated with a diagnosis of severe mental illness, or indeed that associated with suffering from a common mental health problem, has undoubtedly contributed to the inadequate attention paid to mental health services in the past. There are a number of related issues for mental health research; for example, the funding from charitable sources for mental health research is small: there are no wealthy charities such as are associated with the other common conditions, cancer and heart disease. Other issues discussed include the strength of mental health research and the difficulty of mental health as a subject for research.

The National Institute for Mental Health in England (NIMHE) is a product of the concerns relating to lack of co-ordination between policy direction and the mental health services response to implementing the changes necessary to improve patient care. NIMHE, as part of the modernisation of the NHS, takes lead responsibility for mental health programmes and thus has a key role in the future development of mental health services. In the pursuit of effective change in terms of improving services for users, the place that research holds is critical. Chapter 10 provides an insight into the structures that NIMHE has put in place to meet this challenge.

Finally in Part II, clinical governance as a framework for improving quality of care is discussed. As a key policy development in which we might expect research and development to find common territory, it is of crucial importance to understand this policy and its place in models of the NHS. It is seen that clinical governance is a problematic and contentious policy and concept. As such, the authors are cautious about automatically presuming that it is the territory within which research will inform development for local service providers. The argument that clinical governance fits into the context of a range of new external institutions and relationships constituting a strengthening of performance management arrangements is a strong theme that runs throughout this chapter.

It is our intention in this book to bring together key elements of research and development but we cannot maintain that this goal has been achieved without first providing some evidence that the various programmes and service models are making a difference to users of mental health services. In Part III of the book we present insights into actual models within which we might begin to see how research may come together with development to deliver evidence-based service and policy development.

One approach to driving the modernisation of mental health services is the development of Learning, Education, Development Centres (LEDS). The work of the Wolverhampton Dementia Plus Development Centre, which is described in the next chapter, combines the concepts of Dementia Services Development Centres and Learning Education Development Centres to focus on treatment and care of older people with mental health problems in the West Midlands. As a regional centre tasked with being a locus of expertise in mental health for older people, it has an interesting position in relation to the worlds of research and of development.

The first chapter in Part III discusses the positive outcomes that are emerging from the Early Intervention programme. The policy of early intervention in psychosis is one that has been pushed strongly by national policy development. A quick glance at this area of policy may lead one to the conclusion that it is a policy that has developed out of the ether in comparatively recent times. The authors provide historical evidence to the contrary arguing that there is a substantial research and service development activity behind this policy development.

Crisis management is a common concept in the vocabulary of mental health practitioners. It is harder to define what it is and what constitutes a crisis service. In Chapter 14, the authors provide a discussion of the problems relating to aiming for a precise definition and the ramifications of this for research and development in the area. One of the lessons in this chapter is the authors' belief that the 'gold standard' of Randomised Controlled Trial (RCT) research designs is, in the context of complex social systems such as crisis services, at best a malapropism and at worst a chimera. It is argued in this chapter that it is not enough to recognise that treatments are embedded within services but also that services are themselves components of dynamic and complex systems. The authors call for recognition of this, concluding that it is time that systems for planning and managing change within the health sector act as though this were the case.

The next chapter addresses the concept of recovery. The central theme in this chapter is that despite the popularity of recovery as a major approach in empowering service users to play a substantial part in the way their care and treatment is organised and delivered in a growing number of countries worldwide, the take up within the United Kingdom remains low. The author defines 'recovery' as 'the ability to live well in the presence or absence of one's mental illness (or whatever people choose to name their experience). Each person with mental illness needs to define for themselves what "living well" means to them.' Of course there are challenges for mental health practitioners and the service in general in the way it deals with this definition in terms of the impact it has on the current orthodoxy.

Current NHS policy for R&D is to develop a greater strategic alignment with NHS priorities, of which mental health is one. Hence, there are significant efforts underway at national and local levels to develop more and higher quality research programmes in mental health that have relevance to service development needs. In Chapter 16, the importance of local networks as a model that could be used, not only to drive and support research, but also to provide a more direct link between research and development, is explored. The author outlines experiences from an innovative project in Nottingham.

Health care in prisons is a concern for a variety of stakeholders and is a Government priority policy area, and the mental health aspects are discussed in Chapter 17. Most people in a civilised society would accept the fact that a conviction for a criminal offence is not a just cause for the removal of access to the same standards and quality of health care as is available to any other member of the community. However, the mental health care needs of prisoners has largely been overlooked until recently. In a recent survey by the Prison Service, it was found that 90% of those entering prison had a mental health or substance misuse problem. Surveys conducted by the Office for National Statistics in 1997 indicated that nine out of every ten prisoners have at least one of the five disorders considered in the survey (neurosis, psychosis, personality disorder, alcohol abuse or drug dependence). The mental health burden is worse in the women and young offender populations. Clearly, imprisonment provides invaluable opportunities to address some of these health issues. The authors outline the focus of current policy development, which is that the NHS should have direct accountability for the health care needs of prisoners. The authors chart some of the key milestones in providing care to prisoners and some of the implications for this so called 'principle of equivalence'.

Finally, we bring the book to a close with a concluding section gathering together the diverse strands of discussions in the book.

References

Academy of Medical Sciences. (2003). *Strengthening clinical research*. Academy of Medical Sciences, London.

Bioscience Innovation and Growth Team. (2003). *Bioscience 2015: improving national health increasing national wealth*. Department of Trade and Industry, London.

Department of Health. (1999). *National service framework for mental health. Modern standards and service models*. Department of Health, London.

Mental Health Topic Working Group. (1999). *Report to the Clarke R&D Review Committee*. Research and Development Directorate, Department of Health, London.

NSCStHA (2003). Independent inquiry into the death of David Bennett. Norfolk, Saffolk and Cambridgeshire Strategic Health Authority. www.nscstha.nhs.uk.

Showalter, E. (1987). *The female malady women, madness and English Culture, 1830–1980*. Virago, London.

Thornicroft, G., Bindman, J., Goldberg, D., Gournay, K. and Huxley, P. (2002). Researchable questions to support evidence-based mental health policy concerning adult mental illness. *Psychiatric Bulletin*, **26**, 364–7.

Part I

Theory and methodology

1

The research and development strategy in the NHS: incremental evolution?

Michael Clark and David Sallah

INTRODUCTION

In a research and development strategy there is an implicit, if not always explicit, set of assumptions about the interaction of the research and development components. It has not always been clear what these assumptions are in the NHS R&D strategy nor what theory of the interaction underpins the strategy.

In an R&D strategy consuming billions of pounds it is to be anticipated that accountability would be expected in order to show the impact and benefits arising from the investment. Yet the accountability expectations will in part depend upon what is expected of an R&D strategy and the relationship between research and development. Has this always been clear in the NHS?

In this chapter we will discuss various ways of understanding and managing the relationship between research and development and consider their relevance to the NHS and its R&D strategy as it has developed over time. In the process, we shall explore the evolving settlement of NHS R&D. The first perspective that we shall explore is that of *laissez faire* and we then proceed through increasingly active ways of managing the relationship. These include the perspectives we have termed the *strategic commitment, human resources, quality management, dissemination and knowledge-based philosophy, active management of research to fit development, and increased accountability of researchers.*

These perspectives are not mutually exclusive and combinations of them may be in operation at any time. Indeed, different perspectives may be in operation at the *macro* (the Department of Health/NHS as a whole), the *meso* (smaller organisational groups within the NHS) and the *micro* (individual organisations and people) levels. The NHS is far from being a monolithic organisation. There is, however, a likelihood that one perspective will take greater dominance in the overall tone of the R&D strategy.

We will begin, though, with consideration of what has been called 'health research systems' (HRSs) (Pang *et al.* 2003). This is a conceptual framework designed to help with, amongst other things, policy making to ensure that health services have access to, and use, research-based knowledge to improve health service delivery and health.

HEALTH RESEARCH SYSTEMS

Amidst increasing global interest in the relationship between research and addressing health issues, the World Health Organisation supports work to address a deficit in conceptualising 'research systems' in relation to 'health systems' (Pang *et al.* 2003). The framework for a 'health research system' (HRS) is an attempt to describe the 'boundaries, goals and functions' (Pang *et al.* 2003, p. 816) of a model for further conceptual and operational work. The stated aims of the work include to:

> *provide useful information to identify potential policy options to strengthen national HRSs, . . . use scientific knowledge to improve actions within health systems, and ultimately improve health and health equity.'*
>
> (Pang et al. 2003, p. 816)

An HRS is defined as:

> *The people, institutions, and activities whose primary purpose in relation to research is to generate high-quality knowledge that can be used to promote, restore, and/or maintain the health status of populations; it should include the mechanisms adopted to encourage the utilisation of research.*
>
> (Pang et al. 2003, p. 816)

This is an inclusive definition, encouraging consideration of all the (public and private sector) actors involved in health and research and the wide variety of types of research.

Table 1.1 Summary of the functions and operational components of health research systems. (Source: Pang *et al.* 2003, p. 817)

Function	Operational component
Stewardship	• Define and articulate vision for a national health research system • Identify appropriate health research priorities and co-ordinate adherence to them • Set and monitor ethical standards for health research and research partnerships • Monitor and evaluate the HRS
Financing	Secure research funds and allocate them accountably
Creating and sustaining resources	Build, strengthen and sustain the human and physical capacity to conduct, absorb and utilise health research
Producing and using research	• Produce scientifically valid research outputs • Translate and communicate research to inform health policy, strategies, practices and public opinion • Promote the use of research to develop new tools (drugs, vaccines, devices and other applications) to improve health

The goals of the HRS are twofold. Firstly, to advance scientific knowledge. Secondly, and complementary to the first, is using knowledge to improve health and health equity. The model of the functions of an HRS is summarised in Table 1.1. We will now consider each function in a little more detail and related to the NHS R&D system.

Stewardship

There has to be somebody or bodies who take responsibility for overseeing the entire HRS. This is often the government, but probably also involves representation from other key players in the HRS. In terms of the English HRS, the government takes that broad stewardship role and seeks to involve other players including the NHS, universities, research funding councils and the private sector. Scrutiny and analysis of the stewardship function within England would be worthwhile, but is beyond the remit of this chapter. It would be interesting to see how each of the four components of the function have evolved and operate, separately and in relation to each other and the overall HRS.

Financing

This key function ought to be conducted to reflect the overall vision, principles and priorities set out through the stewardship. Again, in the English HRS, a large element of this function is directly conducted through the government, such as through the allocation of funding to NHS R&D and universities. Where the government does not directly manage finance, it has sought to support other research funding (e.g. pharmaceutical research funding), and on occasions to co-ordinate funding from sources such as charities.

Creating and sustaining resources

This refers to the human and physical 'capacity to conduct, absorb and utilise health research' (Pang *et al.* 2003, p. 817). It includes infrastructure, career structures for research, research management, access to research information and opportunities to present and discuss research findings. Clearly, this directly relates to the concerns of this book, namely understanding the relationship between research and development.

Producing and using research

The publication of research findings is seen to be the primary output of the research process, but an effectively functioning HRS also needs to work actively to take those findings into practice. This may be through directly using the knowledge for new 'technology' for health services, and via informing policies, strategies and practices in health systems. Pang *et al.* (2003) comment that a major cause of health systems not fully matching the needs they are meant to meet is because of the problems inherent in synthesising new research knowledge and applying it to improving the performance of the health systems. This is the challenge of relating the research and development components. It is directly related to the previous functions of the HRS. The *stewardship* should be setting research priorities that relate to the overall goal of improving health, hopefully making the research outputs more directly relevant to practice and thus, in theory, more likely to be adopted. *Finances* are required to develop the *resources* for absorbing and using research results. Yet, even if each were operating rationally, it may not necessarily follow that research knowledge would be taken up into practice.

In the rest of this chapter, we will look at various perspectives and approaches for linking research and development which have been employed as the NHS R&D strategy has evolved.

Laissez faire

The *laissez faire* attitude to the relationship between research and development is one in which the two components, and, most notably, their relationships, are left unmanaged through any central means. It is founded on the view that both research and development are best left to the devices of people engaged in them. If there is any explicit consideration of the issue, it is assumed that research will find its way into development through the activities of individuals and that it does not require specific management across the NHS.

The *laissez faire* approach unconsciously characterised R&D in the NHS in the first settlement for the NHS. Medical consultants, chiefly, were allowed to direct their own time for research activity allowing them freedom and implicit trust to use it responsibly (Kirk 2001). This responsibility further implied that they would do the development as well as the research. Such an implicit and individualistic approach was gradually seen to have a number of problems, as summarised by Kirk (2001), including the view that the use of evidence from research was poorer than it ought to be. This was seen to be a key factor in the wide variation in NHS practice and service organisation – and the health of the nation. The House of Lords Select Committee on Science and Technology articulated this concern in 1988 in *Priorities in medical research*. They criticised the NHS for failing to articulate its research needs and attend to the problems of implementation. Arguably, the history of NHS R&D strategy since then has been one of seeking the next rational development to tackle these two criticisms.

Strategic commitment

The strategic commitment approach is characterised by an explicit commitment to R&D at the highest levels of the organisation. It is the explicit commitment to an R&D strategy that distinguishes it from a purely *laissez faire* approach. Of itself, however, an explicit strategic commitment may not necessarily result in significantly greater management of R&D than in a purely *laissez faire* approach.

Within the NHS a major step towards a strategic commitment to research was made when Professor Sir Michael Peckham was made the first National Director of R&D for the NHS – 43 years after its inception. His manifesto and role were grounded in the report *Taking research seriously* (DoH 1990). This articulated the view that research in the NHS had suffered from the worst consequences of the *laissez faire* approach and that as a whole the NHS had not been serious about the role of research within it. From 1991, Professor Peckham began to articulate the case for a strategic approach to relate important health issues and the contribution of interventions to the national research activity. This would require a systematic approach to identifying priorities for research i.e. for a more active management of research to link to national health priorities, with the implied view that this would follow into development and health improvements.

Whilst the emphasis of the report was on a strategic commitment to research, there was some consideration of the links between research and development. For example, the report argued for the commissioning of research with a clear intended use, a strategic approach to research management across the NHS, and better managed dissemination. Professor Peckham also argued for a research approach to the dissemination and application of knowledge and other resources. More explicit consideration of development and its links to research were to emerge later as the NHS R&D strategy evolved.

Another significant step in articulating the view for more active management of research with national priorities and of development activity came with *Supporting research and development in the NHS* (Culyer 1994), the 'Culyer Report'. This better set out principles to define R&D, such as peer review for research. It argued for research to contribute new knowledge to improve the health of the nation, which would require active dissemination of research into development across the NHS.

The Culyer Report also set the grounds for a separation of R&D funding from service funding to NHS organisations, and grounds for them to be more accountable to justify continued research funding. Whilst in large part this was to protect R&D funding from the internal market to the NHS, another step was taken towards central management of R&D activity through an R&D infrastructure.

The R&D strategy thus evolved to this point was a significant move on from *laissez faire*, but:

> *In retrospect it has to be acknowledged that the R&D strategy alone was never going to take the NHS to the brink of a major cultural transformation.*
>
> (Kirk 2001, p. 9)

Management of R&D across the NHS has since evolved to seek this 'cultural transformation'. Further policies, practices and structures have emerged to more directly manage research activity, especially in line with national priorities for health improvements, and to drive research-led development across all NHS organizations. We shall look at the incremental development of this by discussing particular foci for policy activity. We begin by considering the 'human resource' perspective to managing research and linking it with development.

Human resource perspective

Implementing systems and structures for managing R&D in the NHS is pointless without the reciprocal development of staff to work within them. In this respect there are three key focal points for managing human resources. They are:

1. *Staff to undertake research activity.* Developing the skills and experience of researchers was identified as a priority in the Clarke (1999) report. From a mixture of local, regional and embryonic national programmes for providing support to develop researchers in the NHS, we have now moved to a national co-ordinating programme for clinician scientist development schemes (web address: www.acmedsci.ac.uk). This also provides for central control of how these funds are used within the whole of NHS expenditure.
2. *Staff to use research outputs and take them into development.* Whilst this was recognised as important from the early stages of the NHS R&D strategy, it was not given the prominence of the first human resource perspective. There is a need to equip staff to find research information and to apply it to their work (Haines and Donald 1998; Glanville *et al.* 1998). This was largely left to local arrangements and staff education and training. More has developed nationally in this area, closely allied to information technology developments to improve access to research findings. Yet there is a need for a range of perspectives and methods to influence change (Haines and Donald 1998), and these were not systematically addressed in the early NHS R&D strategy – the research approach was not initially systematic in establishing how to influence development and change. More has evolved here quite recently through national co-ordination of activity such as service delivery and organisation research to generate new knowledge on the best ways to organise services and how best to manage change and bridge the gaps between research and development.

3. *Staff to manage R&D across the NHS*. The Clarke report
   recommended that support be given to R&D directors and managers
   as key links in NHS R&D management. This has become clearer the
   greater the drive to manage R&D activity across the NHS. Such
   management requires information and staff to develop local research
   cultures and manage R&D activity. The Clarke report also identified
   local R&D directors and managers as crucial linkages between
   research and development at a local level.

The human resource perspective, then, has shown gradual development
as the national R&D strategy has evolved. Yet there are still areas of
weakness to address.

Quality management

As concern grew with how to improve the quality of NHS care,
especially in terms of its consistency across the country, policy makers
began explicitly to consider how to manage this nationally. Within *A
first class service* the New Labour government set out a framework for
local accountability for quality improvement (clinical governance) within
nationally set standards and frameworks for care, plus inspection of Trusts.
   Within this, one place for research was to be helping to establish
national guidance for local practice. As was stated in *A first class
service* (DoH 1998):

> There is currently no coherent approach to the appraisal of
> research evidence and the subsequent production of guidance for
> clinical practice.
>
> (p. 16)

Further connections were argued with the world research:

> The NHS Research and Development (R&D) strategy is now
> providing access to a rapidly expanding evidence base on health
> care interventions and services, but the development of guidance
> from this is confused.
>
> (p. 13)

The National Institute for Clinical Excellence (NICE) was a new
institution to deliver evidence-based guidance to a nationally set
programme. Where NICE identifies a lack of evidence, it may
recommend that the NHS channel resources to provide it.
   At a local level, Trusts would need to consider the role of 'evidence'
in their clinical governance arrangements. This brings us to the need

for equipping staff to collect and appraise evidence, as seen in the HR perspective.

The policy was not very explicit, however, in the detail of the relationship between R&D and national and local arrangements for clinical governance. To a large extent, the organisations involved are still working through this. For example, there has been more gradual entwining of the research activity support through the Health Technology Assessment (HTA) programme and the requirements of NICE relating to a particular query about care. As NICE draws attention to gaps in the evidence, the NHS R&D programmes are now more likely to identify these as priorities for their commissioning of research. The relationships are, however, yet to be fully clarified.

Having evidence-based national guidelines closes part of the gap between research and development. Yet there is still the issue of implementing the guidelines. This is something NICE does not have direct control over, and if its guidance is not implemented, NICE will be deemed to have failed (Littlejohns 2001). The question of how best to disseminate and implement evidence is itself a topic that is increasingly having a research approach brought to it to ascertain what works (Bero *et al.* 1998; Effective Health Care 1999).

Dissemination of research and a knowledge-based philosophy

In a combined and balanced research and development strategy there needs to be explicit thought given to how to get research findings into practice. In the NHS R&D strategy this has been an area of continuing interest. The way that the R&D strategy emerged and developed over its early years led to 'a sense that the relationship between research and healthcare is optional' (Baker 2001, p. 22). One set of professionals did research and a separate set provided health care as they wished. This was increasingly seen as unacceptable, driven by a number of concerns, including awareness of the following (Haines and Donald 1998, p. 1):

- Disparities between clinical practice and research evidence
- A growth in a sense of need to show clearly that public money spent on R&D results in improvements for the public
- Clearer recognition that passive diffusion of information as a means of research informing practice is doomed given the amount of information published
- Awareness that traditional forms of knowledge dissemination through conferences and courses has little impact on the behaviour of health professionals

- The circulation of guidance without an implementation strategy is unlikely to change practice.

Part of the answer to these concerns includes mechanisms to scan the current state of knowledge, to be able to disseminate research intelligence and to identify research underway. The Clarke report asserted that the Department of Health should develop these mechanisms. Baker (2001) comments that for at least seven years it was a failure of NHS R&D to deal in a systematic manner with the question of dissemination/implementation. Similarly:

> *The UK HTA programme ... has often expressed frustrations that its output did not readily impinge on the consciousness of managers at a local level and policy makers at a national level.*
> (Littlejohns 2001, p. 55)

In its basic conception, the bridge between research output and dissemination would be through the publication of research findings, notably in academic journals. As this has been seen to be insufficient in changing practice, NHS R&D strategists have gradually evolved an infrastructure to take more of an active role in making available research findings to practitioners and managers. Information technology has frequently been central to these efforts. The National Research Register (NRR) and the Research Findings Electronic Register (ReFeR) are electronic databases of, respectively, ongoing research in the NHS and the results of research. There is some thought that the National Electronic Library for Health (NeLH) may develop as the backbone resource to manage the task of co-ordinating knowledge (Baker 2001).

Further dissemination infrastructures are the Centre for Reviews and Dissemination of the University of York and the UK Cochrane Centre at Oxford. Both attempt to take overviews of research findings in an area of health care and to distil them into more accessible forms for clinicians and researchers.

In the managerialist approach to 'knowledge-based' health care there is a move away from reliance upon individual clinicians and teams themselves accessing evidence from research. There is a developing cadre of experts who take responsibility for the clinicians by themselves distilling the results of research into national policy frameworks (e.g. National Service Frameworks (NSFs)) and guidelines (e.g. NICE). It is more of a dissemination and implementation of knowledge by dictat (Baker 2001). As we saw in the previous section about 'quality management', clinical governance and Healthcare Commission inspections emphasise to Trusts that they should have systems for ensuring the implementation of current best evidence. In a sense, the NHS is moving more towards centralised performance management of the take up of research findings. Indeed some of the performance indicators used in 'star ratings' have been direct attempts to influence practice to take up research findings, such as the prescribing of atypical anti-psychotic medication. This developing situation of the relationship between research and other drivers of change has led to the comment that:

> *organisations such as NICE and National Service Frameworks are the drivers for change with the research and development strategy supporting those systems rather than driving change itself.*
>
> (Baker 2001, p. 26)

The move to expect and explicitly seek to develop a knowledge base to support the local delivery of NHS services was a major development that has helped to stimulate something of a culture change across the NHS, but clear evidence of its impact on NHS performance is hard to find (Baker 2001). There is no doubt that the size and diversity of the NHS combined with the complexity of the world of research information make it a very difficult task to co-ordinate all strands of dissemination and implementation. There have been calls for more research into the policy frameworks (clinical governance, etc.) developed by the Labour Government to close the gap between research output and implementation (Baker 2001b; Littlejohns 2001). Yet a managerial perspective seems to be the increasing one being used to frame approaches to bridging the research and development divide through centrally managed dissemination and performance management of implementation. Researchers in the NHS themselves have also been subjected to this approach of increased accountability for justifying through managerialist mechanisms their work and its impact. We shall return to this later, but first we want to discuss the practice of actively managing research to fit with perceived development needs.

This concerns how well the R&D strategy has connected with the NHS at all levels including individuals and organisations for the view has been expressed that:

> *The NHS itself, which is supposedly the customer for the outputs of R&D, appears to have no more than observer status whilst also bearing the responsibility for meeting the costs of NHS R&D.*
>
> (Baker 2001, p. 20)

Active management of research to fit development

The early development of the NHS saw research as an activity done by learned people, directed by themselves, to their own interests and agendas with consolidation of existing research expenditure on this basis (Baker 2001). Observers increasingly noted problems with this approach, including the view that:

> *There needs to be closer links between research and practice so that research is relevant to practitioners' needs and practitioners are willing to participate in research.*
>
> (Haines and Donald 1998, p. 50)

This is another view of how to close the gap between research and subsequent development in practice. Involved practitioners, seeing the outcomes of research and its relevance to them would, in theory, be more inclined to adapt their practice accordingly. Further control over what research activity is undertaken would in theory assist with ensuring that it marries up to the needs of practitioners. These issues were set out in the Clarke report as it called for the research strategy to have a 'sharper focus on NHS needs and priorities'. The Clarke review argued that the government had already identified major priorities for health and established Topic Working Groups to report R&D concerns across these priority areas. The Clarke report began to set out research priorities and needs related to national health priorities, and argued that research activity should be more closely aligned with these priorities. Clarke reported that two-thirds of NHS R&D funding went on own account research within Trusts and that there was variable quality control of this activity. The report argued for the reorganisation of funding towards programmes and centres to improve quality control, with greater emphasis on research in priority areas and the involvement of wider health communities in the research process, including academic partners.

The Clarke report also argued that the NHS could not support all current research activity across its providers. It was argued that there needed to be a more focused approach based upon developing a critical mass of expertise, such as in specialist research units and programmes. The report of the Mental Health Topic Group also recommended establishing research programmes as a means of generating greater stability, improved career development and more coherence of research activity.

The publication in 2000 of *Research and development for a first class service* set a programme of reform for R&D funding to address some of the issues raised by Clarke. Incremental attempts have been made to deliver this agenda. There is now greater central control through various national research programmes which lead in commissioning research to address health needs and priorities. National Portfolio R&D Directors have been appointed to co-ordinate efforts in health priority areas. To support development of this new framework there will be three NHS R&D advisory groups: cancer, heart disease and stroke, and mental health, which will build on the reviews from the relevant Clarke Review Topic Working Groups. The work of these advisory groups will be 'co-ordinated with national service frameworks and other work to develop standards and guidance for the NHS in key areas' (p. 19).

As the NHS continues to move through a 'modernisation' agenda, as set out in such policy documents as the NHS Plan, there is an increasing effort to make research activity across the NHS fit with the perceived development needs of the NHS. Liam Donaldson (2001), the Chief Medical Officer, stated that the NHS faces an agenda of:

- Modernisation
- The need to transform how it manages the quality of care
- Improving public health and reducing health inequalities.

He asserted that:

> *One way of achieving these goals is by making greater use of relevant, high-quality research-based evidence. That is why the NHS R&D programme is so vital and why recent changes to the programme . . . have been so helpful.*
>
> (*Op cit.*)

Amongst the helpful changes was seen to be the establishment of links across the Health Technology Assessment Programme and the National Institute for Clinical Excellence, 'helping to close the loop between research and practice' (*op cit*). Another helpful development was seen to be changes in NHS R&D funding to ensure 'greater transparency and a greater sensitivity to the priorities and needs of the NHS' (*op cit.*)

> *Taken together, these changes will help to ensure that the R&D programme promotes research that is rigorous, relevant and – most important – used by decision makers.*
>
> (*Op cit.*)

As there was a move to align central NHS R&D programmes with the needs and priorities of health care, there has also been an increasing emphasis on, and attempts to co-ordinate, research activity at the level of NHS organisations into programmes that fit national health priorities. In the latest statement of the R&D strategy, *Research and development for a first class service* (DoH 2000), there is a commitment to 'align the management and funding of R&D with the principles of *The new NHS*' (original emphasis) (p. 3). To further this there is a stated plan to target R&D money on the NHS's 'research priorities and needs'. There is a commitment to 'set a **strategic direction** for health services R&D for the benefit of the NHS' (original emphasis) (p. 3). This is justified on the basis of public expectation that R&D funding is made to contribute to the overall goals of the NHS.

Work to increase this alignment includes changes in the R&D funding system in part designed to ensure support to R&D 'to underpin modernisation and quality improvement' (p. 13). Through *priorities and needs* funding to Trusts, research activity will address NHS priorities, such as those embodied in NSFs, the work of NICE and the needs of the NHS in implementing government policy. The Department of Health will see that research activity will lead to improvements in NHS care and that Trusts have appropriate systems to link R&D to clinical practice and organisational development. This is in some part a restatement of previous requirements, but in a more explicit form, with greater managerialist expectations that alignment between research activity, especially in Trusts, can be brought into line with development priorities.

All of this requires more information about research activity, and the annual report system is regularly being radically changed and tweaked to provide this with regard to research underway within Trusts. This is also aimed at greater performance management of research in Trusts receiving R&D funding.

The strategy also includes plans to work with other research partners (such as universities) and engage with areas of health care provision that have not been traditionally so well involved in research, including primary care. The intention is to increase research capacity, activity and engagement, but within a rubric of greater national strategic direction. The emphasis is on greater strategic direction and performance management of research to align it with development needs, as defined nationally. There is some expression given to an allowance for local priorities driving local research activity too, but the emphasis is overwhelmingly on national priorities. Part of the thinking behind the new developments is that programmes and centres will develop critical masses of researchers grouped around specific themes. There are various possible models for such groupings (Bailey 2001), including networks of individually small research providers, centres linked to managed clinical networks, and virtual centres. The approach chosen to operationalise this policy will need to be based upon consideration of how to relate research and development.

On its own, this activity to align research with nationally defined health needs will probably lead to a narrowing of the gap between research and development, but will not close it. Consideration also has to be given to work on the other perspectives discussed above, of how to manage relationships between research and development. Work on any one perspective needs to be coordinated with the others if a holistic health research system is to evolve.

Increased accountability of researchers

Increasing the accountability of researchers and R&D management in the NHS Trusts has been a consistent theme in the R&D strategy. Annual reports of R&D from the Trusts receiving R&D money was a contractual obligation if they wished to continue to receive the money. The early forms of the reports were fairly loosely set, but have since become more tightly defined. They have always included a detailed financial report of where the R&D money has been spent, some description of the research activity undertaken, and an expectation that there would be a report of the outputs (especially publications) and impacts (such as on practice) of that activity. As the reports have been refined there is now more of an attempt to standardise annual reports, in part to allow for central analysis and comparison of data from them.

Another policy for improving the accountability of R&D in the NHS has been that of expecting public involvement in all levels of R&D activity. The Clarke report called for this and it is another policy which has gradually evolved, both centrally and within Trusts.

A further significant step in making research activity more accountable was the introduction of the *Research governance framework for health and social care* (DoH 2001). This sets out requirements on senior managers in all NHS Trusts to have procedures to scrutinise and monitor all research undertaken in their organisations. Individual researchers are made more accountable within institutions for the *quality* of their work, including methodological, topic and ethical scrutiny. Part of a 'quality research culture' in a Trust is that research relates to a need. This is not explicitly required to be a nationally defined need, but the possibility is that it be interpreted thus. This is particularly so as Trusts have to justify their research activity in their Annual Reports. Research outside a programme may be deemed not to be contributing in the best way to the 'quality research culture' and may be discouraged as not being a priority.

To highlight the move of increased managerialism of research further, it is worth noting that the implementation of the Research Governance Framework is itself performance managed. Nationally defined indicators are reported on in the Annual Reports and, now, in Controls Assurance Standards.

There are other perspectives and elements to an R&D strategy for linking the two conceptual halves. These include managing innovation and intellectual property, which the NHS has made significant moves to develop in relation to R&D. A more recent perspective is that of the learning organisation i.e. how to incorporate all kinds of learning into organisational quality improvement. We have, though, outlined above the main perspectives on, and developments in, NHS R&D in terms of a key theme of this book, namely linking research and development. Each perspective and element needs to be considered in relation to the others as a whole strategy and we will now move on to discuss this.

DISCUSSION

The development of an explicit national NHS R&D strategy moving away from the *laissez faire* model was a significant, innovative move. It was agreed to be something that in itself the NHS should be proud of (Clarke 1999). The strategic move was driven by a belief in, and commitment to, a sense of the importance that research plays in improving health. Its continued evolution has similarly been driven by this view.

Yet the settlement for R&D in the NHS has always been uncertain and fluid. Since its instigation, and in its subsequent evolution, the NHS R&D strategy has also been driven by the desire and perceived need to protect research within the NHS. There was the move following Culyer to extract R&D budgets from NHS provision to protect research from the internal market. Now we see a move to justify research in terms of its impact on improving health needs.

The strategy has also evolved driven by learning about its own impact and weaknesses. As it has increasingly come to be realised that research and development do not always automatically connect across the whole NHS, there have been *ad hoc* moves to rectify this. These initiatives have, though, been shaped by a need to adapt in order to keep a foundation for the settlement for R&D in a moving political terrain. This has led to such concerns as that the need to deliver short-term government targets encourages moving money from long-term R&D as this activity often does not immediately deliver improvements in care (Baker 2001).

As a more technocratic and managerialist approach has been brought to bear on NHS management, so the R&D strategy has been obliged to follow some similar routes to justify itself. The desire increasingly to move research to reflect nationally defined development needs is a manifestation of this. This may have happened anyway, without a managerialist turn. The move to manage NHS R&D development by making research-active organisations and individuals more visible and accountable is, though, a direct manifestation of this managerialist philosophy. The managerialist turn leads to the belief in an aspiration to a rationality that can deliver sense and coherence in a complex environment.

There is still space in the interstices of R&D for other activity than that defined nationally. That will always be possible in a research world, but the space within which to do so is becoming more confined, more bounded by an agenda set nationally. As Kirk (2001) comments, it could be 'the apparent end of strategy and its continuation by technocracy' (p. 9). In place of a new strategy document we have in *Research and development for a first class service* a statement of policy and principles and a plan to reform NHS R&D funding. In the foreword we have a statement of Ministerial priorities, which are a reassertion of Peckham's principles but in the language of technocratic analyses (Kirk 2001). The ends (addressing national priorities, especially tackling health inequalities, and modernising health care) are given, and research is seen as the means to these by being responsive to the needs of those using the NHS, its staff and decision makers. A liberal perspective to research and knowledge generation is being subverted to a technocratic one.

Another reason for the incrementalist, reactive development of the NHS R&D strategy has been its innovation and the lack of guiding theory and evidence. Being new can carry a cost, and perhaps the NHS has not learned all that it could from R&D in other sectors. The development of the Health Research System model discussed above and small moves to bring a research approach to developing the R&D

strategy present opportunities to overcome these problems. But we have to wonder if the settlement upon which R&D seeks to find security will be sufficient to give it the space and time to develop and address such issues as the gap between research and development further.

The HRS model presents a guiding framework, but we also need to see the practical and political challenges in the practice of an HRS. The HRS model presents a highly simplified, rational framework which is helpful in stripping down and understanding research and development in their simplest forms and relationships. It is a very helpful contribution to presenting a unifying set of ideas. Clearly, though, more conceptual and operational work is required to build into the model a more sophisticated understanding of the real art of an HRS. This was recognised by the authors of the model.

The competition culture of the NHS in the early and middle 1990s affected R&D by consuming resources and distorting priorities, and the competitiveness of the world of research contributed to this (Baker 2001). The current climate presents an opportunity in its assertion of collaboration, within the NHS and with other partners, such as academia. Yet there is a fear that the nature of political and personnel changes means that 'destabilisation is omnipresent in NHS R&D at the highest levels' (Baker 2001, p. 21). The role of regional offices has been seen as one of providing stability in this change, and a link between determining national and local priorities (Baker 2001), but this level of organisation has been removed. It remains to be seen what impact this will have on R&D in the NHS.

CONCLUSION

The NHS's R&D strategy has always been a careful balancing act between various stakeholders and imperatives. The traditional freedom of health professionals and researchers and local control of R&D is balanced against desires for national strategic direction and control of research. A technocratic and managerialist perspective is currently tipping this balance more in favour of the latter. In part this is driven by increased political concern to demonstrate improvement in the NHS and by the need to improve consistency across it, including the uptake of research evidence into practice. Short-term priorities are managed and a long-term perspective of R&D has been subverted to 'a support mechanism rather than a driver for change' (Baker 2001, p. 14). This technocratic, regulating approach requires more bureaucracy, which may slow the process of knowledge generation. The current situation has led Baker to comment:

> *Compared with its heyday of the early 1990s, the [R&D] strategy seems rather downbeat but its better connections, tighter management and more rational systems of funding will improve the return on investment, make it easier to demonstrate relevance to the NHS and political priorities and stands a better chance of surviving in the long term. But then, in politics, a week is a long time.*
>
> (Baker 2001, p. 27)

There are opportunities for survival for the R&D strategy in the NHS, then, and with that to address the challenges of research and development and connecting the two together. But survival will come at a price, one of serving managerialist, technocratic ends. The impact of this on the R&D strategy and on the freedom of participants to pursue their own R&D is yet to be fully determined.

References

Bailey, C. (2001). Funding NHS R&D: implementing Culyer. In *Research and development for the NHS: evidence, evaluation and effectiveness*, 3rd edition (eds. Baker, M.R. and Kirk, S.), pp. 59–72. Radcliffe Medical, Abingdon.

Baker, M.R. (2001a). R&D in the new NHS. In *Research and development for the NHS: evidence, evaluation and effectiveness*, 3rd edition (eds. Baker, M.R. and Kirk, S.), pp. 13–27. Radcliffe Medical, Abingdon.

Baker, M.R. (2001b). The new national agencies and R&D. In *Research and development for the NHS: evidence, evaluation and effectiveness*, 3rd edition (eds. Baker, M.R. and Kirk, S.), pp. 29–38. Radcliffe Medical, Abingdon.

Bero, I., Grilli, R., Grimshaw, J., Harvey, E., Oxman, A. and Thomson, M.A. (1998). Closing the gap between research and practice: an overview of systematic reviews of interventions to promote implementation of research findings by health care professionals. In *Getting research findings into practice* (eds. Haines, A. and Donald, A.), pp. 27–35. BMJ, London.

Clarke, M. (1999). *Strategic review of the NHS R&D levy: final report to the central research and development committee, Department of Health.* Stationery Office, London.

Culyer, A. (1994). *Supporting research and development in the NHS.* HMSO, London.

Department of Health. (1990). *Taking research seriously.* HMSO, London.

Department of Health. (1998). *A first class service: quality in the new NHS.* HMSO, London.

Department of Health. (2000). *Research and development for a first class service: R&D funding for the new NHS*. Department of Health, London.

Department of Health. (2001). *Research governance for health and social care*. 23553 1P 3K Mar 01 (ABA). Department of Health Publications, London.

Department of Health. (2001) *The NHS as an innovative organisation: a framework and guidance on the management of intellectual property in the NHS*. Department of Health, London.

Effective Health Care. (1999). *Getting evidence into practice*. Volume 5, No. 1, February.

Glanville, J., Haines, M. and Auston, I. (1998). Sources of information on clinical effectiveness and methods of dissemination. In *Getting research findings into practice* (eds. Haines, A. and Donald, A.), pp. 19–26. BMJ, London.

Haines, A. and Donald, A. (1998). Introduction. In *Getting research findings into practice* (eds. Haines, A. and Donald, A.), pp. 1–9. BMJ, London.

House of Lords Select Committee on Science and Technology. (1988). *Priorities in medical research*. HMSO, London.

Kirk, S. (2001). The NHS R&D strategy. In *Research and development for the NHS: evidence, evaluation and effectiveness*, 3rd Edition (eds. Baker, M.R. and Kirk, S.), pp. 1–11. Radcliffe Medical, Abingdon.

Kleijnen. (2001). Information for R&D. In *Research and development for the NHS: evidence, evaluation and effectiveness*, 3rd Edition (eds. Baker, M.R. and Kirk, S.), pp. 73–82. Radcliffe Medical, Abingdon.

Littlejohns, P. (2001). The relationship between NICE and the national R&D programme. In *Research and development for the NHS: evidence, evaluation and effectiveness*, 3rd Edition (eds. Baker, M.R. and Kirk, S.), pp. 39–57. Radcliffe Medical, Abingdon.

Peckham, M. (1991). Research and development for the National Health Service. *Lancet*. **338**, 367–71.

2

Quantitative methods in mental health research

Zaubia Alyas and Kamaldeep Bhui

INTRODUCTION

Mental health research has seen an exponential increase in the quality
and quantity of publications, reflecting a need for an evidence base for
clinically effective practice and service delivery. Alongside this, there
has been a sustained effort to investigate risk factors and interventions,
often with less explicit relevance to health care providers in the short
term, but with the potential for lasting and significant impacts on public
health. Much of the challenge in mental health research has been the
development of discrete and valid outcome measures and verification
that these are clinically relevant. Another element of work is to
elucidate, specify and evaluate complex interventions, which are the
mainstay in mental health care. The emphasis on quantitative research
has been checked recently by demands for more meaningful research
into the values found in mental health settings, user-focused research
and research into the therapeutic value of relationships. This call for a
different form of mental health research seems over-determined where
it seeks to render quantitative research methods to the realms of
meaninglessness, or remoteness from the concerns of the public and of
patients. Complementarity between distinct research traditions has rarely
been achieved, but active debate at the 'edges' of specific research
paradigms is promising. In this chapter we set out the place of
quantitative research of mental health settings and mental health care.
This is not to relegate qualitative research, represented in other chapters,
to a less paramount position, but more to focus attention on the

purpose and limitations of quantitative research, which aims to address specific questions using well-established research designs. Indeed, quantitative research can not be used to answer all questions about practices, and in this regard it faces the same constraints as any research tradition: that its use must be focused to answer the most important questions with pivotal significance for models of mental health care, alongside due reliance on other bodies of evidence including clinical experience to inform wider practice. We present, briefly, quantitative study designs, and then explore clinical trials, the methodology that, according to NICE guidelines and the Cochrane collaboration, yields the 'highest form of evidence'. We discuss the difficulties of undertaking intervention research in mental health care, and present some recommendations that, we hope, will stimulate high-quality research in the next decade.

Public health professionals are now playing a greater role in mental health care, and set the tone for preventive interventions, as well as for providing strategic leadership in evaluating the weaknesses in existing systems of care. This focus on prevention relies on the discipline of epidemiology to study the distribution of disease and investigate the determinants of disease within a population, particularly those determinants that can potentially be manipulated in order to prevent disease or alleviate suffering. One of the major problems with mental health research has been the focus on clinical series, or service-based data. This approach has limited inferential value when considering public health approaches to mental health care. Service-based data are, however, useful for the evaluation of service-level interventions, and for the assessment of individual-level clinical outcomes.

A further complication to mental health research is that it has largely not been strategic; instead it is reliant on the academic interests of the leaders in the field. It has only recently begun to reflect the needs of services (the NHS in the UK), and the public. Furthermore, funding for specific programmes of work cannot, and does not, always reflect disease burden in the population, but the vested interests of fund-givers alongside the prominence given to any condition through the media or charities. For example, the medical products industry funds research that favours their own products and governments tend to support these, as well as the interests of professionals from academic centres. This can lead to the promotion of treatments that patients find unacceptable and believe to be inappropriate, leading to problems with adherence, and ultimately effectiveness. These biases in funding all push the research agenda away from the needs of the consumer that it is meant to serve and compounds the already existent mismatch between the research community and consumers, who differ in their values and life experience, their understanding of science and technology and also their access to decision-making structures. This chapter outlines the principles of evidence-based medicine, describes the strengths and weaknesses of the major study designs in quantitative research, but concentrates on Randomised Controlled Trials (RCTs), and their strengths and weaknesses in mental health research.

EVIDENCE-BASED MEDICINE

There is now a greater recognition of the chronic nature of many conditions, including depression; there are economic arguments for sanctioning the provision of more or less specialist and expensive interventions; clinical practice varies regionally, and even within the same city. Each of these facts has fuelled the move towards Evidence-Based Medicine (EBM) in order to rationalise choice and decision making as much as is possible. EBM aims to:

1. Standardise variations in practice and behaviour in health care
2. Evaluate the rising numbers of new tests, devices and drugs, most of which can be regarded as half-way technologies likely to fall to the wayside when the ongoing revolution in molecular biology starts to pay more concrete dividends
3. Manage the proliferation of half-way technologies that continue to be highly profitable as well as the escalation in production of new tests and devices and drugs.

Thus, hierarchies of study designs that provide the best evidence have been drawn up for therapeutic, diagnostic and prognostic questions. This places RCTs as the gold standard of 'evidence', followed by controlled observational studies, and then uncontrolled trials, followed by expert opinion. The early findings of the Cochrane collaboration and local clinical effectiveness committees were that most interventions, especially complex ones in mental health care, are essentially provided on the basis of expert opinion underpinned with some research evidence. Not all mental health care is provided, nor can be, on the basis of RCT evidence. This reflects not only the volume of interventions that would need to be undertaken, but also the expense of undertaking such experiments. Furthermore, the RCT design has been criticised as not being the most appropriate study design for mental health interventions (Slade and Priebe 2001).

RCTs are still considered the gold standard scientific method for detecting treatment effectiveness and over the past fifty years there has been an explosion in the number of RCTs published in response to calls for evidence for reliable information about treatment efficacy and effectiveness. There is far too much information for the individual clinician to assimilate, and so a clinically more helpful approach is to publish systematic reviews, meta-analyses and evidence-based clinical guidelines to guide practitioners. The Cochrane collaboration assists this process by producing standards of research methodology, data collection and analysis that ensure the highest quality of evidence is now gathered. However, despite these 'good things' there is still a backlash against EBM from clinicians who feel that the over-reliance on these concepts threatens individual patient care and belittles the use of clinical reasoning based on experience and investigation of pathophysiological mechanisms. Critics argue that EBM restricts the use of treatments to ones for which (potentially biased) research evidence exists; some interventions will be overlooked or considered ineffective. Furthermore, this trend is also witnessed by journals which are more reluctant to publish case reports, wishing to gather and report only the highest level of evidence on the most representative samples possible, for example, the new *Journal of evidence-based mental health* only publishes RCTs.

Sackett (2000), proposed a more rounded model for evidence-based decision making using a combination of:

1. Clinical state
2. Patient preference
3. Research evidence form a range of studies from all levels of evidence
4. Clinical expertise.

He argued for the 'Integration of individual clinical expertise with the best available external clinical evidence from systematic research (derived from clinical epidemiology and medical informatics) to make decisions about the care of the individual' (p. 1). Epidemiological studies can be subcategorised most simply into observational and experimental (or interventional studies), differentiated by the way they examine events that (a) occur naturally in the population or (b) have been deliberately arranged or manipulated using an experimental design.

Observational studies

Case controlled studies

These compare characteristics and potential risk factors found in a group of cases defined by the presence of a disease or clinical outcome, with the same characteristics in a control group who are free of the disease or clinical outcome. Essentially this design is efficient if the outcome is rare, and allows inferences about causality through the strength of associations between risk factors and outcome. Confounders can also be adjusted for either in the design stage by restriction or matching, or in the analysis stage using multivariate analytical techniques, for example, logistic regression and stratification. One of the greatest difficulties in this study design is to select controls that are free of the disease outcome and represent the population at risk of becoming cases. Commonly they are selected from groups who share the same environment: for example, the same neighbourhood, socio-economic group or hospital.

One of the hardest tasks of this study design is to ensure controls have the same chance of developing the disease or the clinical outcome, if they were exposed to the risk factor of interest. Thus they have to be as similar as possible in terms of other characteristics. For example, consider a study investigating the number of cases of hypotension following myocardial infarction from the cardiology ward (Schulz 2002). It used hospital controls from the casualty department. However, this group was biased as it included a local population subjected to high local use of a new anti-hypertensive medication that caused drowsiness, had been associated with car accidents and had a higher proportion of injured drivers who were attending the same casualty department.

Case-control studies are also susceptible to recall, selection and information bias. Information bias arises if data gatherers know the case or control status as this can affect how deeply they delve into the cases exposure history; this can be minimised by keeping data gatherers blind to case-control status, and training them to use standardised methods to elicit exposure history from subjects, and by keeping investigators blind to the main hypothesis of study. Case-control studies can yield important scientific findings with *relatively* little time, money and effort. This design was used in the early investigation of the cause of AIDs and identified high-risk groups: homosexual men, intravenous drug abusers and blood transfusion recipients. Public health professionals were quickly able to stop blood donation and put into action fast educational programmes for safe-sex reducing the incidence of HIV infection rapidly. Case-control studies are especially useful if the disease incidence rate is low or there is a long latency period. For example, a cohort study among healthy people to assess the risk of cancer would take a very long time.

Cohort studies

Prospective observational studies follow up individuals over time in order to determine whether exposure to a specific candidate risk factor affects the incidence of the outcome or disease in the future. If an increased risk of disease onset is found amongst the exposed group, it implies that the exposure may have led to the disease as the time sequence precludes reverse causality as an explanation for associations. For example, in a cross-sectional design, where an association is found between depression and life events, it may be that depression leads to poorer inter-personal skills causing life events or that the life events increase the risk of depression. Only a cohort design can address the time sequence issue, although other Bradford Hill criteria (Doll, 1992) must also be considered when inferring a causal relationship.

Exposure status of study participants is best defined at the start as both exposed and unexposed will be at risk of developing the outcome. Exposure status can change with time; for example, the proportion of women using the oral contraceptive pill will change if a proportion of them respond to new data or to media interest by deciding to use IUD instead. An appropriate control (unexposed) is one that is the same as the exposed in all respects except the lack of an exposure experience.

It is important to track participants over time and ensure losses are minimised, as these introduce bias if they are related to exposure or outcome status; attrition also reduces the precision and power of the study. Clear, specific and measurable outcomes should be defined in advance to ensure equal assessment, as knowledge of exposure status (by researcher or participant) can influence ratings of case status. The

Table 2.1   Bradford Hill criteria for a causal relationship
Strength of association
Consistency of findings from other studies
The presence of a dose–response relationship
Plausibility given our understanding of possible underlying biological mechanisms

identification of outcomes needs to be by a comparable procedure irrespective of exposure status. The strength of this design is the clear definition of exposure status that is not biased by knowledge of disease status. It is the only way of determining incidence, natural history of disease and temporal sequence between putative cause and outcome. It also lends itself well to investigation of multiple outcomes after a single exposure: does cigarette smoking cause lung cancer and/or stroke? However, looking at multiple outcomes and then selectively choosing to report only some can introduce bias. This type of study design is vulnerable to 'selection bias' as it is not an option for rare diseases or one that takes a long time to develop. Differential attrition between exposed and unexposed groups also introduces bias. Cohort studies are also relatively expensive due to the duration of follow-up of large numbers of subjects, and the number of interviews necessary. Therefore, the questions to be answered must be sufficiently important, and the study clearly planned to ensure that important research questions are fully answered, whilst any methodological problems are overcome.

Comparing and contrasting observational and experimental studies

Observational studies can yield estimates of treatment effect similar to those provided by experimental (standardised and randomised) studies. But many therapies that originally looked promising in observational studies were later discredited after experimental studies; for example, claims that HRT could reduce the risk of coronary heart disease in postmenopausal women (Sacks 2000). Observational studies do not provide definitive answers to questions about therapeutic efficacy, as there remains the possibility that bias and confounding explain associations. They do identify candidate risk factors, and the possibility of developing interventions to modify, eradicate or prevent the occurrence of risk factors. Furthermore, any intervention must have impact on specific pathophysiological, bio-psychosocial or biosocial pathways. That is, there must be a plausible mechanism, and the intervention must be known to act on that mechanism for there to be confidence in any intervention being safely introduced. Such knowledge also helps identify potential confounders. However, many interventions introduced in mental health care are a result of serendipitous discovery or observation of beneficial effects (ECT, Chlorpromazine as antidepressant) whilst well-thought-out mechanisms of action may later be revised when other interventions acting on different pathophysiological mechanisms are found to be equally effective. For example, the dopamine hypothesis of schizophrenia was, for many decades, considered to explain the mechanism of anti-psychotics. However, the atypical anti-psychotics affect other neurotransmitter systems but are equally, if not more, effective in some cases, with fewer adverse effects.

Observational studies tend to have broader inclusion criteria, a wider spectrum of coexistent illness and disease severity and dissimilarity of concomitant treatments. That is, the experiment is not as pure as is found in RCT designs, where cases and controls, or intervention and placebo groups, are carefully selected according to strict criteria. It is harder to control for confounders and bias with observational methods. In fact without randomisation the decision about treatment allocation would be based on patient characteristics, where the difference in outcome observed may be explained by these factors rather than the treatment. Observational studies do have some advantages over randomised studies. Owing to large sample sizes, some are able to detect very small effects that are not detectable in small randomised studies. They also provide a realistic way to assess the long-term outcome of intervention beyond the time-scale of many trials. Randomised studies have many disadvantages: sometimes a randomised study is too difficult to perform for practical (expense) and ethical reasons; or its results will be clinically meaningless; or, in the case of adverse outcomes, these could be so infrequent that they could only be detected by huge randomised trials that are rarely conducted. In this instance, specific alternatives include observational methods such as post-marketing surveillance of medication. In reality, experimental and observational methods should have complementary not competing roles in the evaluation of health care interventions.

RANDOMISED CONTROL TRIALS

In a randomised controlled study, subjects are randomly allocated into a study group (where they receive the intervention) and a control group (where they may receive a placebo or a comparator intervention). These groups are then followed up to compare their treatment response. RCTs usually have a parallel design where placebo/comparator and active treatment are administered in the same time period to different groups. For rarer conditions it is easier to use a crossover design; in this, during the first period of study, the whole group gets the experimental intervention and then following a washout period the entire group receives the comparator/placebo intervention. The advantages of crossover design include all subjects receiving the experimental intervention and the subjects serving as their own controls. Also, fewer subjects are needed to carry out the study and it is possible to maintain blinding. However, crossover trials present special challenges for mental health care where there are complex interventions, and the concept of a 'washout' period is difficult to sustain.

Analysis of baseline data and covariate adjustment

For unbiased analysis of RCTs, the treatment groups must be well balanced with respect to baseline characteristics. A significant imbalance in baseline characteristics of the two groups will not matter unless the characters that are unbalanced predict outcome. Most trials report simple outcome comparisons between treatments unadjusted for baseline covariates; others include covariate-adjusted results too. Reports vary in their use of covariate-adjusted analyses and this merits clearer guidelines. In a recent survey of research studies, between three and fourteen covariates were included but the reasons for the choice of covariates was not explained (Assmann 2000).

Randomisation

This is the single most powerful element of an RCT study design. It refers to random allocation to intervention groups, and ensures all patients have an equal chance of being assigned to any of the treatment groups. It ensures that all variables that may have an effect on outcome, other than the study intervention are equally distributed between intervention and comparator group(s). This is important to produce groups comparable in respect of known, but more importantly in respect of unknown, prognostic factors at baseline. Any observed effect could then be attributed to the intervention. Any process for randomisation that could be manipulated by researchers may lead to the researcher consciously or unconsciously behaving in a way that could influence the random allocation of the individual. So standard methods exist to generate an unpredictable assignment randomisation sequence by use of random numbers tables and computer-generated lists of numbers.

Statistical methods for randomising are categorised as cluster methods or block methods. In blocked randomisation, patients are assigned to a block on the basis of their characteristics (e.g. age, sex) and then randomly allocated to a treatment group within their block. In this way, the mean value of any potential known confounding factor will be similar in each group, and also the distribution of other characteristics will be identical in each arm of the trial, making any observed differences directly attributable to the intervention.

Sometimes randomisation by group is better than randomising by individual. In certain interventions where the controls' behaviour could be affected by those getting the experimental treatment by sharing information about the intervention, cluster or group randomisation is preferred. Randomisation by GP practice, or ward or clinic will minimise contamination.

Allocation concealment

Allocation concealment refers to a distinct process that protects the allocation sequence before and until assignment, to prevent selection bias. It is important not to confuse this with blinding, although it is sometimes referred to as 'randomisation blinding'.

Blinding

Blinding refers to the degree to which people are kept in the dark about who is randomised to which group. However, blinding can't always be implemented in trials. For example, research with psychological interventions.

Three types of blinding can be discerned on the basis of how many of the three groups of analysers are kept in the dark about intervention assignments (participants, investigators and outcomes assessors). In single blinding only participants are kept in the dark; in double blinding, the participants and investigators; and in triple blind, all three. It is important to monitor maintenance of blinding throughout the course of the trial.

Placebo

Pharmacological studies, define a placebo as an inert substance, usually with no pharmacological effect, matched with thecomparator for colour,

---

Table 2.2   Advantages of blinding

Can improve compliance and retention of trial participants
Can reduce the use of non-standardised supplementary treatment (co-intervention)
Can be used to reduce bias (observational, information and ascertainment)
Prevents those admitting patient to trial from knowing upcoming assignment
Protects sequence after allocation

taste and smell. In some cases an active placebo is used; a placebo with properties that mimics the side-effects that would otherwise reveal the identity of the active drug. Use of a placebo is a good way to get accurate knowledge of the relative tolerability of a new drug. Debriefing patients and investigators to curb overly encouraging behaviours of investigators and overly optimistic patients' assumptions and expectations of outcomes and thinking carefully about the way to present the placebo can reduce some of the psychological placebo effect.

The Declaration of Helsinki (5th Revision, World Medical Association, October 2000) demands individual study patients are assured of the best-proven diagnostic and therapeutic methods, even in the control group. It discards the use of a placebo group as a control group if a proven treatment exists. With respect to informed consent, it raises concerns such as deception and withholding of information by unscrupulous researchers to encourage patient participation. Despite this, the use of a placebo is a necessary obligation imposed by many regulatory authorities involved in appraising new treatments (for example, the US food and drug administration authority). These authorities are effectively endorsing and carrying out medical research violating the Helsinki declaration.

Table 2.3   Factors contributing to placebo effect

Psychological effects	○ Doctor–patient relationship and expectation of both patients and evaluators based on belief that the pill will help ○ Trappings associated with clinical trial, for example: 1. The supplemental attention of enthusiastic appreciative investigators 2. A lowering of anxiety by receiving a definitive diagnosis from trusted and experienced trial doctor 3. An increased sense of mastery and control that comes from a greater understanding of their illness in unhurried, extensive evaluation of research setting
Non-psychological effects	Spontaneous recovery Tendency to seek treatment outside study
Statistical artefacts	Regression to the mean Drift in measurement of response over time

Change to open label (COLA) design

The COLA design was proposed to overcome some of the ethical and organisational problems of the usual design, while preserving its scientific rigour. In this design the patients are randomised on a double blind basis into treatment groups. During the trial the patient or physician can ask for a change from double blind to any open label treatment of choice (experimental or not) if the blinded treatment is not thought to be satisfactory. Then the main outcome variable in COLA design is the time until a patient demands such a change. In trials with a COLA design the patients' personal impression of therapy is the most important factor in its assessment. It has proved to be much easier to get informed consent for this variety of RCT than the standard format of no choice (Hogel 1994).

Attrition

All useful studies need a sufficiently large, long and complete follow-up. In fact, the *Journal of evidence-based mental health* sets a standard and will not publish the results of an RCT unless there has been greater than 80% follow-up. It is important to account for attrition from all sources (Table 2.4).

Intention to treat analysis (ITA)

The advantages of randomisation are lost and bias creeps in if the data analysis is restricted just to completers. Completers are the better prognostic group, are compliant with treatment regardless of whether it is placebo or active treatment, and may have more health-prone behaviour associated with a good prognosis. Non-compliers may have been more symptomatic, developed side-effects or had symptom exacerbation, so may have had a poorer prognosis and leaving them out makes the intervention look better than it really is. ITA requires that all

Table 2.4   Common reasons for attrition
Adverse drug effects
Non-response
Recovery
Death
Loss of motivation
Withdrawal
Concomitant illness/pregnancy

subjects in the initial randomised allocation are included in the analyses, regardless of whether they are compliant with, or completed, the intervention. There are various methods for including these data in the final reporting of a trial (Table 2.5).

Secondary outcomes and subgroup analysis

Some trials report treatment differences in various subgroups of patients subdivided by baseline characteristics. Whilst these subgroup analyses can be informative they can also be potentially misleading. If the overall trial result is significant, almost inevitably some subgroups will, and some will not, show significant difference depending on chance and size of subgroups. Conversely, if the overall difference is not statistically significant, some subgroups may have a bigger observed treatment difference by chance which may even reach significant difference. For example, an intervention trial for mental illness found no overall difference, but if men and women were separated, a significant difference appeared for women (Assmann 2000). The credibility of subgroup analysis is improved if confined to a few predefined subgroups on the basis of biological plausibility hypothesis, or concerns about major adverse effects.

One of the benefits of subgroup analyses is that they can indicate factors that may be used to stratify randomisation. However, subgroup analyses can sometimes adversely affect the benefit observed in clinical

Table 2.5 Three ways to count results of non-completers randomised into the trial

Last observation carried forwards
Modelling
Sensitivity analysis

Table 2.6 Guidelines to decide if apparent differences in subgroup response is real

Did hypothesis precede, not follow, analysis?
Was subgroup one of small number of hypothesis tested?
Was difference consistent across studies?
Is there indirect evidence suggesting hypothesised difference?
Is size of difference clinically important?

trials. In some cases they are the result of a post hoc data dredging exercise to achieve significant results in an otherwise overall negative trial. A conclusion based on subgroup analysis can have adverse consequences both if a particular category of patients denied effective treatment produces a false negative (e.g. duration of symptoms being used as a cut-off post MI for those getting Streptokinase; Lauer 2003) and when ineffective or even harmful treatment is given to a subgroup of patients. Most trials lacked power to detect any but very large subgroup effects. Investigators should recognise if their trial isn't large enough to detect realistic subgroup effects and be particularly wary of claiming a treatment difference in a subgroup when the overall treatment comparison isn't significant; such subgroup rescuers of otherwise negative trials is unwarranted unless evidence is statistically convincing and clinically sensible.

Statistical tests of interaction (that assess whether a treatment effect differs between subgroups) should be used rather than inspection of subgroup p-values that encourage inappropriate subgroup claims. The condition should only be influenced if a statistical interaction test supports a subgroup effect – even then emphasis should depend on biological plausibility, number of subgroup analysis, their pre-specification, and the statistical strength of evidence.

Generalisability
Methodological rigour may lead to biased samples and highly coherent and controlled treatment protocols. This achieves high levels of valid trials at the expense of the trials generalisability. For example, the more rigorously defined the intervention or the control and intervention group's inclusion criteria, the less applicable to routine practice it tends to be. Thus, trials of antidepressants completed on young volunteers who are healthy may not give a good indication of treatment effectiveness, as opposed to efficacy, of the same antidepressant when given to a range of ages, people with co-morbid conditions and different ethnic groups. If the focus of an RCT is 'efficacy', the study tends to be conducted in a centre of excellence, develop stringent eligibility criteria and rigorous study protocols and opt for outcomes that will be sensitive to change. In these conditions closer patient scrutiny reduces adverse events.

If the focus of RCT is 'effectiveness', this assesses interventions in a real-world setting. There have to be liberal eligibility criteria, protocols that can actually be implemented in routine clinical practice, and patient-centred outcomes. Effectiveness research design is weighted to high generalisability but the price paid is a greater threat to internal validity.

Quality in trial design and reporting

There has also been interest in regulating the overall standard of RCTs and reducing restriction of the publication of trials to those with positive results. This results in an unbalanced and often inaccurate summary of evidence when a question is posed. A number of research groups have put together guidelines for the conduct and reporting of RCTs, e.g. Consolidated Standards of Reporting Trials, or CONSORT, Guidelines (Begg 1996).

Registration has been suggested as a way to reduce publication bias (Dickersin and Rennie 2003). Some scientific journals have had RCT amnesty campaigns and the Cochrane project has set up a register. Recently published guidelines call on pharmaceutical companies to publish all their RCTs of marketed products (Wager 2003).

RCTS IN MENTAL HEALTH RESEARCH

In this section we discuss significant challenges in applying RCT designs to mental health care. Illustrated using examples from 'topical' randomised controlled studies of: pharmacological interventions, psychological interventions and complex community interventions.

Pharmacological interventions

The strong influence of the placebo effect in randomised studies of antidepressant efficacy/effectiveness limits the validity of this sort of study to evaluate these drugs. The placebo response can affect the relative efficacy of a drug, reduce trial power and, where placebo responses are linked to other characteristics that are unequally distributed between trial arms, can be an unwanted confounder. Placebo responses are related to a number of influences, including encouragement during the course of therapy. From a strictly pharmacological model of depression treatment, the therapeutic alliance might be considered to be a placebo response rather than a component of the intervention. Depression causes a loss of vitality and motivation. A good clinical care review of what the patient did and didn't do encourages resolving problems and resumption of activity. So history taking, an assessment, verbalising the history and discussing with the clinician may themselves have an impact on the depressive state. Structured problem solving and activity scheduling are approaches proven to help lift depression in randomised controlled trials and can act to confound the effects attributable directly to the drug (WHO 1999). Improvement due to natural history, remission and fluctuating symptom levels can also contribute to the perceived effect of the placebo.

Another criticism of randomised trials of antidepressant efficacy has been the use of an active placebo to compare with the antidepressant. Atropine was frequently used in the past, originally selected to mimic the anti-cholinergic side-effects of antidepressants; using this approach, a difference between the two groups may unblind both subjects and evaluators.

Moncrieff *et al.* (1988), in a small meta-analysis of 9 studies, compared tricyclic antidepressants with an active placebo of low-dose atropine. Moncrieff reported superiority of drug over active placebo, but a diminished effect size in the active placebo group (ES 0.50 in non active placebo trial v ES 0.21 in active placebo).

Janowsky and Overstreet (1995) gave experimental evidence that agents affecting central cholinergic neurotransmitter have a profound effect on mood and suggested atropine itself may be a weak antidepressant (that is, more active compared with a true, neutral placebo).

Placebo responses are dynamic and vary inversely with illness severity (Andrews 2001). Studies also show that while the placebo response declines with increasing severity of depression, antidepressant response increases (Arif 2002).

Thaase (1999) argues that about a third of the published data on antidepressant efficacy fails to demonstrate efficacy. He argues for the recruitment of subjects with moderate and severe illness to reduce the placebo effect. Others suggest a four-week lead-in phase in which subjects receive psycho-education about handling depression, yet this in itself may act as an intervention, but could service as a good comparison group (Arif 2002). There is a significant placebo influence in both arms of trials of antidepressants and also in both studies of short-term antidepressant use during acute episodes and during maintenance treatment (Andrews 2001). Randomisation to maintenance after resolution of an acute episode is not adequate, as controls are not necessarily comparable to the intervention group which has experience of exposure to anti-depressant drugs (Moncrieff 2002). Also it is notoriously difficult to maintain blinding from placebo groups once you discontinue the drug because discontinuation reactions to antidepressants come into play. These occur with all antidepressants and the symptoms can alert patients so that this knowledge affects the assessment of the outcome (Haddad 1989).

Psychological interventions

The economic might of pharmaceutical companies serves to support efficacious pharmacological interventions, whilst advocacy for non-pharmacological interventions is left to overstretched professionals also entrusted to provide clinical care, and patients who also have to contend with debilitating illness. When undertaken, such studies are usually co-ordinated from specialised research units. There has always been a notable lag in non-pharmacological interventions reaching the national research agenda.

Some people continue to hold the view that psychological processes in some forms of psychotherapy are simply too complex, individual in character and multi-factorial for any research evaluation beyond clinical accounts. In fact, Parry and Richardson in a document reviewing strategic policy for psychotherapy research in England proposed abandoning RCTs altogether in favour of naturalistic studies (NHS Executive, DoH 1996). Morstyn (1993) argues that this view inadvertently grants psychological treatments relative immunity from public scrutiny and serves to mystify and compound the stigma of psychotherapies.

Despite this constraining view, some researchers have soldiered on and used the drug metaphor of double blind placebo controlled trial to evaluate psychotherapy as well as they can. Such a tradition can be found in published accounts for at least the last twenty years. However, we view this type of evaluation as fitting, or forcing, a square peg through a round hole, because only 'round holes' are seen as evidence. If the drug metaphor for psychotherapy is adopted and promulgated, *a reductio ad absurdum* leads to questions such as: What are the pharmacokinetic and pharmacodynamic properties of an intervention? How is an interpretation metabolised?

It is virtually impossible to design a double blind study of psychological treatment. It is also difficult to transfer results from efficacy studies to clinical practice, as in a clinical setting people have co-morbidity, enduring symptoms and social disability. Psychological treatments are often second-line in clinical practice, even if recommended as first-line by research, or indeed undertaken as first-line interventions in research projects. Patients with similar symptoms differ in personality, previous life experience, social circumstances and attitudes to psychologists, receptivity and perhaps responsiveness to psychological treatments.

Salkowskis *et al.* (1995) proposed a solution to bridge the gap between research and clinical practice by developing an 'hourglass model' where researchers should first determine efficacy, then do effectiveness studies followed by service evaluation. Salkowskis' group used this model to demonstrate specific effects in Cognitive Behavioural Therapies (CBTs).

Another problem in psychotherapy research is that, in general, controls have fewer sessions of shorter duration, experiencing a different exposure length from those in the intervention group. This has implications for a weaker therapeutic alliance in the control group, perhaps with less mobilisation of the placebo effect, making comparison difficult and potentially flawed. Also, variations of maintenance dose are rarely allowed, or taken account of.

Guthrie *et al.* (2000) identified a number of categories of common myths about how psychotherapies worked that they felt needed to be challenged and factored into evaluations (Table 2.7).

RCTs are only as good as their methods, and rely on well-defined and managed interventions and precise outcome measures. A number of ways have been developed to carry out and evaluate psychotherapy in order to make the square peg fit the round hole.

Manualising an intervention is one method that has gained popularity when trying to achieve uniformity, although it is difficult to imagine this works in practice. It is certainly not possible to manualise every statement or comment or thinking process in therapies; the most obvious example is psychoanalytic therapies where hundreds of sessions may have been spent, and their content is not predictable. Even for manuals of CBT it is likely that the therapist's personality and non-specific factors also influence therapeutic efficacy. Studies challenging this view are those based on trials of virtual-reality-based CBT programmes (Proudfoot 2003). More time limited and structured therapies are now amenable to evaluation by creating 'treatment manuals' which aim to ensure that therapists adhere to specific prescribed therapeutic interventions but in reality, once a therapy has proven value, manuals are rarely consulted.

Psychotherapies can be split into cognitive/behavioural and interpretive/dynamic dimensions. In practice, there is a bias away from the latter as most patients in services are of low social class, 50% have avoidant or dependent personalities and 70% are on psychotropics. The

Table 2.7 Myths about how psychotherapies work		
Myths	Assumption	Reality
Patient uniformity	All treated patients will respond regardless of underlying psychopathology, to any of the various treatments being compared in a similar way	Different pathologies have different predilections
Treatment uniformity	All psychological treatments will effect similar changes within the same time framework	These approaches don't effect changes in the same time frame so cannot be meaningfully compared. Personality change (focus of psychodynamic therapy) takes longer than symptom reduction (focus of briefer therapies with CBT approach) but patients generally prefer symptom reduction not personality change
Therapist–patient dyad uniformity	A similar interest regardless of who is therapist and patient or whether the two fit	Careful matching of patient and therapist is not possible

dynamic/interpretive spectrum show increasingly favourable results if patients are more affluent, better educated and have longer exposure.

Many studies of psychological intervention are comparative studies with patients randomised to different types of therapies, classically one or more of cognitive/behavioural or psychodynamic/interpretive approaches. Researchers have to be wary of reverting to the old exercise of playing off brand A against brand B in order to sustain a collaborative effort between psychotherapists of different persuasions in order to investigate the scope and limitations of psychological treatments available in a typical NHS setting.

There are specific problems with the use of psychodynamic psychotherapy as a research therapy. There is great variability in the short-term response ranging from great improvement to great deterioration. However, the focus is on individual personality management, and possibly change, over long periods of time. This poses the huge problem of determining and measuring outcomes and trying to achieve standard outcomes for inter-study comparison over a time continuum.

To achieve this, psychotherapy researchers have attempted to operationalise interpersonal patterns and intra-psychic changes. For example, Margison *et al.* (2000) defined seven measurement strategies in psychotherapy research (Table 2.8).

Several research teams have set about specifically developing theoretically relevant measures of psychoanalytical constructs and examining their clinical utility. Two main developments have been the Quality of Object Relations score (QoR), rating the persons enduring tendency to establish certain types of relationships (Piper *et al.* 1991) and the Personal Relatedness Profile (PRP), rating psychoanalytical aspects of interpersonal relationships (Hobson *et al.* 1998). There is good corroboration between these two; in fact 22/30 items in PRP correspond to QoR and both have proved useful in a variety of important decision-making methods in psychotherapy (Table 2.9).

Lots of work has gone into the identification of predictable and specific effects of psychotherapy. However, there is also the added problem of trying to identify the standard non-specific effects of

---

Table 2.8   7 measurement strategies in psychotherapy research

1. Verbal response mode – microanalysis of session
2. Case formulation
3. Treatment integrity – adherence, competence and differentiation
4. Performance – synthesis of adherence, competence and skilfulness
5. Treatment definition
6. Therapeutic alliance
7. Routine outcome measures that assess well-being, problems, symptoms and funding

---

Table 2.9   Uses of QoR

Prediction of therapeutic alliance
Prediction of outcome of brief individual therapy
Selection of patients for psychodynamic therapy
Benefits of remaining in day treatment programme
Impact of transference

therapy that contribute to the placebo effect (Gelder *et al.* 1973). Recent studies of eating disorders illustrate this. The comparative approach was adopted in studies of effective psychological intervention for eating disorders. A study by Dare *et al.* (2001) compared routine outpatient care, with cognitive analytical, psychoanalytic, and family therapy groups. It found that experienced therapists delivering therapies of adequate length were a more important variable than the specific therapeutic modality used. A comparative study of cognitive therapy versus dietary counselling in out-patient treatment of anorexia nervosa also found these more non-specific factors to be more important in reducing attrition in the dietary counselling group. They also found fostering therapeutic alliance to be a fundamentally important factor (Serfaty *et al.* 1999). The flaws of using the RCT approach in evaluation of psychological interventions are best illustrated by an in-depth discussion of the limitations of therapies used to treat particular categories of disorder. Using an example of Post Traumatic Stress Disorder (PTSD), we now show in detail the form of controversies in the evaluation of therapies.

Post traumatic stress disorder

Studies evaluating psychological debriefing have been the impetus for much criticism of psychotherapies. The major problem is the loss of historical context of this therapy, which was not originally designed as a stand-alone therapy but as part of 'The critical incident stress management programme' (Mitchell 1983, pp. 36–9), developed as a composite intervention to use for emergency workers shortly after a traumatic event, originally within a group therapy programme (Table 2.10).

Today the term 'psychological debriefing' has been corrupted and refers to a variety of different types of intervention; both individual or group debriefing, with behavioural or cognitive behavioural bias, with

Table 2.10 Components of Mitchell's critical incident stress management programme

Programme including:
1. Pre-incident training
2. Stress inoculation
3. Demobilisation
4. Debriefing
5. Follow up

or without an information-processing component and delivered in a variable number of sessions. There is a body of evidence today that supports the lack of efficacy of psychological debriefing in the individual altogether and suggests that it may actually be harmful and lead to an exacerbation of symptoms (Mayou 1998).

Studies have also shown that psychological debriefing is only valuable when survivors sense their trauma to be over (Bisson *et al.* 1996). Bisson *et al.* (1996) found that their population of in-patient burns victims were exposed to new trauma in an ongoing way; they were dealing with a very heterogeneous group, with their immediate adjustment being affected by factors in the ward environment such as placement in an isolated side-room or an open shared ward. Other confounding factors were differences in burn severity, exposure to previous traumas and involvement with others in the accident. These factors introduced bias within the two groups (psychological debriefing v non-psychological debriefing).

There continues to be evidence that psychological debriefing offered as part of a group therapy is helpful, but there is lack of clarity about which techniques pay most dividends. The Koach project (Solomon *et al.* 1992) examined a population of Israeli war veterans with PTSD. The central treatment component was using a number of behavioural techniques within the framework of a residential group treatment to confront avoidance and deliberate refusal to work through past war experiences. Using their approach, they identified 'habituation of anxiety' as an important confounder. After two years they demonstrated no change in traumatic symptoms but a reduction in phobias and improved social function.

Busuttil *et al.* (1995) also offered a group treatment approach, incorporating a number of behavioural practices, aimed at anxiety habituation and extinction; they had positive results. They also had an additional focus of therapy–information processing. They demonstrated better symptom improvement, 83.5% compared with the Israeli group. They suggested the benefits of information processing and that Pavlovian extinction techniques were additive for PTSD.

Foa *et al.* (1995) added weight to this evidence from their studies of rape victims with PTSD. They noticed therapeutic success was associated with information processing of events, manifest as changes to the rape narratives during the course of exposure therapy. The victim showed evidence of trying to make sense of their traumatic experience by modifying their original narrative in a more adaptive way during the course of therapy.

Complex interventions in community care

Over the last forty years, there has been a trend to introduce treatments for schizophrenia and other Severe and Enduring Mental Illness (SMI) in community orientated settings. Evidence has accumulated for the effectiveness of Community Mental Health Teams as a treatment delivery vehicle for maintaining contact, continuity of care, symptom reduction and improved functioning. However, the hard evidence for community based care stops there.

There is little research evidence looking at the delivery of interventions by community workers. Research in this area would be useful to help determine what roles to assign to multidisciplinary community psychiatric staff. This human resource is one of the most highly trained and valuable commodities in mental health care.

The trend recently has been that community staff are employed to carry out generic case management; certain disciplines, namely psychology, occupational therapy and dual diagnosis workers are assigned smaller caseloads in order to allow space for consultation and to take on complex cases. However, it may be a waste of resources for staff to be delivering interventions that they don't deliver well because of skill deficits. For example, a recent review of mental health nursing for people with schizophrenia (Working in partnership 1994) found 80% of people with schizophrenia were not on the caseload of a CPN. There was speculation that this may be because CPNs were 'indulging' in all sorts of inappropriate alternative interventions in the community; for example, counselling rather than care co-ordination. Gournay and Brooking (1994) compared counselling in GP practices administered by CPNs with standard GP care; they found weak positive results and concluded that CPNs were ineffective counsellors in primary care and better deployed to treat SMI.

A significant proportion of the NHS budget is diverted towards funding training of community staff. This helps retention and personal development but there has been little interest in the evaluation of training to date despite its high cost. Attendance at certain training courses (for example, the THORN course targeted at generic community working) is considered essential for improving the quality of staff. However, capturing the essence of what is done with what is taught and determination of how effective this is at achieving its goal is very difficult. Training evaluation has to consider the impact of training on both staff performance and individual clinical outcomes of patients. The effects of a particular professional will not only depend on skill and knowledge, but also on their individual style of delivery and the therapeutic alliance, as well as patient characteristics. An evidence base looking at the outcomes of training would be invaluable to assist service developers distribute resources efficiently.

Recently there has been a lot of interest in new interventions aimed at different phases of schizophrenia, from early acute onset to after chronic established illness. For example, early intervention programmes are being developed. Evaluating these may prove difficult because of a lack of standard definitions and also because they have developed in specialised centres, with a package of care that is difficult to partition into individual components. Time will tell if such services can be provided in non-academic centres.

The literature does not make the population at whom early intervention is targeted very clear. UK government policy defines early intervention as a service for people who have already developed established recurrent psychotic patterns, whilst in some research centres, services have been set up aimed at secondary prevention, with treatment offered in the prodromal phase (LEO project (Lambeth Early Onset Service), currently underway in South London, 2004).

There has also been recent interest in the literature in assertive rehabilitation of people with schizophrenia immediately after an acute episode, to foster social networks and activity to reduce their level of chronic disability by negative symptoms. Knapp *et al.* (1994) carried out an RCT to evaluate the effectiveness of one such rehabilitation programme, the Daily Living Programme (DLP), as an early intervention. Maudsley in-patients were randomised to the DLP delivered by Community Psychiative Nurses (CPNs) trained in this approach on the THORN (short psychosocial intervention) course or standard care post discharge care. They found a highly significant result at year one, sustained for four years.

A number of methodological weaknesses affected the impact of these study findings. The DLP group was possibly a better prognostic group as they had lower rates of in-patient treatment and analysis was restricted to those who were compliant with assessments. The control intervention was the standard post-discharge care, which was generally of a poor standard and evolving across London. Also, the assessors were not blinded to treatment status. These criticisms are not idiosyncratic to this study and also resonate with general criticism of RCTs of rehabilitation packages.

At present, valuable community-based evidence is being uncovered by a leisurely free-for-all digging endeavour rather than a centralised organised excavation. The ground has been dug a little deeper in some areas, usually in response to political interest. One such area is assertive outreach treatment methods delivered by Assertive Outreach Teams (AOTs).

The AOT literature functions as a minefield against the RCT approach. In some ways it should serve as a historical lesson against the knee-jerk reactions of politicians putting their faith and funding into seductive complex interventions without carrying out further substantiating effectiveness research.

In the UK, AOTs appeared to be the 'quick fix' mental health services needed in order to manage a subgroup of patients with SMI who were risky, difficult to engage and made 'revolving door' use of hospital beds, with CMHTs struggling to meet their needs.

Strong evidence for the efficacy of the AOT model compared with control services came from the Stein and Test (1980) study in the US and a study in Australia (Hoult 1983). One of the positive outcomes was to demonstrate a decrease in bed usage, the most costly component of the British service. Positive practical experience of home-based treatments in north Birmingham also added to the political enthusiasm about adopting this new form of treatment. Assertive outreach became a central part of the British government's mental health policy. In England it became mandatory to develop assertive outreach provision in adjunct to usual CMHT services (National Service Framework for Mental Health (DoH 1999); Mental Health Policy Implementation Guide (DoH 2001)).

Following the original studies, there was a growth of contrary evidence from experimental studies on both sides of the Atlantic, US (Chandler 1996 and McGrew 1995) and UK (UK700 Study, Burns *et al.* 1999 and PRiSM Study, Thornicroft *et al.* 1998).

The UK700 study (Burns 2000) hypothesised that the enhanced outcomes achieved abroad were related to the low caseloads and set out to investigate whether more Intensive Case Management (ICM) was the core element of AOT design resulting in reduced hospitalisation. They set up a multicentred RCT, across four inner city centres (South Manchester, Brixton, Paddington, Wandsworth). Patients with SMI were randomly allocated to receive either ICM with generic workers having a caseload of 1:10–15 or Standard Case Management (SCM), with a caseload of 1:30–35.

Prospective treatment data was collected over a two-year period. The Manchester site was unable to collect SCM data so was excluded from the study, resulting in information bias. We can speculate that perhaps difficulty collating data there reflected other problems in the delivery of case management and the exclusion of South Manchester patients may have served to eliminate a worse prognosis group, who may have responded differently to ICM, which could have affected the study's results. Another criticism was that case managers did their own event recordings; they could not be blinded and the ICM group may have been more diligent with their recording as they had more contact with researchers and more to prove than the SCM group.

The ICM group with reduced caseloads showed a greater contact frequency as measured by care events over 30 days (4.4 v 1.9), greater face-to-face contact, more attempts at face-to-face contact and greater carer contact.

But with respect to number and duration of hospital admissions, UK700 findings agreed with the findings of other British studies of ICM and failed to replicate any advantage over SCM groups. Two main reasons were cited for this consistent lack of advantage observed in the UK studies:

1. Use of different control services. Prior to ACT there had mainly been an office-based service in the US and Australia, whilst the *in vivo*-based (home and neighbourhood) service had already been established in the UK as standard practice and generic workers in SCM provision had always prioritised more ill patients causing the same level of contact as ICM when necessary.
2. Failure to replicate critical components of earlier successful experimental version, i.e. a variation in the fidelity of replication.

The UK700 group also carried out a very revealing parallel study in one of the four centres (St Mary's/St Charles). This was not an RCT but a two-year qualitative investigation of case management examining the 'nature' and 'impact' of 'assertive case working'. The evaluation used a combination of 'thematic interview survey' of the views of case managers and a study of randomly selected longitudinal cases from SCM and ICM groups. The thematic survey revealed consensus amongst case managers about the aims of case management, namely patient engagement, improved health and social function, reduced admission. They also all agreed that a comprehensive needs assessment was fundamental to focus case management. Both groups also viewed casework as an individual, not a team, responsibility.

A surprising finding was that, in practices, the traditional image of persistently non-compliant and elusive patients was rare. In a substantial proportion of study population – over a half – assertive casework was unnecessary and inappropriate as these cases were compliant and had their social needs met.

In the other half of the patients, both sorts of care managers were found to have a similar preferred way of working when consensual management failed. At this point both groups tended to adopt two strategies in varying degrees: firstly, brokerage – negotiating interventions from other individuals/agencies; and secondly, genericism – adopting clinical casework roles not normally associated with their discipline. The case studies identified four challenging patient groups and demonstrated consistent approaches to management among both groups of caseworkers.

There were two groups of patients for whom it was not possible to do assertive work. The first group was of high social functioners with insidious relapse. These people proved difficult to monitor for relapse and a lengthy compulsory admission ensued. The second group was a group with persistent non-compliance, elusiveness and chaotic behaviour. These people were managed as and when crises allowed. The two most challenging groups were:

i) A group with episodic serial non-compliance, who were non-compliant with appointments but taking medication. This group was easily managed by more assertive monitoring.
ii) A group who were also non-compliant with medication – associated with rapid relapse, increasing elusiveness and aggression. The standard case managers managed by having identified early relapse signs and accommodating for the episodic change with an increased frequency of contact, effective time management and displacement of routine casework. Surprisingly, both teams managed this patient group with equal effectiveness.

This finding was contrary to what UK700 had anticipated, i.e that the ICM team would be better able to implement assertive outreach by virtue of their low caseloads. But continual assertive casework with outreach as response to persistent non-compliance was unsustainable for both SCM and ICM because of absence of team-based management.

The study also described a phenomenon called Sensitive Anticipatory Action (SAA) which had a significant impact on the frequency and duration of in-patient admission. It involved action that was sensitive to individual circumstances and anticipated crises and helped prevent some significant psychiatric emergencies from arising. SAA comprised a collection of methods often used with non-symptomatic patients, including techniques promoting engagement, patient-centred medication review, assessment and response to social care needs and development

Table 2.11   Summary of findings of UK700 qualitative study

1. Interdisciplinary tensions of generic work, tend to stick to own role with individual generic work as dictated by individual patient needs, limited brokerage and limited team-based approach
2. In cases where assertiveness is needed, ICM and SCM seem able to practise this equally well
3. Not extensive practice of assertive outreach by ICM; this practice is undermined by lack of team-based management
4. SAA may make ICM more effective than exclusive focus on assertive casework
5. Improved co-ordination of health and social care has an essential influence on frequency/duration of admission – discharge is delayed if reliant on independent social care
6. Enhanced access to social care and team-based management of patients are probably most important elements

of crisis care plans. SAA was found to be carried out more in ICM than SCM patients.

These findings (summarised in Table 2.11), illustrate the value of qualitative and quantitative research in health care delivery, but the findings cannot be generalised to all four centres of UK700.

Some critics felt the lack of fidelity of UK teams to the US assertive community team (ACT) model was responsible for their failure in light of the US success (Marshall 1999).

Several people developed 'fidelity tests' to investigate this, e.g. Dartmouth ACT Scale (DACTS), Teague *et al.* (1998). This was originally developed to test the fidelity of the US replications of Stein and Test. The Pan London AOT study (Priebe 2003) used DACTS to examine the fidelity of the 24 London-wide AOT teams. Priebe, *et al.* characterised the teams into clusters on the basis of variables they thought personally important from a literature review of home treatment team research, expert opinion and their own experiential knowledge of services. Three clusters were differentiated (Table 2.12).

Cluster C teams were found to make up a third of London teams. They managed the highest frequency contacts *in vivo* of all types of teams, largely thought to be related to the lack of any formal administrative binds. They worked with the less risky and severely ill end of the spectrum. Their other idiosyncratic features included that they were associated with less stigma and perceived to be outside controlling mental health services and perceived to be supportive and

Table 2.12 Features of various clusters of London assertive outreach teams	Cluster A	Cluster B	Cluster C
Statutory teams	Yes	Yes	
CPA responsibility	Yes	Yes	No
Integrated health and social care	Yes	Yes	None
Psychiatric input	1 FT Dr / 100 pts	None	None
Dedicated beds	40% dedicated beds	None	None
PT : FT staff ratio	High 2.0 : 5.8		
MDT representation	Wide representation	Less than A	Lowest multidiscipline representation
Out of hours contact	Yes	Less than A	None
Caseload size	Small 9–10	Higher than A	Smaller

provided care for more limited and specific patient groups e.g. Afro-Caribbean and refugee groups.

DACTS was used as a tool to measure the model-fidelity of the teams. It incorporates scales covering three dimensions: human resources, organisational boundaries and service nature. Of 24 teams, only 3 scored more than 4 (high fidelity) and 4 scored between 2 and 2.9 (low fidelity). The majority scored between 3 and 3.9 (moderate fidelity). In fact the mean DACTS score was 3.4, indicating a moderate fidelity overall compared with US models.

DACTS itself was widely criticised as a tool. Some referred to it as a culture-bound instrument and said it was difficult to use it to assess the implementation of assertive outreach within the UK system of care. In fact only 6 out of 14 variables considered important in the cluster analysis used to characterise the London teams were reflected in DACTs. The London teams scored <3 on 8 DACT items suggesting that the London teams were significantly different from the US teams.

Mean scores from DACTS are of limited value and teams can score well because of one good overall feature: for example, provision of a high proportion of services *in vivo* or full social care integration. Overall mean score tells us little about service profile.

In 2002, Tyrer, a prominent and experienced figure in British psychiatry, issued a timely warning. His view, which reflected the findings of the UK literature was that the ACT approach was designed with the deficiencies of US mental health care in mind. He felt that failure to consider the US findings in the context of superior basic psychiatric provision in the UK would lead to unnecessary reorganisation of community services in order to accommodate assertive outreach. He expressed his anxiety that UK community psychiatry was at risk of entering an unhelpful developmental *cul de sac* as a result of this lack of foresight.

Our view is that we are currently in this developmental *cul de sac*, but the past twenty years, the post Stein and Test era, we feel has not been a totally futile venture as we have learnt a lot about the difficulties of trying to evaluate complex composite community interventions. RCTs of AOT in the UK conclude:

1. That case management should not be regarded as a treatment but a care structure to deliver treatment
2. That reduced caseload size achieves an increased level of contact
3. There is an absent outcome difference (continued hospitalisation) despite increased contact.

The focus of British research should now shift to conducting further trials using this increased contact frequency to deliver health gain in the form of evidence-based treatments.

CONCLUSIONS

In fields of medicine such as psychiatry, full of chronic disorders with undetermined aetiologies, choice of interventions is riddled with variance and uncertainty. The search and discovery of harder proof gives clinical decisions more credibility and for the short term offers hope and direction. There is something very powerful about having a strong backbone and the clinicians desire to construct this may yet preserve the dinosaur of the NHS so long as evolutionary processes can be accelerated using information and evidence.

References

Andrews and Jenkins (eds). (1999). Management mental disorder. WHO.
Andrews, G. (2001). Placebo response in depression – bane of research boon to therapy. *British Journal of Psychiatry*, **178**, 192–4.

Arif *et al.* (2002). Severity of depression and response to antidepressants and placebo on analysis of FDA database. *Journal of Clinical Psychopharmacology*, **22**(1), 40–5.

Assmann *et al.* (2000). Subgroup analyses and other mis (use) of baseline data in clinical trials. *Lancet*, **355**, 1064–9.

Begg *et al.* (1996). Improving quality of reporting of RCTs, consort statement. *JAMA*, **276**, 637–9.

Bisson *et al.* (1996). Psychological debriefing for outcome of acute burn trauma. *British Journal of Med Psychology*, **69**, 147–58.

Busuttil *et al.* (1995). Incorporating psychological debriefing technique within brief group psychotherapy programme for the treatment of PTSD. *British Journal of Psychiatry*, **167**, 495–502.

Burns *et al.* (1999). Intensive case management v standard case management in severe psychotic illness – randomised trial, UK700 group. *Lancet*, **353**, 2185–9.

Burns *et al.* (2000). Effects of caseload size on the process of care of patients with severe psychotic illness. *Report for UK700 trial*, **177**, 427–33.

Chandler *et al.* (1996). Client in two model capitated integrated service agencies. *Psychiatric services*, **47**, 175–80.

Dare *et al.* (2001). Psychological therapies for adults with anorexia nervosa: randomised controlled trial with out-patient treatment. *British Journal of Psychiatry*, **178**, 216–21.

Dickersin, K. and Rennie, D. (2003). Registering controlled trial. *JAMA*, **290**, 516–23.

DoH (1999). *National Service Framework for Mental Health: Modern Standards and Service Models for Mental Health*. Department of Health, London.

DoH. (2001). The mental health policy implementation guide. DoH, London.

Doll, R. (1992). Sir Austin Bradford Hill and the progress of medical science. *BMJ*, **305**(6868): 1521–6.

Foa *et al.* (1995). Changes in rape narratives during exposure therapy for PTSD. *Journal of Traumatic Stress*, **8**, 675–91.

Gelder *et al.* (1973). Specific and non-specific effects of psychotherapy. *British Journal of Psychiatry*, **123**, 445–62.

Gournay and Brooking. (1994). Counselling and CPNs. *British Journal of Psychiatry*, **164**, 231–8.

Guthrie *et al.* (2000). Psychotherapy for patients with complex disorders and chronic symptoms need for a new research paradigm. *British Journal of Psychiatry*, **177**, 131–7.

Haddad *et al.* (1989). Antidepressant discontinuation reaction. *British Medical Journal*, **316**, 1105–6.

Hobson *et al.* (1998). Objectivity in psychoanalytical judgements. *British Journal of Psychiatry*, **173**, 172–7.

Hogel *et al.* (1994). Change to open label design. Proposal and discussion of a new design for clinical parallel group double masked trials. *Arzneimittezforschung*, **44**(1), 97–9.

Holloway *et al.* (1997). Intensive case management for severe mental illness: controlled trial. *British Journal of Psychiatry*, **172**, 19–22.

Hoult *et al.* (1983). Psychiatric hospital v community treatment: the results of a randomised trial. *Australia and New Zealand Journal of Psychiatry*, **17**, 160–7.

Janowsky and Overstreet. (1995). The role of acetyl choline in mood disorder. In *Psychopharmacology: the 4th generation of progress* (eds Bloom and Kupfer), pp. 945–56. Raven Press, New York.

Knapp *et al.* (1994). Service use and costs of home-based versus hospital-based care for people with serious mental illness. *British Journal of Psychiatry*, **165**(2), 195–203.

Lauer *et al.* (2003). Clinical trial – multiple treatments, multiple endpoints and multiple lessons. *JAMA* (editorial), **289**(19), 2575–7.

Margison *et al.* (2000). Measurement and psychotherapy evidence-based practice and practice-based evidence. *British Journal of Psychiatry*, **177**, 123–30.

Marshall *et al.* (1991). Assertive community treatment for people with severe mental illness. *Schizophrenia nodule of Cochrane database of systematic reviews.*

Mayou *et al.* (1998). Psychological debriefing for road traffic accident victims, 3 year follow-up of RCT. *British Journal of Psychiatry*, **176**, 589–93.

McGrew *et al.* (1994). Measuring fidelity of implementation of a MH program model. *Journal of Consulting and Clinical Psychology*, **62**, 670–8.

Mitchell, J.T. (1983). When disaster strikes . . . the critical incident stress debriefing process. *JEMS.* **8**(1), 36–9.

Moncrieff *et al.* (1988). Metanalysis of trials comparing antidepressants with active placebo. *British Journal of Psychiatry*, **172**, 227–31.

Moncrieff *et al.* (2002). The antidepressant debate. *British Journal of Psychiatry*, **180**, 193–4.

Morstyn *et al.* (1993). Some fallacies of statistical inference about psychotherapy. *Australia and New Zealand Journal of Psychiatry*, **27**, 101–7.

Parry and Richardson. (1996). Psychotherapy services in England review of strategic policy. NHS Executive, DoH, London.

Piper *et al.* (1991). Quality of object relations v interpersonal functioning as predictors of therapeutic alliance and psychotherapy outcome. *Journal of Nervous and Mental Disease*, **179**, 432–8.

Priebe *et al.* (2003). AOTs in London: patient characteristics and outcomes. Pan London AO study part 3. *British Journal of Psychiatry*, **183**, 148–54.

Proudfoot *et al.* (2003). Computerized, interactive, multimedia cognitive-behavioural program for anxiety and depression in general practice. *Psychol Med.* **33**(2), 217–27.

Sackett. (2000). Evidence-based medicine; how to practise and teach EBM, 2nd edition. Churchill and Livingstone.

Sacks *et al.* (2000). Observational studies and randomised studies. *NEJM* (correspondence), **343**(16), 1194–7.

Salkowskis *et al.* (1995). Hourglass model. In *Research foundation for psychotherapy practise*, (eds Shapiro and Aveline). Wiley, Chichester.

Schulz *et al.* (2002). Case control study: research in reverse. *Lancet*, **359**, 431–5.

Serfaty *et al.* (1999). Cognitive therapy v dietary counselling in out-patient treatment of anorexia nervosa: effects of treatment phase. *European Eating Disorder Review*, pp. 334–50.

Slade and Priebe. (2001). Are RCTs the only gold that glitters? *British Journal of Psychiatry*, **179**, 286–7.

Solomon *et al.* (1992). The Koach project for treatment of combat related PTSD: rationale, aims and methodology. *Journal of Traumatic Stress*, **5**, 175–95.

Stein and Test. (1980). Alternative to mental hospital: conceptual model, treatment programme and clinical evaluation. *Archives General Psychiatry*, **37**, 392–7.

Teague *et al.* (1998). Program fidelity in ACT; development and use of a measure. *American Journal of Orthopsychiatry*, **68**, 216–32.

Thaase *et al.* (1999). How should efficacy be evaluated in randomised controlled trials of treatment of depression? *Journal of Clinical Psychiatry*, **60**, suppl 4, 25–31.

Thornicroft *et al.* (1998). From efficacy to effectiveness in community mental health service: PRiSM psychosis study 10. *British Journal of Psychiatry*, **173**, 423–37.

Tyrer *et al.* (2003). Assessing value of assertive outreach: dual study of process and outcome generation in UK700 trial. **183**, 437–45.

Tyrer *et al.* (2000). Are small caseloads beautiful in severe mental illness? *British Journal of Psychiatry*, **177**, 386–7.

Wager *et al.* (2003). Good publication practices for pharmaceutical companies. *Current Medical Research and Opinion*, **19**, 149–54.

3

Qualitative methods in psychiatric and mental health research

John R. Cutcliffe

INTRODUCTION

Qualitative research, by comparison with the quantitative paradigm, is
a relative newcomer. This may be one of the reasons for the historical
predominance of quantitative studies in mental health. Yet, even a
cursory examination of the number of recent psychiatric-nursing-related
studies that use qualitative approaches indicates that the number is
growing. For scholars and researchers who recognise and espouse a
pluralistic approach to research and knowledge generation, it is most
heartening to see that the impact of qualitative studies is increasing
and qualitative studies are starting to receive major funding. This
chapter provides an overview of the purpose of qualitative inquiry.
It then outlines some of the key differences in the underpinning
philosophies of qualitative/quantitative methods. Following this,
the chapter then attempts to dispel some common myths and
misconceptions of qualitative methods and provides an overview of
the more common methods. In order to demonstrate the use and
application of such methods, the chapter draws on examples from the
growing literature (and then highlights some common pitfalls that often
show in reports of qualitative research). The chapter concludes by
reiterating the need for a new paradigm of research and by considering
the role of qualitative research methods in the future of mental health
research.

AN OVERVIEW OF THE PURPOSE OF QUALITATIVE INQUIRY

All research is important to the development of knowledge within, and across, disciplines. In addition, arguments have been made that show the value and role of research to the wider community (Morse and Field 1995). However, no one single research paradigm can provide all the different knowledge that is required for a discipline, neither can it meet all the knowledge needs of the community. What qualitative research does then is attempt to understand, describe, explain and make sense of the social world. According to Morse and Filed (1995) qualitative research is 'the primary means by which the theoretical foundations of a social science may be constructed and re-examined' (p. 1). Accordingly, qualitative research is necessary for the knowledge, practice, education and policy-related goals of some mental health professionals and the formal area of mental health care. Qualitative research is concerned with phenomena as they occur and 'play out' in everyday life, and thus qualitative research is primarily concerned with descriptions and explanations of observed phenomena in order to induce solid theory (Sandelowski 1997). One crucial difference though between qualitative and quantitative approaches is that quantitative approaches are concerned with testing (existing) theory and qualitative approaches are concerned with the construction or induction of theory. Thus, qualitative inquiry is indicated when little or nothing is known about a phenomenon whereas quantitative studies are indicated when there is already an existing body of knowledge about a phenomenon. It is therefore incumbent upon the researcher to select the approach that is indicated by the current extent of knowledge/theory regarding a phenomenon and not be drawn into methodological 'turf wars'.

Having indicated that qualitative approaches are concerned with generating theory, it should be pointed out that all qualitative approaches do not have this aim. There are some methods, phenomenology for example, that aim to uncover the essence of a lived experience, describe and interpret key insights into these experiences and lived moments and thus produce a description. An often stated edict of qualitative research is that it is most useful when the researcher wishes to access and understand the phenomena from the point of view of the person who is in the experience, from the emic perspective, from the native's point of view (Schwandt 1994). As a result, qualitative inquiry is most often carried out in natural or 'naturalistic' settings, and this leads Morse and Field (1995) to point out that, 'the context in which the phenomenon occurs is considered a part of the phenomenon itself' (p. 10). The purpose of qualitative approaches is to answer certain types of questions, just as the purpose of quantitative approaches is to answer certain other different types of questions. Qualitative research cannot answer questions related to causality, questions relating to quantification or measurement. But qualitative research can answer questions relating to how processes occur, what an experience is like, how a culture contributes to and influences behaviour, how people live, cope, process and experience their daily lives. Within mental health care then, qualitative research is necessary to answer questions such as: What is it like to live with certain forms of mental health problems? How does one care for such individuals? How does the particular culture of a community relate to and influence certain health-related behaviours? More specific examples would then include: What is the lived experience of living day-to-day with schizophrenia? How do mental health practitioners form relationships with schizophrenic clients? What cultural norms exist within an acute mental health in-patient unit that serve to normalise 'outrageous' and 'shocking' behaviours? Just from this very short section it can be seen that qualitative research has much to contribute to the knowledge base of mental health care and practice.

THE KEY DIFFERENCES IN THE UNDERPINNING PHILOSOPHIES OF QUALITATIVE/QUANTITATIVE METHODS

It is perhaps a redundant point[1] that if qualitative studies are judged according to quantitative criteria and the philosophical underpinnings of quantitative studies, then they are likely to be seen as invalid, methodologically unsound and flawed. In order to understand the value and subsequent application of qualitative approaches it is necessary to point out the key differences in the underpinning philosophy when compared to quantitative approaches. Lincoln and Guba (1985) have pointed out that a variety of adjective labels have been coined to capture the philosophical underpinnings of the qualitative paradigm including naturalistic, interpretivist, postpositivist and hermeneutic. These approaches each incorporate the view that acknowledges a 'real world' where 'concrete phenomena' exist. Nevertheless, and importantly, the experience of that real world, the symbolic meanings ascribed to it, and how one subsequently behaves and acts in it, are determined by a

---

[1] However, a criticism that is still common in some places today.

Table 3.1 Major philosophical differences between the qualitative and quantitative paradigm

Qualitative	Quantitative
Subjective	Objective
Naturalistic	Positivistic
Interpretive	Empiricist
Concerned with uncovering shared, intersubjective meanings	Concerned with uncovering universal laws
Concerned with identifying and explaining life from the emic perspective; from the insider's point of view	Concerned with objective 'truth'
Idiographic 'generalisations'	Nomothetic generalisations

web of factors made up of language, symbol, culture, history and individual situatedness. Consequently, in terms of culture, human behaviour, experience and process, qualitative researchers purport that there is no 'objective truth'. Truth is contextual, temporal, locally located and constructed as a result of shared intersubjective meanings. The qualitative researcher then acknowledges that in undertaking such inquiry, he or she is a product of the same contextual web, his or her understandings and even the tools to undertake the inquiry also stem from the same contextual web (see Lincoln and Guba 1985; Schutz 1994; Schwandt 1994; Morse and Field 1995; Walters 1995). Furthermore, the qualitative researcher has no aspirations towards nomothetic generalisations, moving the specific to the general. Instead, if they aspire to generalisable findings, they wish to uncover idiographic generalisations. Or to rephrase, contextually based truths, essences or universals that are understood in terms of the particulars of various cases. A summary of these key differences is provided in Table 3.1.

DISPELLING SOME COMMON MYTHS AND MISCONCEPTIONS OF QUALITATIVE METHODS

In this section of the chapter I will identify and attempt to dispel some commonly occurring myths and misconceptions of qualitative research.

Qualitative research is incomplete if it does not lead to a deductive, theory testing, quantitative study

According to Sandelowski (1997) this inappropriate (and inaccurate) conception of qualitative research as *only* the preliminary, forerunner of a quantitative study is one of the key factors bedevilling the utilisation of qualitative methods. The view that qualitative research is incomplete by itself and the view that qualitative methods are only able to describe (Morse 1996), only serves to undermine the contribution of such studies and serves to reinforce the binary opposite (Derrida 1976), dominant discourse debate surrounding the hegemony of quantitative studies. (This will be addressed in more detail below.) There exist some theories, admittedly with a noted vintage, that describe levels of theory and posit qualitative studies as producing lower level theory than quantitative studies (Dickoff and James 1968). Additionally, it is entirely appropriate to follow an inductive with a deductive study, particularly if the research strategy has been designed this way. But that in no way suggests that every qualitative study *must be* followed by a quantitative study, or that a qualitative study on its own is incomplete.

Qualitative research is quick and cheap

Good qualitative research takes time and it costs money! The days of the single researcher forging ahead into the clinical area with a notebook and pencil are now, thankfully, consigned to the annals of history. The collection of data can be time consuming; the management and subsequent analysis of copious amounts of unwieldy data takes further time; the emergent nature of the design of qualitative studies often means that they evolve in the undertaking, change and evolve and thus need additional responsive thought and action. As a result, it is little surprise that qualitative studies usually take longer to complete than quantitative studies (Morse 2002). These days qualitative research is often conducted in teams, and most often is undertaken with the assistance of a variety of technologies.[2] As a result, the costs are increased exponentially. Technology is expensive, but more expensive is the time of the principal investigator, the graduate student (e.g. financial support for the student), the research assistant, and the secretaries. Interestingly, Morse (2002) points out that qualitative studies are still disproportionately 'under funded' in comparison to quantitative studies.

[2] Such as audio recording with sensitive microphones, video recording, laptops, software for data analysis, software for audio voice recognition, web access.

Consequently, there is a need for all qualitative researchers to be aware of the realistic time frame for a study and make clear, cogent budgetary arguments when applying for funds.

Qualitative research is a simple matter of categorising respondents' answers to a number of questions

All too often, inexperienced[3] qualitative researchers posit qualitative findings as the simple matter of grouping the responses to a number of questions. Unfortunately, there is ample evidence of such 'studies' in the associated literature. Such 'studies' have more in keeping with journalism and may bear only a passing resemblance to qualitative enquiry. Indeed, the most illuminating qualitative findings go far further than crude descriptions of clusters of similar statements; they interpret, they predict, they explain, they solve problems. This is perhaps a key feature of 'expert' qualitative researchers' work that sets them apart from less experienced researchers. Expert qualitative researchers go beyond the words, see past the obvious, access the underlying and hidden language, the often present yet invisible process/culture/ experiences. Qualitative researchers are not concerned with searching for the same word or phrase. Indeed, awkward attempts to count the frequency of the same word in qualitative data analysis have been strongly criticised as inappropriate. Morse (1995) makes this point most clearly when she states, 'I repeat: The **quantity** [original emphasis] of data in a category is not theoretically important to the process of saturation. Richness of data derived from detailed description, not the number of times something is stated. Frequency counts are out' (p. 148).

Additionally, 'Frequency of occurrence of any specific incident must be ignored. Saturation involves eliciting all forms of types of occurrences, valuing variation over quantity' (p. 147). Perhaps some of these methodological limitations would be addressed by ensuring that novice qualitative researchers are given adequate supervision from a senior, experienced qualitative researcher, and by addressing the associated myth that a training and education in quantitative methods will equip the researcher to undertake a qualitative study without having had additional qualitative training.

[3] Or qualitative researchers who have not undergone a formal research training.

The results of qualitative inquiry cannot be generalised

Qualitative researchers do not seek to generalise their findings in the same way that a quantitative researcher might. That is, they do not seek *nomothetic* generalisations relating to universal laws and absolute 'truths'. They do seek, however, to produce *idiographic or naturalistic* generalisations. That is, generalisations about, and drawn from, cases (Sandelowski 1997). Generalisations drawn from purposeful samples who have experience of the 'case' and are thus applicable to similar 'cases', problems and questions, irrespective of the similarity between the demographic group (Morse 1999a). In nursing studies for example, each 'case'[4] of nursing will bear a clear resemblance to nursing as a 'whole' and any related, similar 'cases'. Denzin and Lincoln (1994) make this point most cogently when they state: 'Every instance of a case or process bears the general class of phenomena it belongs to' (p. 201). Thus, a process that is identified in one setting, group or population (i.e. one case), can be similarly experienced by another related setting, group or population. For example, a grounded theory concerned with credentialising that was induced from a sample of nurses is likely to be generalisable to, and bear similarity with, any population that shares the process of credentialising.

Qualitative studies are invalid, non-rigorous, unsystematic and unscientific

Often-levelled accusations at qualitative research include the statement that qualitative research is unsystematic, it lacks rigour and as a result is 'unscientific'. This may in part be a response to some of the badly designed studies that have been published within the associated literature. But to judge the entire paradigm on the basis of a limited number of poor studies would be analogous to suggesting that all people with mental health problems should be maintained in secure facilities just because a tiny minority of people do present with a degree of dangerousness. This is simply wrong! While qualitative research may lack the level of prescription relating to design issues and indices for calculating issues such as sample size, reliability and validity, good qualitative research is always systematic and rigorous (Morse 1999b). This myth, again, appears to be grounded in the practice of judging qualitative studies according to criteria developed for the quantitative

---

[4] Microcosm, experience, process or culture.

paradigm. Qualitative inquiry has a different form of systematic rigour, most notably in the form of data collection/analysis, the observation of patterns, the questioning of data, the process of internal verification and conjecture and, not least, the rigour of systematic writing (Morse 1999b).

AN OVERVIEW OF THE MORE COMMON QUALITATIVE RESEARCH METHODS

There exist a wide range of approaches or methods all of which can be described as qualitative, e.g. phenomenology, grounded theory, ethnography, discourse analysis, ethnoscience, narrative analysis. Furthermore, new or adapted methods are being published regularly within the relevant methodological literature. However, in order to give the reader some understanding it is necessary to focus on the three principle approaches.[5]

Phenomenology

Phenomenology is a human science whose purpose is to describe and understand particular phenomena as lived experience. It is the rigorous, critical and systematic study of 'essences'; the purpose of which is to explicate the structure or essence of the lived experience of a phenomenon in the search for the 'unity meaning' which is the identification of the essence of the phenomenon and its accurate description through everyday lived experience (Rose *et al.* 1995). While a range of methods exist under the broad banner of phenomenology (see Colazzi 1976; Gadamer 1976; Giorgi 1985; Van Manen 1997) and these methods draw upon a range of phenomenological philosophy (e.g. Satre 1943; Heidegger 1962; Merleau Ponty 1962; Husserel 1964), each asserts that phenomenology is inductive. Furthermore, lived experience in the everyday world is the central focus of phenomenological inquiry (Schultz 1972). Or to rephrase, those experiences that are central to human life are appropriate for phenomenological study, if not required

[5] While contemporary qualitative methodology orthodoxy recognises that none of the terms phenomenology, grounded theory and ethnography refer to a single, unified approach, in order to provide this overview the terms will be used to represent the collection of methods included within these more capacious terms.

to be studied using phenomenological methods. There is utility in understanding behaviours as a result of a person's life, his/her experiences and the situated contextual meaning that the person attributes to these experiences (Heideggar 1962).

According to Morse and Field (1995), phenomenological researchers ask questions of participants in order to answer the question: 'What is it like to have a certain experience?' Van Manen's (1997) writings are more specific in stating that the phenomenological researcher needs to try to access the 'pre-reflexive' moment. In other words, to capture the moment as it is lived; as it is experienced, not as one reflects and thinks about the moment *ex-post facto*. To do so would be to move into the reflexive and as a result he purports the need for certain types of questions. Examples of such questions are included in Table 3.2.

Phenomenologists draw upon the 'life world' of the participants as the primary source of data; however, this can be supplemented by literature, poetry, art or artefacts (Sandelowski 1994). Further, these participants are drawn upon 'purposefully' as they can speak to the lived experience in the greatest depth, and accordingly, phenomenological researchers use 'purposeful' rather than random sampling selection. Consequently, the axiomatic position of phenomenological research is that there is always bias (Morse 1998); bias that is both necessary and purposeful. There is deliberate bias in the decisions made about which literature to access, in the choice of setting and selection of participants. The product of a phenomenological study should be a text, an accurate description (and in some cases interpretation) of the phenomena (or experience) being studied. Morse

Table 3.2 Examples of questions used in a phenomenological study of the lived experiences of suicidal Alberta males (adapted from Van Manen, 1997)

- Can you describe your experience of attempting suicide or being on the very cusp of attempting suicide as you live(d) through it?
- Can you try and describe the experience from the inside as it were, almost like a state of mind: your feelings, your mood, your emotions, your thoughts?
- Can you focus on a particular example or incident; can you describe specific events, particular happenings?
- Could you focus on an example of the experience that stands out for its vividness?
- Could you describe how your body felt at that time, how things smelled, how they sounded?

and Field (1995) point out that, in this way, phenomenology is different from grounded theory (see below) as it does not attempt to induce a theory; accurate, rich description, sometimes with interpretation, in the form of text, is thus the product of phenomenological inquiry. Examples of such studies in the formal area of psychiatric nursing are included below.

Grounded theory

Glaser and Strauss (1967) first developed the method(ology) of grounded theory and published this in their now seminal text, *The discovery of grounded theory: strategies for qualitative research*. As a reaction to the then overzealous pre-occupation with the verification of theory, grounded theory is concerned with generating theory (Glaser and Strauss, 1967). Its basic and central theme is generating theory from data that is systematically obtained from social research; consequently, grounded theory is an inductive process. It is a method(ology)[6] for developing or inducing a theory that should provide clear enough categories and hypotheses that explain and aid understanding of the basic (psycho)social[7] process being studied. Thus, it needs to induce explanatory theory. Glaser (1998) points out that a researcher who wishes to undertake a 'pure' grounded theory study would not commence with existing literature but begin instead with an identified area of study. Then as data are collected, the process of constant comparative analysis occurs whereby each item or label of data is compared with every other item or label. Thus, data collection, sampling and data analysis each occur simultaneously. Furthermore, the methodological choices of where to go for the next data and what questions to ask are driven by the emerging theory, not by an *a-priori* research design decision; such a process is called 'theoretical sampling' (Glaser 1978). This process of theoretical sampling means that participants need to be selected according to their knowledge and

[6] Grounded theory is described as both a methodology and a method. It therefore provides both the philosophical underpinnings to the method, the tenants upon which the method is built, and the 'nuts and bolts' of operationalising the method in a study.

[7] While their 1967 work described the need to discover social processes, this is not surprising given the sociological background of the authors. This was later amended to include psychosocial processes in Glaser's 1998 *Doing grounded theory* work.

experience of the (psycho)social process under study. While similar to 'purposeful sampling' that would be associated with phenomenology, ethnography and other qualitative methods, it is important to point out that it is not the same.[8]

Grounded theory concentrates on the interactional processes at work within the world, provided by the perspective of the participants, and these perspectives are then replaced by theoretical conceptualisation. Grounded theory usually occurs when there is little or no research into the research subject or area. Consequently, research questions in grounded theory (if present at all) are markedly different to research questions postulated at the start of a quantitative study. The questions need to be flexible and open-ended enough to allow freedom for the theory to develop.[9]

The theory can be seen to originate from 'ground level', from the social world where the data originates. As Stern (1985) suggests, grounded theory scientists construct theory from the data rather than applying a theory constructed by someone else from another data source. Thus, the theory remains connected to, or grounded in, the data, and in that way grounded in reality; the specific reality of where the data originated. As a result, a grounded theory should therefore 'fit' the situation being researched. To sum up: 'A well-constructed grounded theory will meet its four most central criteria: fit, work, relevance, and modifiability' (Glaser 1992, p. 15).

Ethnography

Ethnographic research in health care related matters has its roots in cultural anthropology (Morse and Field 1995). It is appropriate and congruent with this origin then that these studies and others related to health care are always informed by the concept of culture (Boyle 1994). Furthermore, while acknowledging the variations within the different types of ethnography, typical ethnographies attempt to be holistic, reflexive and contextual (Boyle 1994). Ethnographies attempt to account

---

[8] For further reading on this matter, readers are directed to Cutcliffe, J.R. (2000) Methodological issues in grounded theory. *Journal of Advanced Nursing* 31(6), 1476–84.

[9] Indeed, Glaser's (1992) position is that the researchers approach an area with a 'general wonderment' and no clearly defined research question. Though it has been argued recently that there are a number of processes and issues that may inhibit such an approach (Cutcliffe, in press).

for human behaviours from the 'emic' perspective; from the perspective of those who are on the inside, those who participate in the behaviour. Ethnographers attempt to elucidate the particular beliefs, nuances, idiosyncrasies and practices[10] that exist within certain cultures, yet these understandings have to be obtained by the researcher observing and maybe participating in the context (and culture) in which they occur. Accordingly, the ethnographer will use a variety of data collection methods. Most often some form of observation (participatory or otherwise) and field-note-taking will occur, and this can be augmented by additional methods.[11] Morse and Field (1995) argue that the information obtained from ethnographic studies is critical to understanding the provision of health care, for without this information how can one understand and thus account for the particular culture of the health care recipients?

Ethnographic researchers ask questions such as: This community of First Nation Canadians has a higher than average rate of completed suicide – how do members of this community and culture activity construct their world? What is it like for a person living in this community? What health care beliefs, nuances, idiosyncrasies, and behaviours exist within this community and culture that may influence this suicide rate? Thus, ethnographers wish to determine if and how people can actively shape their lives within these cultures; they wish to identify and determine if there are environmental factors which are contributing to these health related behaviours. Importantly, in place of studying people, ethnographers learn from people and this allows for the 'emic' perspective, the 'insiders' view to emerge (Boyle 1994). The product of an ethnography will involve description, but Morse and Field (1995) argue that it should move beyond description. The ethnographer needs to identify and explicate social patterns and observed conduct. According to Geertz (1973), the product of an ethnographic study is, typically, *thick description*, the search for shared meaning within the cultural norms, the patterned behaviour that is indicative of the culture and the cultural context.

---

[10] And thus within health care related studies, the particular health beliefs, health related nuances, health related idiosyncrasies and health related practices.

[11] Such as the interrogation of appropriate and relevant records, accessing life histories, examining artifacts.

THE NEED FOR A 'NEW' RESEARCH PARADIGM?

Previously, I have drawn on the work of Benner (1984), Pearson (1989), Morse (1991) and McKenna (1997) and reiterated the argument for a 'new' research paradigm (Cutcliffe 1998; 2003b). Acknowledging the increased credibility that qualitative research appears to have achieved within many academies and funding bodies might mean that it would be inaccurate to suggest the need for a 'new' research paradigm. Yet, as stated earlier, qualitative studies are still disproportionately 'underfunded' in comparison to quantitative studies. The majority of the studies that are published in nursing and related journals have a quantitative method and/or research design. Similarly, in order to enter postgraduate courses in many countries, the aspirant student is required to take a statistics course, and yet there is no such mandatory requirement to undertake a qualitative data analysis course.[12] Consequently, it appears that the case for equal standing or status for qualitative studies needs to continue to be made. What I find particularly difficult to understand is that nursing, and mental health nursing in particular, has much in common with the philosophical underpinnings with qualitative research. Yet, despite the fact that nursing has certainly embraced qualitative methods far more than many disciplines, there remains a quantitative predominance. This is all the more difficult to understand given the common phenomenon in nursing which is referred to as the 'theory-practice divide' or sometimes 'theory resistance.'

There is a well-established argument that purports how the 'theory resistance' is most understandable, when the theory has not been derived from practice, and has produced predominantly 'know that' knowledge (Cutcliffe 1998; 2003b). Yet qualitative research produces 'know how' knowledge, by accessing the implicit knowledge embedded in clinical expertise and the subsequent theory produced from this knowledge is central to the advancement of nursing practice and the development of nursing science. Uncovering the knowledge embedded in expert practice, as Benner (1984) argues, then leads to new theories which have their foundations in the 'know how' knowledge of the practitioners themselves.

Accessing the knowledge embedded in such practice requires qualitative research designs concerned with describing and interpreting

[12] Even if the student intends to use a qualitative method for the research component of his/her Masters degree.

the intentions, expectations, meanings and outcomes of expert practice (Benner 1984). Such methods may create the situation where nurse researchers, practitioners, and users of services are involved collaboratively in uncovering this knowledge, and a consequence of this may be that nurse researchers are viewed with less suspicion by practitioners (McKenna 1997). Additionally, since the theory would be constructed from within nursing practice and not passed down from 'on high' to the practitioners, perhaps the research and the theory produced by the research is then much more real, vibrant, alive and applicable to the practitioners (2003) and the 'theory resistance' is diminished.

THE FUTURE RESEARCH DIRECTION

The argument concerning which paradigm of research should be embraced by nursing has been one of the most widely and commonly debated issues in the associated nursing and methodological literature. An examination of the contemporary nursing and methodological literature indicates that the arguments appear to have abated recently. Indeed, for some, this 'old chestnut' is increasingly seen as pointless conjecture and the question is regarded as a bit sterile. For others, the issue is 'alive and well' and the case for qualitative methods still needs to be made. While there is less evidence of this debate in the relevant contemporary literature, recent published papers that have focused on this matter have produced a volley of passionate and assertive commentaries and responses.[13] Furthermore, an alternative view posits that while the issue may be less often openly debated, maybe the issue has 'gone underground' so to speak and is now manifest in a different guise. In place of 'open' declarations and debates about what methods to focus on, we now have the 'evidence-based practice' movement as the dominant discourse and the implications arising out of hierarchies of evidence wherein there is most often implicit and oblique references to what types of evidence are 'real', 'best' or 'most useful' and accordingly, which methods are therefore needed to produce this evidence.

Ironically, in some ways, this argument can never be resolved. The enlightened researcher will always recognise that both research

---

[13] See the multiple responses to Rolfe's (2002) recent paper in *Nurse Education Today*, and the multiple responses to Burnard and Hannigan's (2000) paper in the *Journal of Psychiatric and Mental Health Nursing.*

paradigms are needed to advance the knowledge base of the discipline. One research paradigm is not better or worse than the other and to attempt to place these paradigms (and the evidence they produce) in some artificial and linear hierarchy only serves to confuse and obfuscate (Cutcliffe and Ward 2003). The research paradigms enable different questions to be asked and answered, consequently the 'best' paradigm is the one that offers the highest chance of reaching the most complete understanding of the particular issue or even dimension of an issue. In adopting this pluralistic approach to research, the different paradigms and methods within them become equally valuable 'tools' within a tool kit. Accordingly, the enlightened researcher selects the tool (the method) that will best help get the job done (uncover and access the knowledge).

In conclusion, qualitative research studies are needed in order to advance the unique knowledge base of mental health practice. The methods these studies use are no better or worse than quantitative studies, they just allow different questions to be asked and answered and produce different knowledge. There are a growing number of studies in the relevant empirical nursing-related literature which have utilised a qualitative approach. Yet, there is still a great deal we do not know about mental health care and practice. Thus, there is a clear need for additional, well-designed, systematic studies and the particular forms of knowledge they produce.

EXAMPLES OF THE CONTRIBUTION TO THE KNOWLEDGE BASE OF MENTAL HEALTH CARE MADE BY QUALITATIVE STUDIES: A GROWING LITERATURE

In order to give the reader an idea of the contribution that qualitative studies have made to the formal knowledge base of mental health care I will focus on certain contemporary issues and practices. There is not enough room in this chapter to list, let alone describe, all such studies. Therefore, what follows is a cross-sectional representation of the contribution that studies using the three methods described in this chapter have made. The reader is encouraged to access these and other texts in order to comprehend more fully the findings of these studies.

Nurses use of 'traditional client management' techniques such as control and restraint, seclusion and PRN medications – see Mason (1997); Alty (1997).

The use and limits of 'observations' (special observations, close
observations), particularly as a means to care for suicidal clients –
see Pitula and Cardell (1996); Fletcher (1997); Caedell and Pilutal
(1999); Jones *et al.* (2000a; 2000b).

Nurse prescribing in P/MH nursing – see Kaas *et al.* (2000).

Dealing with violence and aggression – see Morrison (1990); Cutcliffe
(1999); Carlsson *et al.* (2000).

Clinical decision making – see Carpenter (1991); Pugh (2002).

The nature of P/MH nursing practice – see Barker *et al.* (1999).

Building relationships with clients who have severe and long-
term mental health problems – see Repper *et al.* (1994); Thomas
(1998).

Clinical Supervision – see Scanlon and Wier (1997); Cutcliffe and
Burns (1998); Hyrkas *et al.* (2002).

User involvement – see Anthony and Crawford (2000).

Caring for the suicidal client – see Long and Reid (1996); Talsteth
et al. (1997; 1999); Cutcliffe *et al.* (2003).

Issues of empowerment – see Tilley *et al.* (1999).

Working with clients who are undergoing Electro-convulsive therapy
– see Gass (2003).

Inspiring hope in the bereaved, elderly – see Cutcliffe and Grant
(2001); Cutcliffe (2003a).

(Adapted from Cutcliffe and Ward, 2003)

References

Alty, A. (1997). Nurses' learning experience and expressed opinions regarding
seclusion practice within one NHS trust. *Journal of Advanced Nursing,* **25**,
786–93.

Anthony, P. and Crawford, P. (2000). Service *user involvement* in care planning:
the mental health nurse's perspective. *Journal of Psychiatric and Mental
Health Nursing,* **7**, 425–34.

Barker, P., Jackson, S. and Stevenson, S. (1999). What are psychiatric nurses
needed for? Developing a theory of essential nursing practice. *Journal of
Psychiatric and Mental Health Nursing,* **6**, 273–82.

Benner, P. (1984). *From novice to expert: excellence and power in clinical
practice.* Addison-Wesley, New York.

Boyle, J. (1994). Style of ethnography. In *Critical issues in qualitative research
methods* (ed. Morse, J.M.), pp. 159–85. Sage, Thousand Oaks.

Burnard, P. and Hannigan, B. (2000). Qualitative and quantitative approaches in
mental health nursing: moving the debate forward. *Journal of Psychiatric
and Mental Health Nursing,* **7**(1), 1–7.

Cardell, R. and Pitula, C.R. (1999). Suicidal inpatients' perceptions of therapeutic and non-therapeutic aspects of constant observation. *Psychiatric Services*, **20**(8), 1066–70.

Carlsson, G., Dahlberg, K. and Drew, N. (2000). Encountering violence and aggression in mental health nursing: a phenomenological study of tacit caring knowledge. *Issues in Mental Health Nursing*, **21**, 533–45.

Carpenter, M.A. (1991). The process of ethical decision making in psychiatric nursing practice. *Issues in Mental Health Nursing*, **12**, 179–91.

Colaizzi, P.F. (1975). Psychological research as the phenomenologist views it. In *Existential phenomenological alternatives for psychology* (eds. Valle, R. and King, M.), pp. 48–71. Oxford University Press, Oxford.

Cutcliffe, J.R. (1998). Is psychiatric nursing research barking up the wrong tree? *Nurse Education Today*, **18**, 257–8.

Cutcliffe, J.R. (1999). Qualified nurses' lived experience of violence perpetrated by individuals suffering from enduring mental health problems: a hermeneutic study. *International Journal of Nursing Studies*, **36**, 105–16.

Cutcliffe, J.R. (2000). Methodological issues in grounded theory. *Journal of Advanced Nursing*, **31**(6), 1476–84.

Cutcliffe, J.R. (2003a). *The inspiration of hope in bereavement counselling.* Jessica Kingsley, London.

Cutcliffe, J.R. (2003b). A historical overview of psychiatric/mental health nurse education in the United Kingdom: going round in circles or on the straight and narrow? *Nurse Education Today*, **23**(5), 338–46.

Cutcliffe, J.R. (in Press) Adapt or adopt: developing and transgressing the methodological boundaries of grounded theory. *Journal of Advanced Nursing.* In press.

Cutcliffe, J.R. and Burns, J. (1998). Personal, professional and practice development: clinical supervision. *British Journal of Nursing*, **7**(21), 1318–22.

Cutcliffe, J.R. and Grant, G. (2001). What are the principles and processes of inspiring hope in cognitively impaired older adults within a continuing care environment? *Journal of Psychiatric and Mental Health Nursing*, **8**, 427–36.

Cutcliffe, J.R. and Ward, M. (2003). *Critiquing nursing research.* Quay Books, London.

Cutcliffe, J.R., Stevenson, C., Jackson, S., Smith, P. and Barker, P. (2003). Meaningful caring responses to people at risk of suicide: how do P/MH nurses care for suicidal clients? *Report for NHSE Trent*, University of Northern British Columbia and University of Teeside.

Derrida, C. (1976). *Grammatology.* Gayatri Chakrovorky Spivak (trans). Johns Hopkins University Press, Baltimore.

Fletcher, R.F. (1999). The process of constant observation: perspectives of staff and suicidal patients. *Journal of Psychiatric and Mental Health Nursing*, **6**(1), 9–14.

Gadamer, H.G. (1976). *Philosophical hermeneutics.* (trans and ed. Linge, D.E.) University of California Press, Los Angeles.

Geertz, C. (1973). *The interpretation of cultures.* Basic Books, New York.

Gass, J. (2003). Perspectives of electroconvulsive therapy: the work of mental health nurses. *Ph.D. Thesis*, University of Aberdeen.

Giorgi, A. (1985). Sketch of a psychological phenomenological method. In *Phenomenology and psychological research* (ed. Giorgi, A.), pp. 8–22. Duquesne University Press, Pittsburgh.

Heideggar, M. (1962). *Being and time.* Harper Row, New York.

Husserl, E. (1964). *The idea of phenomenology.* (trans. Alston W. and Nakhikan G.) The Hague, Nijhoff.

Hyrkas, K., Appleqvist-Schmidlecher, K. and Paunonen-Ilmonen, M. (2002). Expert supervisors' views of clinical supervision: a study of factors promoting and inhibiting the achievements of multi-professional team supervision. *Journal of Advanced Nursing*, **38**(4), 387–97.

Jones, J., Lowe, T. and Ward, M. (2000a). Inpatients' experiences of nursing observation on an acute psychiatric unit: a pilot study. *Mental Health Care*, **4**(4), 125–9.

Jones, J., Ward, M., Wellman, N., Hall, J. and Lowe, T. (2000b). Psychiatric inpatients' experiences of nursing observation: a United Kingdom perspective. *Journal of Psychosocial Nursing*, **38**(12), 10–19.

Kaas, M.J., Dehn, D., Frank, K., Markley, J. and Herbert, P. (2000). A view of prescriptive practice collaboration: perspectives of psychiatric-mental health clinical nurse specialists and psychiatrists. *Archives of Psychiatric Nursing*, **14**, 222–34.

Lincoln, Y.S. and Guba, E.G. (1985). *Naturalistic Inquiry.* Sage, Newbury Park.

Long, A. and Reid, W. (1996). An exploration of nurses' attitudes to the nursing care of the suicidal patient in an acute psychiatric ward. *Journal of Psychiatric and Mental Health Nursing*, **3**, 29–37.

Mason, T. (1997). An ethnomethodological analysis of the use of seclusion. *Journal of Advanced Nursing*, **26**, 780–9.

Merleau-Ponty, M. (1962). *Phenomenology of perception.* (Smith, C. trans) Humanities Press, New York.

Morrison, E. (1990). The tradition of toughness: a study of non-professional nursing care in psychiatric nursing settings. *Image: Journal of Nursing Scholarship*, **22**, 32–8.

Morse, J.M. (1995). The significance of saturation. *Qualitative Health Research*, **5**(2), 147–9.

Morse, J.M. (1996). Is qualitative research complete? *Qualitative Health Research*, **6**, 3–5.

Morse, J.M. (1999a). Qualitative generalisability. *Qualitative Health Research*, **9**, 5–6.

Morse, J.M. (1999b). Myth number 19: qualitative inquiry is not systematic. *Qualitative Health Research*, **9**, 573–4.

Morse, J.M. (2002). Myth number 53: qualitative research is cheap. *Qualitative Health Research*, **12**, 1307–8.

Morse, J.M. and Field, P.A. (1995). *Qualitative research methods for health professionals* 2nd Edition. Thousand Oaks, London.

Pitula, C.R. and Cardell, R. (1996). Suicidal inpatients' experiences of constant observation. *Psychiatric Services*, **47**(6), 6491–651.

Pugh, D. (2002). A phenomenologic study of flight nurses' clinical decision-making in emergency situations. *Air Medical Journal*, **21**(2), 28–36.

Repper, J., Ford, R. and Cooke, A. (1994). How can nurses build trusting relationships with people who have severe and long-term mental health problems? *Journal of Advanced Nursing*, **19**, 1096–104.

Rolfe, G. (2002). Faking a difference: evidence-based nursing and the illusion of diversity. *Nurse Education Today*, **22**(1), 3–12.

Sandelowski, M. (1994). Towards a poetic for qualitative inquiry. In *Critical issues in qualitative health research* (ed. Morse, J.M.), pp. 46–63. Thousand Oaks, London.

Sandelowski, M. (1997). 'To be of use': Enhancing the utility of qualitative research. *Nursing Outlook*, **45**(3), 125–32.

Satre, J.P. (1943). In *Six existentialist thinkers* (Blackham, H.J. 1986), pp. 58–79. Routledge, London.

Scanlon, C. and Wier, W.S. (1997). Learning from practice: mental health nurses' perceptions and experiences of clinical supervision. *Journal of Advanced Nursing*, **26**, 295–303.

Schutz, S.E. (1994). Exploring the benefits of a subjective approach in qualitative nursing research. *Journal of Advanced Nursing* **20**, 412–7.

Schwandt, T.A. (1994). Constructivist, interpretivist approaches to human inquiry. In *Handbook of qualitative research* (eds. Denzin, N.K. and Lincoln, Y.S.), pp. 118–37. Sage, Thousand Oaks.

Talseth, A.G., Lindseth, A., Jacobson, L. and Norberg, A. (1997). Nurses' narrations about suicidal psychiatric inpatients. *Nord Jour Psychiatry* **51**, 359–64.

Talseth, A.G., Lindseth, A., Jacobson, L. and Norberg, A. (1999). The meaning of suicidal in-patients' experiences of being cared for by mental health nurses. *Journal of Advanced Nursing* **29**(5), 1034–41.

Thomas, S. (1998). It hurts most around the heart: a phenomenological exploration of women's anger. *Journal of Advanced Nursing*, **28**, 311–22.

Tilley, S., Pollock, L. and Tait, L. (1999). Discourses on empowerment. *Journal of Psychiatric and Mental Health Nursing*, **6**(1), 53–60.

Van Manen, M. (1997). *Researching lived experience: human science for action sensitive pedagogy*. State University of New York Press, New York.

Walters, A.J. (1995). The phenomenological movement: implications for nursing research. *Journal of Advanced Nursing*, **22**, 791–9.

4

The pursuit of inquiry in mental health care

Peter Nolan

INTRODUCTION

Despite the many criticisms levelled at mental health research, including low levels of activity, the limited resources available for it, poorly designed studies and an even greater failure to translate findings into practice than is apparent in other fields of health care, a remarkable amount is known about the causes and treatment of mental illness. Indeed, compared with three or four decades ago, there is far greater optimism today in mental health care, largely owing to new ways of engaging with people with mental health problems so as to make use of their own resources and experiences. More is known about what constitutes supportive environments and relationships and how they can help people in the acute phase of mental health problems.

Where the focus of research was once determined by the sometimes idiosyncratic interests of the individual health professional – usually a doctor – now it is determined by central government and reflects the areas that it considers central to its programme of NHS modernisation. Recent policy statements indicate that research should be undertaken close to where clients and patients are being cared for, rather than by academics in academic settings whose research often takes a generation or longer to get into practice. The theory/practice divide might be illustrated by the case of Thomas Arnold who was Superintendent of the Leicester Asylum in the mid-nineteenth century and who formulated three principles of mental health care. These were:

- Early detection of illness
- Appropriate interventions
- Good social support once the patient was discharged (Carpenter 1989).

Such aspirations have a very contemporary feel to them, and the fact that we are still trying to put them into practice today indicates the challenge of moving theory into the clinical arena.

This chapter aims to show the range of research that has been carried out into mental health care, with a view to improving our understanding of why research does or does not influence practice, and to describe the various descriptive and investigative approaches that have been used through the centuries. Reference is made to creative thinking and innovative treatments and to the impact they have had on mental health care. Analysis of the evolution of mental health research can facilitate a better understanding of how effective research might be undertaken today.

PHILOSOPHICAL ENQUIRY AND ITS APPLICATION IN MENTAL HEALTH CARE

How do we set about assessing mental health research and determining what has been helpful to those engaged in service delivery? Theorists and critics suggest different epistemological starting points for the study of mental health and illness. De Chardin (1979) argued that an understanding of human beings is best achieved by being thoroughly grounded in the natural sciences because men and women are essentially matter, although matter which has become conscious of itself. All branches of science have the power to illuminate who we are and why we behave as we do, but De Chardin regarded brain biochemistry as the 'queen of the sciences' without which other explanations of human experience and behaviour are merely conjectural. During the nineteenth century, the observation and careful description of the behaviour and symptoms of people with mental illness were the precursors to research based in biochemistry. A startling extension of De Chardin's thinking can be found in the very recent work of Horrobin (2001) who draws on his knowledge of evolution, medicine, psychiatry and nutrition to generate the hypothesis that much behaviour labelled as mental illness could be rectified by devoting more attention to what people eat and the constituents of *a healthy lifestyle*.

Horrobin also claims that the special attributes of the human race can be attributed to schizophrenics who have introduced into the genotype the exceptional skills and creativity which distinguish us from our nearest primate relatives.

Critics argue that De Chardin's position results in pathology-led health care which fails to locate the person within his or her socio-economic context. By looking only at the biological changes within the body, we overlook the links between people's life-styles, their domestic, cultural and social circumstances and their illnesses. Nettleton (1995) opposes De Chardin and indicates the direction of much current research by showing how patterns of morbidity and mortality are related to factors other than biology including gender, race/ethnicity, education, income and age.

Ryle (1976) believes that an understanding of people as individuals and as members of society is best achieved through philosophical inquiry, which explores the nature of thought, its origins, its expressions and why it sometimes becomes dysfunctional and pathological. Clifford Beers, the author of *A mind that found itself* (1908), noted that insight into how people think was generally lacking in the doctors and nurses who cared for him during his time in a psychiatric institution:

> *My attendants were incapable of understanding the operations of my mind and what they could not understand they would seldom tolerate.*

Sacks (1983) has progressed Ryle's standpoint by arguing that patients need to tell their stories in their own way in their own time, and that health care personnel should aim to understand how their problems are affecting their lives. Recent research (Makoul *et al.* 1995) in the wake of Sacks' ideas has investigated whether GPs allow patients time to talk and has shown that doctors prefer to control consultations by using closed questions and technical language which the patient does not understand. Open questions to enable the patient to reveal more information about himself and which would help the doctor to understand his beliefs about his illness are avoided, apparently through fear of prolonging the consultation time.

Handy (2001), too, has invited us to consider people's biographies and the narratives they provide of their lives. He argues that by appreciating the meanings and values that people attribute to their experiences, we can come to understand them better. It is clear, however, that in our own times, patients do not feel that health professionals try to understand their problems. Dobson (2003) estimates that approximately a quarter of the people suffering from life-diminishing neurotic disorders do not seek the help of health professionals either because they feel that these professionals have nothing to offer them, or through fear of being reproved for taking up their 'valuable' time.

Makoul *et al.* (1995) showed that doctors spend just one minute in twenty giving information, although they believe that they spend approximately half the consultation doing this. Yet Broody (2003) states that patients are more likely to improve when things are explained to them and when their experiences are altered in positive directions. Mutual discussion of treatment options and goals leads to fewer referrals and fewer investigations as the patient feels in control of the action being taken and therefore more satisfied with their care. Patient-centred consultations make it more likely that doctors will prescribe drugs or treatment regimes to which the patient will adhere, thus reducing the problem of non-adherence which currently eats up scarce NHS resources with approximately 50% of patients either not taking their medication correctly or not at all.

The thinking of eminent writers such as those mentioned above has certainly been influential in mental health care. Yet it is not clear what channels of communication exist between those who do research, those who manage evidence-based health care and those who deliver it. Consider the following anecdote.

> *A senior health services manager declared recently at a team meeting that there was no need for any more research into mental health care and that she would not support any of 'her staff' wasting valuable time on research projects.* We have the National Service Framework for Mental Health and a raft of policy documents; what more do we want? *she demanded.*

This manager spoke with a conviction equal to that of Fukuyama (1992) when he said that our social evolution has advanced as far as it can go and that we have reached the end of history. Her ensuing comments seemed to deny the importance of having a curious, questioning and flexible workforce committed to ongoing appraisal of what they do. Her steadfast affirmation that what needs to be done in mental health care is self-evident was read by many attending the meeting as displaying an astonishing ignorance of the complex nature of mental problems and of the multiple ways in which people can be helped.

Establishing what exactly constitutes mental illness and how it should be dealt with has challenged some of the most intellectually able and creative thinkers. Conflicting theories are still being put forward about the nature and causation of mental illness; some authorities such as Szasz (1970) even deny that it exists. He argues that psychiatry has no place in the pantheon of medical specialities. In his opinion, it is a *pseudoscience*, akin to alchemy and astrology. Seedhouse (2002) contends that mental health and mental illness are artificial categories, and that the distinction between the physical and mental realm is unreal and unhelpful. Nonetheless, he accepts that classifications enable us to think about the world we inhabit and to act in it and that unless we draw a demarcation line between acceptable behaviour and antisocial behaviour, between normal thinking and abnormal thinking, and between illness and health, we are powerless to negotiate our personal and social environments. Yet it is the difficulty in defining illness states that makes mental health care so problematic, and renders establishing appropriate care pathways so challenging. Schon (1983) refers to a messy swamp of symptoms that are often hard to disentangle and rarely conform to disease categories. In addition, health care professionals use varied approaches to establish the nature of the mental health problem, and are more or less skilled in helping users to describe their symptoms while users present their problems in individual and sometimes idiosyncratic language (Goldberg *et al.* 1993).

Our knowledge of how the brain functions and of what the mind comprises is certainly in its infancy. Down the centuries, researchers and policy makers have looked in different places for answers to the problem of 'what or where is the mind'? It must be appreciated that understanding how best to care for and treat people with mental health problems is still very much work in progress and that what has been achieved during the last three or four decades is a mere footnote to history.

EARLY IDEAS ABOUT MENTAL ILLNESS

In 441 BC, Sophocles wrote in his play, *Antigone,*

> *Your laws today were not the laws of yesterday nor will they be the laws of tomorrow.*

When exploring the history of ideas and practices, it is important to be mindful that different era may have adhered to different concepts of mind, health and illness and used terms differently from those we work with today. Researchers, thinkers and health carers may have held different attitudes from those that we now consider acceptable. We must also remember that those who have chronicled ages past, and those who chronicle the present have many and varied agendas. There is not one history of human inquiry into mental health and care; there are many histories.

At the beginning of the seventeenth century there were no mental hospitals, neither were there any specific mental health services even though the experience of mental disorder was clearly widespread. Szasz (1995) feels that this presents us with two problems. Firstly, where do we start our inquiry into what it was like to be mentally ill in centuries gone by? And secondly, without the existence of, and records relating to, institutional care, how can we begin to understand why certain treatments were developed, considered to be likely to be effective and then fell into disrepute?

Before 1780, academic institutions appear to have taught little, if anything, about the state of mind of the mentally disordered person, the provenance of mental illness, or its management and treatment. The closest academics came to addressing such questions was to speculate about *the good life,* how it should be lived and how those who strayed from the straight and narrow could be reformed and redeemed. The realm of such inquiry was inhabited by students of philosophy, theology, literature and history and these disciplines frequently provided frameworks of thought and practice as opposed to scientific theories about the nature and progress of illness.

Many ideas about madness originate from antiquity and although the terminology in which they are expressed may have changed, they persist even in our own day. Such ideas include the belief that mental illness is an infantilising condition, rendering people dependent and desiring therapy as a substitute for parent figures in their lives. Madness has often been seen as a metaphor for a war taking place within oneself, for the conflict of the self with the self. Until the last fifty years, there has been little agreement about diagnostic categories. Berrios (1996) points out that from the seventeenth to the early twentieth centuries, medical personnel were regularly confronted with mental problems generated by organic disorders often predicated upon venereal diseases. The death of patients apparently from mental illness was a common occurrence and alienists (early psychiatrists) used the post-mortem as a means of diagnosis. The result was to foster a line of enquiry regarding the origins and aetiology of mental illness that was dependent on dissection. Here we have the start of research whose logical culmination is the approach of De Chardin as described in the opening section of this chapter.

NINETEENTH-CENTURY ASYLUMS AND THE CONSEQUENCES OF SEGREGATION FOR UNDERSTANDING MENTAL ILLNESS

Much of what passed for clinical practice in the seventeenth and eighteenth centuries was based on assumptions drawn from the observation of patients and post-mortem dissections. It was then suggested that institutions specially dedicated to the care of patients with mental disorders would create ideal laboratory conditions for the study of the symptoms and progress of mental illnesses, and of the effectiveness of various types of interventions. This thinking was novel but flawed because, as Berrios (1996) comments, confining patients for long periods of time in an artificial environment inevitably changed the manifestations and course of their conditions and thereby made it difficult to establish which interventions were effective, and to what any improvements or deterioration could be attributed.

Kraepelin (1904) believed that the national asylum programme, which commenced in the 1830s, was motivated less by a desire to care for sick people than by the demands of aspiring psychiatrists for a captive group of patients who could be studied at leisure. He also believed that the asylums were built to remove the mentally ill from the public gaze and allay fears regarding their potential dangerousness. Scull (1979) is largely in agreement with this opinion. He argues that from the Middle Ages, mad people were generally treated as moral and physical deviants and those who did not conform to social mores were treated as mad. The poor, vagrants, minor criminals and the physically disabled could all be thus conveniently labelled and removed to workhouses or in the nineteenth century, to asylums. Scull concludes that the original purpose of psychiatry was not to discover scientific solutions to mental illness, but to exercise control and surveillance over individuals thought to be a risk to the social order. Porter (2002) does not fully endorse this position, but recognises that any therapeutic function, which the asylums might once have been designed for, was soon lost in the crises brought about by severe overcrowding and unsatisfactory bureaucracies.

The segregation in asylums of people with mental health problems from the rest of the community, and the persistent location of investigation into human behaviour, health and illness in academic institutions allowed, or certainly did not hinder, the emergence of the eugenics movement in the late-nineteenth century. Perhaps too little attention has been given by historians of mental illness and mental health care to the influence of this movement in determining attitudes towards, and the treatment of, people with mental health problems (Gejman and Weilbaccher 2002). The belief that people with mental illness would adversely affect the physical stock of the nation was held by many leaders, especially in countries which had strong nationalistic tendencies. In Germany, nurses and doctors were actively involved in the euthanasia programme at the Hadamar Centre, near Frankfurt, where 10,000 mentally and physically disabled patients were murdered. In total, over 100,000 patients were deliberately killed in Germany during the Second World War. Although there is no comparison in terms of scale or severity, it should not be overlooked that the way in which people with mental illness have been treated in the UK led, in the second half of the twentieth century, to eighteen public inquiries into the running of psychiatric institutions. This can only be interpreted as indicative of neglect bordering on wilful indifference. Benedict (2003) has observed that we urgently need to deepen our understanding of how such a situation could have arisen and Miller and Rose (1986) argue that mental health services require constant surveillance through research and other scrutinising measures.

ACADEMICS AND CLINICIANS FROM THE NINETEENTH TO THE TWENTIETH CENTURIES

In the early-nineteenth century, academics at the prestigious University at Leipzig offered lectures on the structure of the nerves and the pathology of the soul alongside lectures on moral philosophy and the nature of reason (Steinberg and Angermeyer 2002). They were dedicated to theories of how societies should be governed, how individuals might be prepared to fulfil a responsible role in society, and how the weaker members of the community should be treated. Gradually, theory started to incorporate a more practical element and in 1806, Johann Christian August Heinroth (1773–1843) was appointed specifically to teach the newly emerging subject of psychiatric medicine. He was the first academic in Europe to hold such a post, although beyond dealings with a few wealthy patients, he had little experience of treating the mentally ill. What knowledge he laid claim to was based on his interpretation of Christianity. He considered all mental disorders to be endogenous and the consequence of guilt (original sin). This naturally led him to the belief that it was the approach used by doctors, rather than the medication they prescribed that determined patients' recovery. Despite his limitations as a clinician, he seems to have been an inspirational teacher who encouraged his students to explore how real life affected patients rather than argue about what constituted the ideal life. He also convinced the authorities that new subjects related to clinical practice should be introduced into the University and as a result, Wilhelm Wundt, one of the founding fathers of modern psychology was appointed in 1879. Wundt's most famous student was Emil Kraepelin who had studied anthropology and physiology and who was destined to make a seminal contribution to the study of mental illness through his work on schizophrenia and manic disorder (Kraam 2002). Kraepelin, however, made no secret of his preference for laboratory work rather than dealing with patients and was dismissed from his hospital post because of his complete lack of attention to the appalling hygiene on the wards, and the inadequate food given to patients.

In England, one of the first to be appointed as Lecturer in Experimental Psychology at Cambridge University was William Halse Rivers who was born in Luton in 1864, the son of a man who was both a Church of England vicar and a speech therapist who treated Lewis Carroll for his stammering problem. After training as a doctor, William joined the Royal Army Medical Corps and observed at close quarters soldiers' behaviour in war conditions. He spent the summer of 1893 at Heidelberg working with Kraepelin to measure the effects of fatigue on people. During the First World War, he transferred to Craiglockhart War Hospital near Edinburgh where he treated many shell-shock victims, including the poet, Siegfried Sassoon. Rivers vigorously opposed the common belief that soldiers who experienced shell-shock were cowards and should be punished. Instead, he tried to understand how they saw the war and their part in it (Slobodin 1997). He could be confrontational and often dismissed the explanations given to him by his patients and students as facile and needing more consideration. Nonetheless, research and practice in mental health care are indebted to his ability to create an environment that was both caring and inquiring. Rivers' influence was very much to the fore when the Tavistock Clinic opened in 1920 with a brief to examine the effects of prolonged exposure to stress and its management. Dr Hugh Crichton-Miller, its first director, aimed to research treatments which could form part of a programme of social prevention and to teach mental health promotion skills to health care professions allied to medicine. The Tavistock attracted eminent thinkers such as Wilfred Bion who worked on group dynamics and stress, and Michael Balint and John Bowly whose interest was in attachment disorders. Mental health care has benefited considerably from the work that has been conducted there on the psychodynamics of individuals and organisations, marital relationships, interpersonal relationships and group functioning (Dicks 1970). In June, 2001, the Tavistock joined Middlesex University in creating a new Centre for Mental Health Nursing based on psychodynamic principles.

MEDICAL RESEARCH UNITS IN MENTAL HEALTH

The lack of any co-ordinated or coherent approach to research into mental illness and its treatment was clearly exposed by the scandal around insulin coma therapy. This was introduced as a treatment for schizophrenia by Manfred Sakel who told a conference in New York in 1937 that he was achieving a 70% remission rate. The conference accepted his claim. Shepheard (2002) suggests that even though delegates were highly suspicious, none of them felt able to challenge Sakel either on clinical or scientific grounds. Not for the first time was there widespread acceptance of a belief purely because no one was able to refute it. Insulin coma therapy therefore continued until the publication of Harold Bourne's paper, *The insulin myth*, in the *Lancet* in 1953. Although Bourne incurred the wrath of senior members of the psychiatric profession, his paper stimulated a heated debate and gave confidence to those psychiatrists who felt that insulin therapy had no basis either in theory or in clinical practice. Bourne exposed a fad, which had been accepted enthusiastically by a profession not educated to test its validity. Within five years, insulin coma therapy virtually disappeared only to be replaced by the new treatment/fad of ECT. Fierce debate still persists as to the efficacy of ECT and many studies into its long-term therapeutic effects have proved inconclusive.

The absorption of mental health services into the NHS in 1948 promised better treatment for people with mental illness based on properly funded research. However, although psychiatry gained equal status with other branches of medicine, it did not receive the same level of resources as acute medicine. It was not until the early 1960s that the Medical Research Council (MRC) started to fund Mental Health Research Units although it had long been funding investigations into other kinds of illness. Rather than targeting areas in which research was needed, the MRC tended to target doctors whom it considered to have research expertise. Little effort was made to avoid mental health research being seen as elitist, mostly irrelevant and the concern of the few. One of the first MRC Units was at Graylingwell Hospital where Martin Roth was appointed to oversee the research programme. His contribution to psychiatry was to classify the disorders of old age and to increase understanding of mood disorders. Peter Sainsbury replaced him and the Unit's focus of research interest then switched to suicide. Myer Gross worked at the Uffculme Unit in Birmingham where he did some pioneering work on mental illnesses in old age. Alec Jenner was appointed to the MRC's Unit at Hollymoor Hospital in Birmingham, Ivor Batchelor worked at Dundee and Morris Carstairs in Edinburgh where his Unit specialised in epidemiology and social psychiatry. Alex Coppen and David Shaw did some pioneering work in the MRC Unit at West Park Hospital, Epsom, on the effects of lithium as a prophylactic against depression. While some outstanding members of the psychiatric profession thus received monies to pursue their personal research interests, there was still no coherent approach to identifying which were the issues around mental illness and mental health care of greatest interest to patients, and funding those. Some of the psychiatrists mentioned above made a significant contribution to mental health practice but it must be concluded that overall, their work had a negligible impact on services nationally (Freeman 2003).

While some attempt has been made since the middle of the twentieth century to evaluate and develop medical interventions in mental illness, Repper (2000) argues that nurses' contribution to mental health care has never been properly evaluated. Because their work underpins all services, it is easy to overlook it when the contribution of other professional groups is being assessed. There has been a tendency to attribute successful mental health outcomes entirely to medical, psychological or social interventions; indeed, the design of some studies has been constructed intentionally to confirm this. However, it may be that clients' relationships with carers, the manner in which information is imparted to them, and the encouragement and assistance they are given to draw on their own resources have the greatest impact on their recovery. Repper (2000) points out that although nurses form the largest group in mental health care, they are relatively powerless to define the research agenda because they are divided by ideological debates about what they should be doing and where they should be working.

RECENT INQUIRY IN MENTAL HEALTH CARE

The quantity of mental health research has increased substantially since the 1970s; some has been driven by the interest and commitment of individuals, but the majority by the Department of Health. Despite efforts to ensure that the processes by which studies are funded are transparent, there remains the suspicion that research serves the interests mainly of doctors and policy makers and does not always address the issues which are of main concern to users and carers. Mental health still receives less funding than other fields of health care, and biological research into mental illness, carried out in collaboration with genomic and neurological researchers, commands much larger financial support than other aspects of mental health care. Nonetheless, the types of interventions provided by mental health services are a central focus of research. Arguably the most prolific contributors to mental health research have been psychologists. Individual disciplines still tend to research their particular interventions even though interdisciplinary research is warmly encouraged by policy makers and funding bodies. The *National Institute of Mental Health for England* (1999) notes that the lack of integrated research perpetuates the tradition of disciplines in mental health working in isolation from each other. Interdisciplinary research will be hard to achieve while there remains considerable variance in research competence and protected time between mental health disciplines.

Lester (2003) testifies to the considerable variation in research quality within the field of mental health. She reviewed 650 research papers relating to research in primary mental health care published between 1997 and 2002, and classified them using the hierarchy of evidence adopted by the *National Service Framework for Mental Health* (1999):

CLASSIFICATION OF MENTAL HEALTH RESEARCH PAPERS 1997–2002

Types of Evidence	No of Papers
Type 1: includes at least one systematic review and at least one randomised controlled trial	8
Type 2: represents at least one randomised controlled trial	14
Type 3: represents one well-designed intervention study without randomisation	7
Type 4: represents at least one well-designed observational study	17
Type 5: represents expert opinion including the opinion of users and carers	55

The majority of studies fall into categories which are well below the 'gold standard' of research. Lester's findings do not support the claim of the manager who featured in the anecdote described earlier in this chapter that there is ample research being undertaken in mental health. However, the manager may have a point if she intended to suggest that what we now need is more research on how to implement the findings we already have and research to help us understand why some organisations are better than others at implementing progressive practice; why some health care teams are more open than others to challenge and change. We know that one of the effective ways of improving mental health care is to nurture a workforce that is curious about what they do and has the freedom to challenge their practice and initiate changes. Although more personnel are now active in research than ever before, why is it that the type and quality of services available continues to vary so much nationally?

In order to help us move the research agenda forward into the twenty-first century, it makes sense to examine why mental health research has to date had so little impact. The brief analysis provided in this chapter shows that, in the past, mental health research has:

- Tended to be undertaken by a small number of senior people in the medical profession who followed their own agenda
- Changed direction according to the whims of individuals rather than in response to identified needs
- Tended not to be applied in practice because researchers did not see this as part of their responsibilities.

In addition:

- It is difficult to assess how rigorously studies were conducted because they tended to be reported as commentaries
- Researchers and practitioners rarely collaborated, thus perpetuating the theory/practice divide
- Research was often focused on an individual 'case' and was not extended beyond the individual patient.

Historically, therefore, research has been ineffective because:

- It was not linked to policy and did not take into account the resources available to implement findings
- It felt no obligation to demonstrate efficacy in practice rather than merely under research conditions.

SOME REFLECTIONS ON RESEARCH IN ORGANISATIONS

This brief overview of the history of thinking about, and research into, mental health care illustrates how they have tended inevitably to locate in academic institutions where philosophical enquiry into the nature of mind, reason and human behaviour has flourished since universities came into being. This divorce between the theory of mental illness and the practice of caring for sufferers has been sustained down the centuries by society's fear of the mentally ill which has led to their segregation, culminating in the massive asylum programme of the nineteenth century. Such segregation tended to diminish the status of those working with the mentally ill, and to make research more difficult as the manifestations of illness were distorted by prolonged incarceration in a clinical environment. Difficulty in defining the nature of mental illness – a problem which continues today with authorities still in disagreement – has, in more recent times, made funding agencies reluctant to fund research, preferring to target money at projects that are able to demonstrate outcomes that can be clearly described.

Nonetheless, today research into mental health care is more vigorous than it has ever been, and involves members of various health care professions as well as users and carers. Attention has been given to how to identify relevant research, for example, by involving users and care providers from the earliest stages of defining and planning a project. Their involvement makes it much more likely that research will be implemented in practice.

Clifford and Murray (2001) discuss the importance of the project leader working in the practice area to ensure that staff have ownership of research and that their insights are valued and utilised. Clinical staff need support if they are to develop and sustain an environment in which research can flourish – support to use existing knowledge, to collect data that will improve understanding of care and the care environment, and to take a lead in clinical research. It is vital that those with research training and skills are highly visible within the clinical arena and are prepared to help students and staff who want to evaluate and improve their work. When researchers work regularly with clinical colleagues on research and development initiatives, the quality and relevance of research are improved and its findings stand a much better chance of being implemented in practice.

For research to be effective within organisations, ideally there should be:

- A supportive organisational culture that encourages and values inquiry into what is being done and how it is being done
- A drive to foster critical, reflective thinking in all staff, carers and service users
- A culture of openness to new ideas
- Support for those involved in research and resources to ensure maximum research quality
- Opportunities for all disciplines and departments to become involved in the learning community
- Means of communicating across the whole organisation what individuals have achieved
- Organisational events where work that has been successfully implemented can be discussed and celebrated
- A culture where staff are encouraged to challenge practice, rather than each other.

Equally a research culture will not flourish if:

- Research is seen by staff as an elitist activity involving only a few individuals
- Research is undertaken by people who are unable to communicate with service-based colleagues about the relevance of the work they are doing
- Senior managers do not understand or value what research can achieve
- It is thought to be possible to do good quality research 'on the cheap'
- Researchers are used for the prime purpose of generating income
- Researchers are given short-term contracts and have uncertain futures
- There is no investment in an educated workforce who can see the relevance of research and collaborate in the implementation of findings
- Individuals are permitted to undertake research solely for the purpose of advancing their careers
- The composition of health care teams changes frequently
- There is a 'free for all, anything goes' attitude towards research where the need for rigorous design and methodology is undervalued.

Tyrer (2003) acknowledges that, historically, research has tended to take a long time to get into practice, but is wary of rushing findings into the clinical arena. He considers that the major problem facing researchers and practitioners today is that there are far too many findings and a shortage of skills to evaluate findings critically and consider their usefulness in the context in which they are going to be applied. The kind of large population studies favoured by cancer and coronary care specialists look impressive but are of limited use in determining how we care for individuals who present with unique and multiple problems. In mental health, there is a need for longitudinal studies, which map the effects of mental health problems over the life span of a person. Shooter (2003) considers that we should step back and look at why we are doing research by asking ourselves the question: What *is* an advance in mental health care? Is it the case that by reconfiguring services in the name of modernisation, we are losing more than we are achieving? He contends that much research is directed towards the acquisition of technical knowledge rather than improving the ability to understand distress and work with people in need of someone to listen to them and befriend them during turbulent periods in their lives. The pressure to undertake research to meet targets set by universities or health care trusts may have serious repercussions for the quality of research. The emphasis on quantity undermines both the range of research that can be carried out and its credibility and leads to many researchers becoming disillusioned (Lagnado 2003).

Healy and Cattell (2003) argue that all mental health workers must be assisted to develop research awareness as a crucial dimension of their work. When the workforce is aware of potential bias in research, and willing and able to ask questions about how research is funded, it is better able to judge where evidence may be flawed. The influence of research funders, especially the pharmaceutical industry, on the conduct and dissemination of research, must be considered. Being selective about inclusion criteria, the types of data collected, and the kinds of analysis undertaken so that results are skewed to show certain interventions in a favourable light may be far more prevalent than is realised. In the final analysis, the best guarantee of high-quality, relevant research is an educated and critical workforce that demands excellent evidence on which to base its practice.

References

Beers, C. (1908). *A mind that found itself.* Doubleday, Doran & Co. Inc., New York.
Benedict, S. (2003). Killing while caring: the nurses of Hadamar. *Issues in Mental Health Nursing,* **24**, 59–79.

Berrios, G.E. (1996). *The history of mental symptoms.* Cambridge University Press, Cambridge.

Bourne, H. (1953). The insulin myth. *Lancet,* **ii**, 964–8.

Broody, H. (2003). *Stories of sickness.* Oxford University Press, Oxford.

Carpenter, P. (1989). Thomas Arnold; a provincial psychiatrist in Georgian England. *Medical History,* **33**, 199–216.

Clifford, C. and Murray, S. (2001). Pre- and post-test evaluation of a project to facilitate research development in practice in a hospital setting. *Journal of Advanced Nursing,* **36**, 685–95.

De Chardin, T. (1979). *The human search.* Collins, Glasgow.

Department of Health. (1999). National service framework for mental health: modern standards and service models. Department of Health, London.

Dicks, H. (1970). *Fifty years of the Tavistock Clinic.* Routledge & Kegan Paul, London.

Dobson, R. (2003). A quarter of patients with neurotic disorders don't seek help. *British Medical Journal,* **326**, 1056.

Freeman, H. (2003). Former editor of the Journal of Psychiatry – personal communication.

Fukuyama, F. (1992). *The end of history and the last man.* Penguin Publications, New York.

Gejman, P.V. and Weilbaccher, A. (2002). History of the eugenic movement. *Israeli Journal of Psychiatry and Related Sciences,* **39**, 217–31.

Goldberg, D.P., Jenkins, L., Millar, T. and Faragher, E.B. (1993). The ability of trainee general practitioners to identify distress among their patients. *Psychological Medicine,* **23**, 185–93.

Handy, C. (2001). *The elephant and the flea.* Hutchinson, London.

Healy, D. and Cattell, D. (2003). Interface between authorship, industry and science in the domain of therapeutics. *British Journal of Psychiatry,* **183**, 22–7.

Horrobin, D. (2001). *The madness of Adam and Eve.* Bantam Press, London.

Kraam, A. (2002). The legacy of Kraepelin. *History of Psychiatry,* **13**, 475–80.

Kraepelin, E. (1904). *Lectures on clinical psychiatry* (translated and edited by Thomas Johnstone). Tindall and Cox, London.

Lagnado, M. (2003). Increasing the trust in scientific authorship. *British Journal of Psychiatry,* **183**, 3–4.

Lester, H. (2003). *Cases for change, primary care.* National Institute for Mental Health in England: The Modernising Agency at the Department of Health, London.

Makoul, G., Arntson, P. and Schofield, T. (1995). Health promotion in primary care: physician–patient communication and decision making about prescription. *Medication, Social Science and Medicine,* **41**, 1241–54.

Miller, P. and Rose, N. (1986). *The power of psychiatry.* Polity Press, Cambridge.

Nettleton, S. (1995). *The sociology of health and illness.* Polity Press, London.

Porter, R. (2002). *Madness, a brief history.* Oxford University Press, Oxford.

Ryle, G. (1976). *The concept of mind*. Penguin Books, Aylesbury.

Sacks, O. (1983). *Awakenings*. Dutton, New York.

Scull, A. (1979). *Museums of madness, the social organisation of insanity in nineteenth-century England*. Allen Lane, London.

Seedhouse, D. (2002). *Total health promotion*. John Wiley & Sons, London.

Shepheard, M. (2002). Neuroleptics and the psychopharmacological revolution: myth and reality. *History of Psychiatry*, **13**, 224–32.

Shooter, M. (2003). On Pushto, principles and passion: just what is an advance in psychiatric treatment. *Advances in Psychiatric Treatment*, **9**, 239–40.

Slobodin, R. (1997). *W.H.R. Rivers*. Sutton Publishing Ltd, London.

Steinberg, H. and Angermeyer, G. (2002). Two hundred years of psychiatry at Leipzig University: an overview. *History of Psychiatry*, **13**, 267–83.

Szasz T. (1970). *The manufacture of madness*. Dell, New York.

Szasz, T. (1995). The origin of psychiatry – the alienist as nanny for troublesome adults. *History of Psychiatry*, **vi**, 1–19.

Tyrer, P. (2003). Entertaining eminence in the British Journal of Psychiatry. *British Journal of Psychiatry*, **183**, 1–2.

5

Researching 'race' and mental illness

Frank Keating

▌INTRODUCTION

'Race', ethnicity, and mental illness/health have received growing interest in the literature of the last three decades. These constructs are shrouded in complexity and fraught with contradictions. Subjectively, these topics evoke a variety of emotional responses that could range from fear to denial and prejudice. Utilising these constructs in research therefore brings us to one of the most contentious spheres of knowledge construction as well as that of policy and service development in mental health.

This chapter will explore how researchers in general have addressed the issues and concerns for Black and Minority Ethnic (BME) communities. Grouping these communities in this way does not imply that the heterogeneous and dynamic nature of these communities are being overlooked or denied. Some of the epistemological considerations that should be taken into account when researchers investigate 'race' and mental health will be reviewed. I will highlight some of the dilemmas inherent to this arena of work by making reference to an example from my own practice. I will not discuss methodological issues in any depth as these have been reviewed elsewhere (see, for example, Sashidharan and Francis 1993; Ndegwa 1998; Patel 1999; Boushel 2000; Gunarutnum 2003). The historical trajectory of research on 'race' and mental health will not be reviewed here due to limited space, but suffice it to say that it is characterised by a multifaceted and contentious history in the creation and generation of knowledge

(Centre for Evidence in Ethnicity, Health and Diversity, 2003; Fernando, 2003).

I start from the premise that BME communities have not taken an active role (or indeed been allowed to) in setting the research agenda or leading research about their lives and the issues that affect them. I firmly believe that the beneficiaries of research should be actively and meaningfully involved in developing and carrying out research, and monitoring whether that knowledge is being used or applied in their interests. I propose that all research activities concerning BME communities should be framed in the context of their lived experiences; that is, understanding how 'race' and ethnicity function as signifiers in their social interactions and the meanings they have in relation to group and individual identities (Gunaratnam 2003). However, this has to be understood in the framework of the inter-relatedness of 'race' and ethnicity with other social divisions. This would require researchers to take full account of the historical and contemporary contexts for BME communities and the pervasive racism and levels of disproportionate disadvantage they experience in service delivery.

THE RESEARCH AGENDA

Research practice in health and social care reflects the power relations in service provision, that is, a hierarchical relationship where power rests with professionals (Oliver 1992; Zarb 1992). Knowledge production in these spheres is also marked by, for example, racial, class, gender and age hegemonies (Stanfield II 1993). Traditional research in its very nature re-invokes fixed hierarchical relationships where the researcher ultimately holds the dominant position over 'the researched'. However, I do acknowledge that there are emerging research paradigms that aim to redress the power imbalances between the researcher and the 'researched'. Participatory research methods and the small but growing body of user-led research projects are examples of this. Service users have particularly become engaged in research activity to ensure that their narratives are heard and presented in ways that reflect their lived experiences (Faulkner and Thomas 2002).

The Department of Health's (DoH) draft second edition of the guidelines for research governance (2003a) suggests that researchers should take full account of the multi-cultural nature of society and that research evidence should reflect the diverse nature of the population. It proposes closer collaboration and consultation with communities under study, a recommendation previously made by Patel (1999). Consultation with communities under study is advantageous because it can ensure that the concepts and methods that are adopted are culturally valid and sensitive to the population concerned. Credibility in the community can also be attained in this way. Macaulay *et al.* (1999) suggested that it could maximise lay and community involvement. Progress in relation to these recommendations, however, is slow.

Another factor that plays a role in how the research agenda is set is the fact that the research community in the UK is predominantly white, largely male and mainly work in academic institutions that are removed from the communities they are researching (Fenton *et al.* 2000). There are growing numbers of BME researchers who essentially seem to enter the research arena to promote and advance a focus on issues of 'race' and ethnicity. It is hoped that the recent moves by the Higher Education Funding Council for England (HEFCE) to widen participation in higher education may ultimately lead to an increase in the number of BME researchers.

The main focus in research on BME communities and mental health has been on what I would term as an obsession with establishing pathology in these communities and seeking causal explanations for it. Explanations are frequently located within these communities or groups and linked with theories of migration, culturalist explanations, genetic predisposition or deficits within these communities (Sharpley *et al.* 2001). These frameworks mean that the lived experiences of BME communities are explained in terms of cultural differences and their 'otherness' and usually equating this with pathology (Ahmad 1993).

There is an emerging body of research that attempts to shift the research paradigm from pathology to examining and analysing how health and social care is structured in terms of inequality and disadvantage (Stubbs 1993). However, this research seems to remain at the margins and does not appear to influence policy and service developments. The National Institute for Mental Health in England (NIMHE) (Department of Health 2003b) has recently launched a framework for delivering race equality in mental health services and there is some optimism that this will produce changes in how services are delivered to BME communities. There has more recently been a move towards locating the problems for, and concerns of, BME communities in a broader context, i.e., societal and institutional racism and social inequality (Fernando 1998; Thornicroft 1999; Williams 1999; Sashidhuran 2001; McKenzie 2003). However, there is still a great deal of resistance to consider the racism paradigm as a possible explanation for psychiatric morbidity in BME communities, or indeed, for their negative experiences and poorer outcomes in mental health services.

McKenzie's (2003) hypothesis that racism is a causal factor in mental illness evoked a flood of critical responses (see the January 2003 issues of the British Medical Journal). Racism should be considered as a possible variable in the aetiology of psychiatric morbidity, and in service experience and outcomes for BME communities. However, accepting the racism paradigm as the only explanatory framework is not entirely unproblematic because it can lead to determinism. According to Stubbs (1993) racism as a 'catch-all' category has limited analytical value. Viewing racism as the only causal factor for mental health problems in BME communities reduces their life experiences solely to the domain of racial and ethnic identity. It can also lead to a denial of other forms of oppression in these communities. Stubbs (1993) further suggests that researchers need to take account of the different ways in which communities experience racism and of the differential impact it may have on them.

Research pertaining to BME communities and mental health has also centred on organisational concerns such as over- and under-representation and seeking culturally appropriate models of care (Bhugra and Bhui 2001). However, models of practice in the BME voluntary sector in general have been excluded from research enquiry: a reflection of the fact that black-led voluntary sector agencies are on the margins of mainstream service provision. To date there has been no large-scale study to document or evaluate the contributions of black-led organisations to mental health service provision (Keating 2002). A recent survey (Joseph Rowntree Foundation 2001) examined the role of BME voluntary sector organisations, but did not specifically include mental health.

It is thus clear that there is a need to change the research agenda before it can have relevance to the needs and interests of BME communities. In a multi-ethnic society, issues of ethnicity, culture and racism are important dimensions of everyday life and should therefore receive careful consideration in defining research problems and agendas. I will return to this in the final section of this chapter.

IDEOLOGY AND CATEGORY CONSTRUCTION

Knowledge production is ideologically determined and culturally based (Foucault 1977). In relation to how research problems evolve, Stubbs (1993) argued that they are shaped within particular social, economic, professional, theoretical, ideological and historical contexts. Patel (1999) suggests that the difficulties in mental health research involve the underlying concepts behind the research and the methods selected for carrying out the research.

Even though the field of 'race' and health research is an ideological minefield, there is little evidence that the role of ideological considerations in research involving BME communities has received attention (Ahmad 1993). This glaring omission in research involving issues of 'race' and culture is informed by the notion that research is a value-free and neutral activity because of its reliance on the principles of scientific logic. A field of social inquiry with such an inherent emotive dimension requires a different paradigm. The naturalistic paradigm offers the practice of reflexivity, that is, the practice of incorporating an evaluation of the research process, and in particular the role of the researcher in it (Adamson and Donavan 2002). We need to search for ways in which this practice can be incorporated into the positivist framework; specially since the National Service Framework for Mental Health espouses the positivist paradigm as the preferred method of generating knowledge in their hierarchy of evidence (Department of Health 1999).

Researchers have to acknowledge that what they 'see and interpret' when doing research will be influenced by their own consciousness about 'race', culture and ethnicity and how they identify themselves. Marks (1993) suggests that researchers need to consider their own life histories and how this influences their choice of design and study methods. Adopting the positivist paradigm, which is premised on principles of objectivity and scientific logic, is insufficient to overcome this dilemma. Any attempt at knowledge construction pertaining to BME communities is in essence of its own nature a subjective activity regardless of the methods chosen. Researchers therefore have to engage intellectually and emotionally with the subject under investigation.

Category construction is an important aspect of social inquiry, particularly in what Stanfield II (1993) refers to as 'race-centred societies' such as the UK. He suggests that in these societies citizens have been socialised to view self and others in terms of race and ethnic categories. These categories are, for example, reflected in vocabulary, everyday discourse, how individuals describe themselves, and the assumptions we make about others. A logical conclusion is that social scientists will be no different from the general population in their assumptions about a racialised society because they too have been socialised to accept racially constructed stereotypes and assumptions about the world (Stanfield II 1993). To address this they need to be reflexive about its implications for their world views and activity as researchers.

Defining 'race', ethnicity and culture as variables in research has been an area of continuing debate. The term 'race' has been rejected based on scientific evidence that human races do not exist (Lee *et al.* 2001). Therefore, it has become accepted practice to write the term in inverted commas. Moreover, these constructs are rarely defined and used uncritically, thereby conflating issues of biology, culture, and social and environmental factors (Patel 1999). Ethnicity as a term to define group definitions is now widely preferred when making reference to minority groups. However, using ethnicity to define groups has its own limitations.

Firstly, there is what Stanfield II (1993) refers to as the 'fallacy of homogeneity' where minority ethnic groups are treated as undifferentiated communities with shared internal identities. The result is that these groups are cast into fixed identities and categories, so that if someone looks a certain way s/he is assumed to possess the characteristics associated with that group. A classic example in psychiatry is schizophrenia, which has become strongly associated with African and Caribbean people.

Secondly, Bhugra and Bhui (2001) suggest that another difficulty with using ethnicity as a category arises from the fact that it is linked to history and a distinct culture. Unfortunately this has meant that the concerns for, and of, these communities tended to be articulated as an issue of culture or cultural complexity (Keating *et al.* 2002). Conceptualising ethnicity in this manner means that culture is invoked as the major explanatory framework for the experiences of BME communities in mental health services and, according to Aspinal (1998), ignores the fact that these groups are racialised. Differences between and within groups are not being disputed or minimised, but cultural approaches have a tendency to homogenise communities and reinforce stereotypical views of individuals. It is important to bear in mind that groups are differentiated by gender, age, class, sexuality, ability and that these intersect in complex ways (Keating 1997; Bowes and Dar 2000). Smaje (1996) argues that research should be aimed at establishing and analysing the complex connections between ethnicity and these other forms of differentiation. Issues and concern for individuals from these communities should be understood and analysed in their wider social, historical, economic and political context.

Thirdly, the way in which ethnic identity is assigned or ascribed to individuals is a crucial factor. Some authors suggest that the most preferable practice is to use group categorisations based on self-identified ethnic categories rather than assigning individuals to categories based on observed features and characteristics (McKenzie and Crowcroft 1996; Aspinall 2001). Not only should this provide more accurate information, but could help to overcome stereotypical views of BME communities. Aspinall (2001) further suggests that we need to seek additional identifiers, for example, religion, to reflect the complexity and broad nature of ethnic diversity. For some groups these identifiers may be more significant sources of identity. However, Aspinall (2001) cautions that a multidimensional measurement approach to ethnicity involves a number of problems such as time, resources and respecting the privacy of the respondent. I would argue that if ethnicity data is vital to the issue under investigation, it is crucial that these problems are given careful consideration prior to the start of the study.

Another factor that adds to the complexity of the arena of category construction is the tools and frameworks used for identifying and categorising mental illness. According to Bhugra and Bhui (2001), the adoption of bio-medical explanations for mental illness and the universal application of a concept that may not have validity, as an illness, disease or disability in other societies. Fernando (2003) suggests that there is an over-reliance on diagnosis as a basis for categorisation of research participants. He posits that diagnoses as they are currently used have little scientific value in a multi-cultural society. It is further argued (Fernando 2003) that one has to bear in mind that psychiatric data derived from diagnosis are transient and can therefore fluctuate over time. The issue of relying on diagnoses is further compounded by the fact that these systems of classification have been developed in western contexts (mono-cultural) and can not therefore summarily be applied to other cultural and social contexts. Kleinman (1977), for example, highlighted the danger of 'category fallacy' when categories are used to yield homogenous and undifferentiated groups. Fernando (2003) suggests that we need to, '. . . shift from categories to dimensions in measuring symptoms, . . . and such measures must always be supplemented by other ways of identifying mental health problems' (p. 204).

Aspinall (2001) succinctly summarised the challenges related to measuring ethnicity, and I would add that these relate to measuring mental illness as well, by suggesting that:

there is no true measure of ethnicity that can be applied in a wide variety of contexts and consequently no way in which it can be fixed or easily measured. Rather, its contingent, complex and labile nature demands that the means of measurement should be related to the purpose of the research.

(p. 452)

Given all the complexities around ethnicity, researchers should bear in mind that as a construct it is contextual, i.e. it takes many forms depending on associated conditions. Defining ethnicity and mental illness is also deeply interactive, because they are closely intertwined with political and economic events and social processes (Nazroo 1997).

ETHNIC MATCHING

The importance of matching researchers with research participants has been highlighted elsewhere (Modood *et al.* 1997; Adamson and Donovan 2002; Papodopoulus and Lees 2002). It has been argued that this practice can minimise the cultural distance between the interviewer and the research participant (Aspinall 2001). Additionally, it has been suggested that the practice of ethnic matching encourages a more equal context for interviewing and allows for more accurate and sensitive data collection (Papodopoulus and Lees 2002).

Ethnic matching can be beneficial in certain circumstances. For example, in situations where language is an issue this practice can overcome the likelihood of misunderstanding. It also seems to yield positive results when there are additional characteristics that the researcher shares with research participants. For example, I was co-facilitating a focus group with families and carers. When I introduced myself there was a great deal of scepticism about participating in the research and mistrust about the intentions of the research. However, when the co-facilitator introduced herself and disclosed the fact that she too was a carer, the levels of mistrust dissipated significantly and it was much easier to engage the participants in fuller and more open discussions. What we therefore learnt was that shared ethnicity was not adequate to gain support and participation. Shared experience seemed to have been a more beneficial attribute of the researcher than ethnic background. The challenge is to be alert to the subjectivity of the researcher and to guard against influencing the discourse on the basis of the interviewer's experiences.

Matching researchers and study participants on ethnic background is good and valuable practice, but there are inherent tensions. Given the complexities and contentious nature of ethnicity outlined above, one cannot automatically assume that ethnic matching will engender trust, rapport and commonality between the researcher and research participants. Such practice also assumes or suggests that 'outsiders' cannot appreciate and understand the issues and concerns for BME communities, which raises the issue of whether white researchers should be involved in research with BME communities. Douglas (1992), for example, holds the view that racism is paramount for BME people and as white researchers do not experience racism, this limits their ability fully to comprehend the experiences of these communities. This view has its own limitations, because it assumes that white groups as a category is undifferentiated and ignores the fact that some minority white groups such as the Irish also experience significant levels of disadvantage and discrimination in mental health services, albeit differentially to other BME communities (Tilki 1998). Bhavnani (1993) recommends that white researchers can be involved in research with black people, provided they embrace an anti-racist perspective. This requires challenging stereotypes and racism and contextualising the experience of black people in the wider structures of social life.

Bhavnani (1993) critiques the 'insider only' perspective on the basis that shared experience cannot be held as truth as it 'silences and ends the right to argue with it' (p. 42). Arguments for ethnic matching can be in danger of producing essentialist standpoints where racial identity and/or shared experience of the researcher come to be seen as the major criterion for validity and truth (Bhavnani 1993). More appropriate criteria for validity in research on 'race' and health should be clarity and openness about the ideological framework that is being used to inform the research and a conscious analysis of the power relations throughout the process.

A further tension when 'insiders' are carrying out research is that there is likely to be other social divisions that can create a distance when the research participants are disadvantaged along those dimensions. Bhavnani (1993) posits that matching strategies often fail to take account of the power relations and the imbalances between the researcher and research participants. Ethnic matching can also obscure other differences such as gender, class, age, disability and sexuality (Gunaratnam 2003). It is therefore important that researchers take account of the fact that no social category exists in isolation and the impact of this on the research relationship needs to be examined and addressed. BME researchers are also guided by the principles of science and evidence, which often may limit how they 'give voice' to the concerns of BME communities. Balancing these tensions presents a challenge for BME researchers when, ultimately, the aim of many of them is to highlight the plight of Black people. Furthermore, these issues should not be relegated to those researchers whose work specifically focuses on these issues: it is the responsibility of the entire research community (Gunaratnam 2003).

ETHICS AND GOOD PRACTICE

A range of bodies has published codes of ethical and/or good practice. The guidance on research involving BME communities is varied and may not always be adhered to. The Royal College of Psychiatrists published a code of ethics in 2001. It is surprising to note that given the well-documented evidence about the over and under-representation of individuals from various ethnic communities in mental health services (Bhugra and Bahl 1999; Bhui and Olajide 2001; Fernando 2003), that the code does not include specific guidance for research involving BME communities. The code makes one reference to working with communities in general as is illustrated in the following guiding principle:

> *It is good research (and ethics) practice to consult members of the community to be studied when planning studies. As appropriate to the individual study, such consultation might involve consumers, professionals, community members of ethnic/religious groups.*
> (Royal College of Psychiatrists 2001, p. 20)

The British Psychology Society (BPS) has paid greater attention to the issues of diversity and gives specific guidance in this area. These guidelines (BPS 2000) recommend that any investigation should be considered from the perspective and views of all participants. More specifically, it suggests that:

> *Investigators should recognise in our multi-cultural and multi-ethnic society and where investigations involve individuals of different ages, gender and social background, the investigators may not have sufficient knowledge of the implications of any investigation for the participants. It should be borne in mind that the best judges whether an investigation will cause offence may be members of the population from which the participants in the research are drawn.*
> (BPS 2000, p. 8)

The Transcultural Psychiatry Society (UK) (TCPS) in collaboration with Mind published a set of guidelines for ethical mental health research involving issues of 'race', ethnicity and culture (Patel 1999). This document was developed after TCPS engaged in a critical discussion of the value and impact of research for BME communities. The publication addressed the need for developing ethical practice in the design, conduct and use of research and provides a set of guidelines for ethical practice. These guidelines are offered to facilitate good practice and improve the ways in which BME communities are treated in research. Patel (1999) suggests that ethical practice should begin with the formulation of research questions and continue throughout the research process. She further posits that this can be achieved through collaboration with the communities whose members are potential research participants.

   Ethical guidelines for good practice are necessary, but the challenge lies in how these are implemented. The DOH guidelines (2003a) for research governance set standards for good practice in research. It unfortunately recommends that failures to meet these standards should be addressed through normal management channels and disciplinary procedures. I suggest that all ethics committees should be assigned the task of monitoring and implementing these guidelines if we expect research to reflect the multi-cultural nature of society.

BREAKING THE CYCLE: AN EXAMPLE FOR PRACTICE

Given the long-standing concerns of BME communities about mental health services and research, the Sainsbury Centre, in 2000, launched a study to examine and analyse the relationship between mental health services and African and Caribbean communities (Keating *et al.* 2002). These communities were selected because of the compelling evidence that shows that they are massively over-represented in mental health services and in terms of negative experiences and indicators. It was felt that special attention was required to be given to this subject. It was also decided to break from the tradition of bringing together all concerns relating to ethnicity and culture under the rubric of 'black and ethnic minorities'. Moreover, it was felt that unless there was a focus on a specific community to devise dedicated strategies, a clear health care and social policy opportunity would be missed.

   The subjective notion of 'fear' framed the study because there is ample evidence that this emotion permeates so much of the social context surrounding a community whose profile within political debate and social policy is disproportionate to its size within the general population. This is true whether we look at policing, education, social work or health.

The approach of this study differed from the numerous epidemiological studies and instead focussed on the experiences and views of service users, families and carers and staff working in the various mental health sectors. A naturalistic enquiry approach (Guba and Lincoln 1989) was adopted to seek the views of service users, families and carers and professionals in all sectors. This ensured that organisationally defined issues and concerns did not purely frame the study. Moreover, a participatory approach was taken to seek ways of working which did not reinforce exclusionary processes. This practice is in line with recommendations by Patel (1999) that researchers should consult members of communities to be studied throughout the research process. This ensures that the concepts and methods used are culturally valid and sensitive to the population concerned. Participatory methods can also help to establish credibility in the community. Macaulay *et al.* (1999) suggested that participatory methods can maximise community and lay involvement in research.

A group of facilitators comprising service users, families and carers and mental health workers were recruited to develop data collection instruments, carry out focus group interviews and analyse data. Four training workshops were run to brief the facilitators about the aims of the study, develop an interview schedule and provide training in interviewing techniques. A striking feature of these sessions was an awareness of the differences in terminology used, so a great deal of space and time were devoted to identify shared interests and to develop a common language to guide the research.

We learnt a few lessons from this experience. Firstly, a clear ideological framework ensured that the research activity was relevant to the lives of service users, families and carers and to the practical concerns of mental health workers. Secondly, that a collaborative and participatory approach engendered trust. Thirdly, that shared understandings and meanings between all researchers and interviewers were vital to the success of the data collection and analysis processes. Fourthly, power (not statistical) was a significant dimension of the research process. For example, in focus groups participants were asked to develop solutions for change. Service users, families and carers found it incredibly difficult to participate in this activity. On reflection I concluded that it is unfair to ask individuals in relative positions of powerlessness to comment on issues that require considerable organisational and personal power. Lastly, shared ethnicity and shared background was beneficial, but not entirely unproblematic, as described earlier.

GAP BETWEEN RESEARCH AND PRACTICE

Given the growing body of research on 'race' and mental health there is little evidence to show that research has made a difference to practice (Ahmad 1993). Numerous other research reports over the last decade have highlighted these concerns, yet it seems that policy makers and service planners have not taken these messages on board. In the study discussed above (Keating *et al.* 2002), participants shared a view that research has not made a difference to how they experience mental health services. Therefore, this study was viewed with a great deal of suspicion and mistrust and a great deal of effort was needed to overcome this high level of understandable resistance to participate.

The reasons for failing to get research into practice have been identified (Berro *et al.* 1998; Haines and Donald 1998; Kerrick *et al.* 1999). These include a lack of a clear and active dissemination strategy and a lack of attention to organisational and social barriers to change. A more significant reason for the failure is offered by Kernick *et al.* (1999) who posited that research continues to provide answers that are irrelevant to everyday practice and, more importantly, to the concerns of service users, families and carers. I suggest that research can better influence practice when, firstly, the communities under investigation are actively involved in setting the research agenda and carrying out the research; secondly, clear dissemination and implementation strategies have been outlined at the conceptualisation of the research programme; and thirdly, an effective change strategy informs the process.

RESEARCH INTO PRACTICE

The biggest challenge for any researcher is to ensure that their findings can be applied to practice. Reason (1994) posited that emerging paradigms in research such as participatory research are offering the potential to democratise the research process. He suggests that the research community stand a better chance of translating research into practice by adopting some of these frameworks.

Following this lead, I propose that research findings will have greater likelihood of influencing service development for BME communities when the following issues have received careful consideration:

- An acknowledgement of the subjective nature of inquiry when issues of 'race' culture and ethnicity are research variables
- Attention to how categories are constructed and defined
- An assessment of the instruments and tools for measurement of sensitivity to the needs and issues of these communities and to develop appropriate and relevant tools where necessary
- Reflection on the power dimensions in the research process
- Active involvement of the communities under study throughout the research process
- Situating the study in the lived experiences of the communities under study.

SUMMARY

This chapter has reviewed some of the methodological issues around researching 'race' and mental illness. It is clear that these constructs are controversial and pose particular problems for the research community. The evidence seems to suggest that research on these issues has not contributed significantly to changes to the way in which mental health services are organised and delivered. If research is to be relevant to the lives of individuals with mental health problems in these communities, then we need an overhaul of the orthodoxy of research. The overhaul should be in terms of how we theorise research, how we conceptualise 'race' and mental illness and how we involve BME communities in commissioning, designing and carrying out research. In this way we can ensure that research pays attention to their agency and views (Bowes 1996).

References

Adamson, J. and Donovan, J.L. (2002). Research in black and white. *Qualitative Health Research*, 12(6), 816–25.

Ahmad, W.I.U. (ed.) (1993). 'Race' and health in contemporary Britain. Open University Press, Buckingham.

Aspinall, P.J. (2001). Operationalising the collection of ethnicity data in studies of the sociology of health and illness. *Sociology of Health and Illness*, 23(6), 829–62.

Bero, L.A., Grilli, R., Grimshaw, J.M., Harvey, E., Oxman, A.D. and Thomson, M.A. (1998). Closing the gap between research and practice: an overview of systematic reviews of interventions to promote the implementation of research findings. *British Medical Journal*, **317**, 465–8.

Bhavnani, K. (1993). Talking racism and the editing of women's studies. In *Introducing women's studies: feminist theory and practice* (eds. Richardson, D. and Robinson, V.), Macmillan, London.

Bhugra, D. and Bhui, K. (2001). African-Caribbeans and schizophrenia: contributing factors. *Advances in Psychiatric Treatment*, **7**, 283–93.

Boushel, M. (2000). What kind of people are we? 'Race', anti-racism and social welfare research. *British Journal of Social Work*, **30**, 71–89.

Bowes, A.M. (1996). Evaluating an empowering research strategy: reflections on action–research with South Asian women. *Sociological Research Online*, **1**(1), 1–21.

Bowes, A.M. and Dar, N.S. (2000). Researching social care for minority ethnic older people: implications of some Scottish research. *British Journal of Social Work*, **30**, 305–21.

British Psychological Society. (2000). *Code of conduct, ethical principles and guidelines*. British Psychological Society, Leicester.

Centre for Evidence in Ethnicity, Health and Diversity. (2003). *Concepts of diversity*. http://users.wbs.ac.uk/group/ceehd/homeconcepts_of_diversity. Accessed 25 July 2003.

Department of Health. (2003a). *Research governance framework for health and social care (draft second edition)*. Department of Health, London.

Department of Health. (2003b). *Delivering race equality: a framework for action*. Department of Health, London.

Department of Health. (1999). *National service framework for mental health: modern standards and service models for mental health*. Department of Health, London.

Douglas, J. (1992). Black women's health matters: putting black women on the research agenda. In *Women's health matters* (ed. Roberts, H.), Routledge, London.

Faulkner, A. and Thomas, P. (2002). User-led research and evidence based medicine. *British Journal of Psychiatry*, **180**, 1–3.

Fenton, S., Carter, J. and Modood, T. (2000). Ethnicity and academia: closure models, racism models and market models. *Sociological Research Online*, **5**(2), http://www.socresonline.org.uk/5/2/fenton.html.

Fernando, S. (2003). *Cultural diversity, mental health and psychiatry: the struggle against racism*. Brunner-Routledge, Hove.

Foucault, M. (1977). *Discipline and punish: the birth of the prison* (translated by A. Sheridan). Vintage, New York.

Gunaratnam, Y. (2003). *Researching 'race' and ethnicity: methods, knowledge and power*. Sage, London.

Joseph Rowntree Foundation. (2001). *The role and future development of black and minority ethnic organisations.* Joseph Rowntree Foundation, York.

Keating, F. (1997). *Developing an integrated approach to understanding oppression.* CCETSW, London.

Keating, F. (2002). Black-led initiatives in mental health: an overview. *Research, Policy and Practice,* **20**(2), 9–20.

Keating, F., Robertson, D., Francis, E. and McCulloch, A. (2002). *Breaking the circles of fear: a review of the relationship between mental health services and African and Caribbean communities.* Sainsbury Centre for Mental Health, London.

Kernick, D., Stead, J. and Dixon, M. (1999). Moving the research agenda to where it matters. *British Medical Journal,* **319**, 2006–7.

Lee, S.S., Mountain, J. and Koenig, B.A. (2001). The meanings of 'race' in the new genomics: implications or health disparities research. *Journal of Health Policy, Law & Ethics* **1**, 33–68.

Macaulay, A.C., Commanda, L.E. and Freeman, W.L. (1999). Participatory research maximises community and lay involvement. *British Medical Journal,* **319**(7212), 774–8.

Marks, C.C. (1993). Demography and race. In *Race and ethnicity in research methods* (eds. Stanfield II, J.H. and Dennis, R.M.), Sage Publications, London.

McKenzie, K. (2003). Racism and health. *British Medical Journal,* **326**, 65–6.

McKenzie, K. and Crowcroft, N.S. (1996). Describing race, ethnicity and culture in medical research. *British Medical Journal.* **213**(7038), 1054.

Modood, T., Berthoud, R., Lakey, J., Nazroo, J., Smith, P., Virdee, S. and Beishon, S. (1997). *Ethnic minorities in Britain: diversity and disadvantage.* Policy Studies Institute, London.

Oliver, M. (1992). Changing the social relations of research production. *Disability, Handicap and Society,* **7**(2), 101–14.

Papadopoulos, I. and Lees, S. (2002). Developing culturally competent researchers. *Journal of Advanced Nursing,* **37**(3), 258–64.

Patel, N. (1999). *Getting the evidence: guidelines for ethical mental health research involving issues of 'race', ethnicity and culture.* TCPS & Mind, London.

Royal College of Psychiatrists. (2001). *Guidance for researchers and ethics committees on psychiatric research involving human participants.* Gaskell, London.

Sharpley, M., Hutchinson, G., McKenzie, K. and Murray, R.M. (2001). Understanding the excess of psychosis among the African-Caribbean population in England: review of current hypotheses. *British Journal of Psychiatry,* **178** (supplement 40), s60–s68.

Stanfield II, J.H. (1993). Epistemological considerations. In *Race and ethnicity in research methods* (eds. Stanfield II, J.H. and Dennis, R.M.), Sage, London.

Stubbs, P. (1993). 'Ethnically sensitive' or 'anti-racist'? Models for health research and service delivery. In *'Race' and health in contemporary Britain* (ed. Ahmad, W.I.U.), Open University Press, Buckingham.

Tilki, M. (1998). The health of the Irish in Britain. In *Transcultural care for health professionals* (Papadoulos, I., Tilki, M. and Taylor, G.), Quay Books, London.

Williams, J. (1999). Social inequalities and mental health. In *This is madness: a critical look at psychiatry and the future of mental health services* (eds. Newnes, C., Holmes, G. and Dunn, C.), PCCS Books, Ross-on-Wye.

Zarb, G. (1992). On the road to Damascus: first steps towards changing the relations of disability research production. *Disability, Handicap and Society.* **7**(2), 125–38.

6

Women and mental health research: methodological issues and recent progress

Alison Longwill

CONTEXT

Women constitute over half of the general population, play a significant role in the workforce and provide the majority of care for our children and other dependent family members. Thus, mental ill health in women has profound individual and societal consequences. However, women frequently have less access than men to resources, opportunities and decision making and hence, unsurprisingly, mental health care has not been developed or delivered in a gender-sensitive manner.

BACKGROUND

In her book, *The female malady*, Showalter (1985) details how cultural ideas about 'proper' feminine behaviour have shaped the definition and treatment of female mental disorder over the last two hundred years. Women have typically been represented on the side of 'irrationality, silence, nature and body, while men are situated on the side of reason, discourse, culture and mind' (Showalter 1980, p. 30).

Even radical critics of traditional psychiatry have paid scant attention to gender as a determinant of mental ill health and have preferred to concentrate on issues related to social class and ethnicity in a 'gender blind' context for the most part. Thus, the most powerful sources of challenge to mainstream constructions of 'women's madness' derive from very different cultural sources such as asylum inmate narratives, diaries, memoirs and novels written by women.

FEMINIST APPROACHES

In the 1960s, the feminist movement was immensely influential in raising consciousness regarding the pervasive nature of women's oppression within society and highlighting the social and political forces which maintain gender-related social inequalities in relation to power, income and status. Gülçür (2000) states that economic dependence, lack of decision-making power, conflicting gender roles, disproportionate domestic responsibilities, and violence are closely linked to mental health problems in women and this is a problem of global significance, linked to the violation of basic human rights.

Wright and Owen (2001) explore feminist conceptions of 'madness' which view psychiatry as a method of socially controlling women and medicalising women's unhappiness. A linked development related to the development of feminist psychotherapies where recovery of well-being is associated with reframing common 'health symptoms or problems' and empowering women to make healthy choices for themselves. For instance, Susie Orbach's work *Fat is a feminist issue* (1978) and *Outside-in inside-out* (Eichenbaum and Orbach 1982) enabled many women to confront their problems with eating in a new and liberating way.

Feminist theorists viewed women's mental ill health from a social constructionist perspective linked to the interactions of women within their specific social context (see Webb (2002), Miers (2002) for reviews with respect to gender-sensitive nursing care and therapy (Finfgeld (2001)). Pugliesi (1992) argues that feminist scholarship on mental health has followed two lines of inquiry. The first, a social causation approach, examines the features of women's lives that enhance or undermine well-being. The social constructionist perspective involves critical analyses of methodology and conceptions of mental health and illness. This body of literature suggests that the findings of gender differences in mental health are artifactual and focuses on the sexism of psychiatry. Although these bodies of work have remained largely distinct and have been criticized as contradictory, both are important ingredients of a general feminist perspective on mental health. Feminist therapy is used as a model for a synthesis of approaches.

Characteristics of feminist mental health research (Bunting 1997) include: (a) perceiving the purposes of the study as benefiting women, (b) demonstrating an awareness of the structures and policies that oppress women, (c) sensitivity to issues of diversity, (d) commitment to social change, and (e) recognition of the female participants' strengths. Feminist research is also reflexive and considers the standpoint and emotions of the researcher in this process (Campbell 2002).

In more recent years, a more insidious concept of 'post-feminism', predicated on the idea that women's equality has been achieved, has tended to deny the impact of societal factors and has suggested to women that an individualistic quest for mental and physical well-being can be achieved by consuming various products and services in the marketplace.

BIOMEDICAL APPROACHES

Feminist theorists (e.g. Contratto 2002) have often been deeply critical of biological determinist or evolutionary psychology approaches to understanding mental ill health as their underpinning theoretical models are associated with maintenance of the status quo and do not empower women as actors who can influence and change their environment. Horwitz (2002) argues provocatively that the formulation of mental illness as disease benefits various interest groups, including mental health researchers and clinicians, drug manufacturers, and mental health advocacy groups, all of whom promote disease-based models. Modern psychiatry can be characterised by the quest for a 'pill for all ills'. Women receive approximately twice as many prescriptions for psychotropic medication and there has been a tendency to expand the territory of misery for which medication appears to offer a solution. Advertisements for pills to combat depression emphasise 'serotonin deficiencies' and other biomedical constructs which tend to individualise the cause of the 'depression epidemic' in western society. This construction ignores the root causes of depression in terms of multiple and conflicting societal roles for women as, for example, mother, carer, worker, partner and sexual athlete, combined with less access on average to the material and financial resources typically enjoyed by men.

Biomedical treatments of mental ill health have the markers of 'hard science' such as large-scale randomised control trials – often conducted at large expense by major pharmaceutical companies. However, there is substantial evidence that the trial populations consist of predominantly male college students. Professor Dora Kohen and colleagues (2000) state that this bias has led to patterns of psychotropic prescribing in dosages which are too high for the majority of women and to insufficient attention to gender issues in responsivity to these medications – for instance at different stages of the female reproductive cycle.

Blehar (2003) also notes that the course of mental disorders in women in relation to reproductive transitions remains an important but under-researched issue for the mental health field because the burden of mental disorders such as depression and anxiety, fall disproportionately on women of child-bearing and child-rearing age. This links to a pervasive failure to analyse and segment research data by gender routinely. In this way, important differences in presentation and response between men and women are routinely ignored.

Women are more likely to be prescribed certain psychotropic drugs such as antidepressants, anxiolytics and hypnotics than men. However, they may require lower doses of these drugs than men and may experience more problematic side-effects (e.g. weight gain, effects on foetal and perinatal child development).

Sramek and Frackiewicz (2002) detail aspects of the pharmacokinetic profile of antidepressants and conclude that sex differences in depression may result from the interaction of multiple factors, including social and environmental factors, genetics, and the organisational and activational effects of hormones on the central nervous system. Ettorre and Riska (2001), in a study of long-term psychotropic drug users, found that men tended to attribute their usage to 'external stressors', whereas women were more inclined to attribute this to their 'internal state' or 'nerves'.

CURRENT CONTEXT

The Department of Health published a document detailing the strategic development of mental health care for women, 'Women's Mental Health: Into the Mainstream', in September 2002, followed by 'Mainstreaming Gender and Women's Mental Health: Implementation Guidance' (Department of Health 2003). This guidance was developed as part of the UK Government's broader policies to tackle inequalities, improve public services and promote social inclusion.

The Mental Health National Service Framework, published in 1999 (supplemented by much subsequent detailed policy implementation guidance) focuses on key issues in modernising mental health services including:

- Mental Health Promotion: NSF Standard 1
- Primary Care and Access: NSF Standards 2 & 3
- Effective Services for People with Severe Mental Illness: NSF Standards 4 & 5
- Caring about Carers: NSF Standard 6
- Preventing Suicides: NSF Standard 7.

The Women's Mental Health Strategy should be 'mainstreamed' in the context of the NHS Plan and its associated NHS Priorities & Planning Framework which sets out key expectations for Local Delivery Plans within NHS Trusts over consecutive three-year investment periods. Targets for more detailed monitoring between 2003 and 2006 include:

- Early intervention for young people
- Crisis resolution/home treatment
- Assertive outreach
- Carer breaks
- Improving prison mental health care
- Improving care and management of older people.

The aims and intentions of the strategy are:

- To develop local gender-awareness training initiatives on a partnership basis, so that staff working in specialist mental health and primary care services can participate
- To ensure that formal and informal staff support structures are sensitive to gender
- To enhance the ability of practitioners to develop effective therapeutic relationships with service users to promote the emotional health of the workforce
- To ensure that women and men, with a clear commitment to addressing gender (and ethnicity) and the specific needs of women, are in leadership and mentoring roles within organisations
- To ensure that managers and practitioners actively and equally value female and male staff, as well as service users
- To include gender (and ethnicity) formally in all governance arrangements including reporting procedures and relevant council reviews and consequent actions

- To review all service monitoring and evaluation processes to ensure a gender (and ethnicity) underpinning
- To develop and implement service standards for women service users in order to monitor and evaluate the effectiveness of services for women (mixed and single-sex) against these standards, across specialist mental health and primary care services.

EPIDEMIOLOGY OF WOMEN'S MENTAL HEALTH PROBLEMS

Mental ill health is common in the general population. However, anxiety, depression and eating disorders are significantly more common in women, whereas substance misuse and personality disorders are more common in men. Women comprise two-thirds of the adults living in the poorest households or amongst those dependent on income support and there is a strong association between poverty and mental ill health.

Elliott (2001) found a complex relationship between gender and social context in that women are more exposed to stressors than men, but are not more vulnerable to them. Positive social relationships do have more beneficial psychological effects for women than for men.

SURVEY OF NEEDS: WHAT WOMEN WANT

As part of the DoH Women's Strategy development some large-scale national consultation/listening exercises were undertaken and several consistent themes emerged about what support women want in dealing with their mental distress:

1. Offer safe, women-only alternatives to psychiatric hospital admission
2. Recognise that experiences of sexual and physical abuse are shared by many women with mental distress, and train staff to work with these issues
3. Create opportunities for women to share with, and learn from, others who have had similar experiences
4. Recognise and work with the diversity of women in respect to culture, ethnicity, parenting, sexuality, age and ability
5. Provide culturally sensitive services, including for women who are refugees or asylum seekers

6. Ensure that voluntary sector initiatives, self-help groups and advocacy and service-user organisations play a full and resourced role
7. Provide secure and stable funding to ensure consistent support
8. Promote less reliance on medication and more access to talking and complementary therapies
9. Provide more information to women about medication
10. Provide services for older women with mental health needs
11. Provide services for black and minority ethnic women with mental health needs
12. Provide services for lesbians with mental health needs
13. Develop mental health promotion or prevention activities explored from a gender perspective
14. Develop an understanding of women's mental distress in the context of their lives as a whole, including how it may relate to their experiences as mothers and carers
15. Provide services which are responsive to daily family, social and economic realities and which recognise women's roles as mothers and carers
16. Provide practical responses to the diversity of women's concerns, e.g. housing and financial issues, support with child-care
17. Enable women to have a say in their care and treatment, and be involved in service planning and delivery
18. Work in ways that involve women in plans and decisions made about their treatment and recovery
19. Acknowledge that behaviour such as self-harm or abuse of food or substances has meaning for the women concerned and be prepared to work with women to understand and explore this
20. Provide choice of gender of key worker
21. Promote access to education, training and meaningful employment
22. Promote a 'whole person' approach and 'whole systems approach' which recognises that one's need for any one aspect of mental health services is determined by the capacity or effectiveness of other aspects and which emphasises multi-agency partnership.

SERVICE DELIVERY

Delivery of mental health services for women needs to recognise and respond to differences in relation to:

- **Childhood and adult life experiences**: e.g. women are more likely to experience violence and abuse
- **Day-to-day social, family and economic realities** e.g. poverty, lone parenthood and part-time work
- **Different expressions and experiences of mental ill health** e.g. women are more likely to self-harm or present with depression and anxiety whereas more men have diagnoses of antisocial personality and present with earlier onset of more disabling schizophrenia
- **Pathways into services which may differ**
- **Treatment needs and responses to treatment which may differ** e.g. women are more likely to seek talking therapies and self-help and may respond differently to psychotropic medication.

Gender differences need to be explored in the assessment of mental ill health, drafting and reviewing care programmes in accordance with good practice guidelines for the Care Programme Approach. For instance, a number of research studies have indicated that around half of the women presenting to mental health services have significant histories of violence or sexual abuse. There is a need to train staff in sensitive but routine enquiry about these issues to avoid perpetuating a cycle of abusive neglect (Creedy *et al.* 1998; Romito and Gerin 2002).

The Women's Strategy emphasises the need:

- To ensure that, in all assessment and care planning, key components are included which are particularly relevant to women
- To ensure that women service users are prescribed appropriate medication only if and when required (to address the concerns of women service users that there is an over-reliance on medication).

Gatz *et al.* (1983) also consider the 'myths and counter myths' concerning various aspects of older women's lives pertaining to poverty, intellectual incompetence, illness, tranquility, bereavement through loss, loneliness and sexlessness, outlined in terms of their impact on the health of older women and unhelpful distortions of focus in relation to research regarding older women's mental health. Many of these issues are comprehensively reviewed by Trotman and Brody (2002) in their book, *Mental health and older women*.

Similarly, contrary to widely held beliefs, menopause is not associated with an increase in psychiatric illness (Robinson 2001). Although just prior to menopause there is a slight increase in minor psychological symptoms, prevalence rates of depression fall post menopause. The relationship between hormonal changes and depression is complex and poorly understood at present.

The Women's Strategy recommends that women service users have access to a range of appropriate psychological therapies in the assessment and treatment of their mental health problems.

PRIMARY CARE ISSUES

The primary care team has an important front-line role in relation to:

- Assessment and treatment of common mental health problems (Weintraub *et al.* (1996) advocate for an enhanced role of primary care nurses in this area)
- Early recognition of depression, including post-natal depression, anxiety and eating disorders – depression tends not to be accurately identified and treated in primary care settings (Van Hook 1999)
- Appropriate use of medication alongside prompt access to psychological therapies
- Detection and management of conditions that often remain hidden, for example, self-harming behaviour, alcohol and substance misuse in women, including the abuse of prescription medication
- Recognition of the high proportion of women who have experienced violence and abuse, in child and/or adulthood, which is a significant contributory factor to many forms of mental distress and physical ill health, particularly as a result of childhood sexual abuse
- Recognition of the increased risk of domestic violence during pregnancy and/or after childbirth
- Review of long-term prescribing, particularly benzodiazepines, anti-psychotic and antidepressant medication
- Provision of information on, and facilitation of access to, relevant community support services largely provided by the voluntary sector e.g. benefits or housing advice, child care facilities, day services, local learning opportunities, counselling, support groups and helplines particularly for women survivors of violence and abuse and those who self-harm
- Identification and support for women in their role as mothers and carers and recognition of the physical and mental stresses that caring can cause.

WOMEN-ONLY COMMUNITY DAY SERVICES

The Department of Health has introduced a new target in relation to the provision of women-only day services. This might involve services and support by women staff in women-only settings (e.g. abuse survivors, older women, lesbian women, women from particular religious or cultural groups, women-only provision for women with problems of depression, anxiety, social isolation).

There is general recognition that the most innovative services have been developed and delivered by a variety of voluntary sector organisations – often with core funding from the statutory sector, but there is a need to ensure funding is sustainable and included in Local Delivery Plans. The aim of these services should be to improve and promote mental health and well-being, to help prevent mental ill health or relapse by supporting women in their own homes and communities. The range of provision should include:

● Educational programmes
● Therapeutic interventions and activities (on an individual and group basis), self-help and support groups
● Crisis support
● Information
● Parenting support
● Workshops and activities
● Art and complementary therapies.

SUPPORTED HOUSING

There is a need to provide women-only supported housing which is integrated with primary care, specialist mental health services and other aspects of community support. The primary target group for such services should include:

● Hidden homeless e.g. those in abusive relationships, staying with friends
● Women offenders with mental health problems
● Women being discharged from secure MH settings.

A variety of safe and supported housing provision is needed including:

● Short-term shared housing
● Permanent tenancies in self-contained flats

- Short-term crisis housing to provide assistance to support and sustain tenancies during periods of greater illness or pressure
- Help to sustain existing tenancies in illness periods
- Support for child-care responsibilities.

Key features of such services should include:

- Accommodation for children and employment of nursery nurses
- Women-only staff including recovered service users
- 24 hour opening
- Homely/non-institutional environment
- Fewer than ten residents.

WOMEN-ONLY IN-PATIENT SERVICES

A number of studies have highlighted significant problems in terms of safety and appropriateness of mixed-sex psychiatric wards (Batcup 1997). In-patient services should address the wish of many women service users to be cared for in a women-only in-patient environment by providing a self-contained women-only ward/unit in every acute in-patient service or by reconfiguring existing services (or provision of a new-build facility if one is planned).

Women-only crisis houses provide an alternative to acute in-patient admission and respite houses, as an intervention to avoid women's mental ill health deteriorating to an acute or crisis phase.

WOMEN-ONLY COMMUNITY BASED ACUTE CARE SERVICES AND TEAMS

Alternatives to psychiatric admission need to be developed such as community based residential acute care settings that can accommodate women's children as appropriate, women-only crisis and respite housing for all women including those with learning and associated disabilities.

It is essential that existing and emerging teams – community mental health, assertive outreach, crisis resolution/home treatment and early intervention in psychosis – deliver a gender sensitive service (as outlined in the DH Policy Implementation Guidance) and meet the specific needs of their female clients as recommended in this guidance (e.g. choice of a female key worker). There needs to be recognition that for some women, time away from home and their domestic and caring responsibilities may be therapeutic; but for others, the possibility of being treated in the community for acute mental ill health problems may be preferable, ensuring that their family remains intact and dependent children are not removed into Local Authority care.

WOMEN'S SECURE SERVICES

The Women's Strategy states the following aims for women's secure services:

- To provide safe and effective, secure mental health services for women with learning and associated disabilities; to provide safe and effective low secure services for all women patients
- To provide high-support community residential settings for women with complex needs who may have a diagnosis of borderline personality disorder, be recovering from severe trauma with attendant risk and/or offending behaviours
- To ensure that women service users on mixed-sex wards are protected from intimidation, coercion, violence and abuse (including rape) by other patients, visitors, intruders or members of staff.

WOMEN'S SECURE SERVICES – HIGH-SUPPORT, COMMUNITY RESIDENTIAL SETTINGS

Therapeutic community provision has proven efficacy in assisting women who have experienced severe abuse and trauma and includes the following components:

- Safe, validating environment to recover from severe abuse and trauma (1–3 years)
- Therapeutic context – with high-relational security, trust and openness
- Appropriate level of environmental/physical security
- Integration with broader mental health care system

- Safe and effective low-secure services for further rehabilitation and recovery
- Inclusion of women with learning and associated disabilities
- High-support community residential settings for women with borderline personality disorder, recovering from trauma and who present with risk/offending behaviours.

WOMEN WITH SEVERE AND ENDURING MENTAL ILL HEALTH

Kulkarni (1997) notes that there is very little gender-specific research in relation to the treatment of schizophrenia and hence very little understanding of the specific impact of schizophrenia on women. Repper *et al.* (1996, 1998) advanced the view that in research, as in services, the abilities of women with serious mental health problems appear to be underestimated, and there is almost a total absence of research into the views and experiences of women with severe and enduring mental ill health. A series of focus group interviews with such women revealed that their mental health problems led to numerous losses: loss of homes, jobs, relationships, children and loss of 'normality', yet the women retained hopes and aspirations for the future. The women clearly identified aspects of the service that they valued, in particular the support and company of women workers and other women service users. This type of research provides valuable information for service planning and development.

WOMEN WHO HAVE EXPERIENCED VIOLENCE AND ABUSE

A number of studies have shown that women's experience of abuse and violence in childhood and adult life is extremely high (Humphries *et al.* 2001):

- 20–30% of women have been sexually abused as children
- Domestic violence accounts for 25% of violent crime
- 50% or more of women in mental health system are survivors.

The mental and physical health impacts of intimate partner violence are extremely significant (Campbell and Lewandowski 1997) and childhood sexual, emotional or physical abuse is associated with a greatly increased incidence of depression in adult life (Mullen *et al.* 1988; Hall *et al.* 1993). Nyamathi *et al.* (2001) found that homeless women victimised through abuse in their adult lives were more likely than others to have a history of childhood sexual and physical abuse, lifetime substance use, greater mental health symptomatology, and current risky sexual activity.

Mental health providers and other professionals generally have a low awareness and training in handling these issues which need to be routinely assessed in care planning (e.g. Helfrich *et al.* 2001). In a qualitative study of women who had experienced sexual abuse in childhood, Perrot *et al.* (1998) found that abuse characteristics did not predict outcome but women who 'deliberately suppressed' the abuse incidents were more likely to have low self-esteem and women who 'reframed' were significantly less likely to have a psychiatric diagnosis.

However, many of the criticisms of Koss (1990) regarding the lack of empirical data to support various interventions for assisting women survivors are still relevant today. Nonetheless, some key features necessary to improve services for women survivors of violence and abuse include:

● Lead person addressing these issues in each mental health provider organisation
● Links with safe housing, police and criminal justice
● Community support available to survivors
● Support to staff
● Acknowledging and addressing the links between violence and abuse and women's mental ill health, in the delivery of mental health services in in-patient and community-based settings.

WOMEN FROM BLACK AND MINORITY ETHNIC COMMUNITIES

There is a dearth of well-conducted studies regarding the mental health of women from black and minority ethnic communities. However, the level of mental distress is likely to be high – particularly where women live in isolated or socially deprived communities. Maziak *et al.* (2002), in a study of low-income Syrian women, found that illiteracy, polygamy and physical abuse were the strongest determinants of mental distress leading to the worst outcomes.

There are a number of issues which are particularly pertinent to women from black and minority ethnic communities:

- Self-harm/suicide in Asian women
- Refugee and asylum seeker issues e.g. post-traumatic stress disorder and cultural isolation (e.g. Davis 2000).

The Race Relations (Amendment) Act places a general duty upon public authorities and those carrying out public functions to promote race equality and positive community relations. New service developments need to link with the Black and Minority Ethnic (BME) mental health strategy and framework for action. The following actions are essential to improve access and quality of provision of services for BME communities:

- Make information on services accessible in all community languages and at appropriate venues
- Monitor workforce by ethnicity and ensure that it reflects the local population
- Ensure that single-sex services are also culturally competent. It should not be assumed that gender sensitive or single-sex services automatically meet the needs of women from these communities or that discrimination and racism against them will not occur in these settings.

Lam and Sue (2001) confirm the paucity of research on the efficacy of psychotherapy for various culturally diverse groups including black and minority ethnic people, gay, lesbian and bisexual and lower socioeconomic status people. Trotman (2000) confirms the need to respect diversity in terms of issues in psychosocial development in her review of psychotherapy with African-American women.

Burman *et al.* (2003) describe a development project, Sanjhe Rang, offering psychotherapy in a range of South East Asian languages in Rochdale, Lancashire (UK) and suggest some implications for ways of thinking about culturally autonomous, cross-community and cross-disciplinary collaborations around mental health. Gibbs and Fuery (1994) emphasise the need to identify empowering strategies which recognise the strengths as well as the needs of black women to develop culturally appropriate mental health services. Porter (2000) emphasises the need to respect heterogeneity within minority ethnic groups as well as shared experiences of racism and oppression and this should inform therapeutic intervention.

LESBIAN WOMEN

The service needs of lesbian women is an under-researched area. Bernhard and Applegate (1999) found lesbians reported more stress due to sexual identity, being female, and mental problems, and heterosexual women reported more stress due to parents and children. Welch *et al.* (2000) found that while the mental health of lesbians is influenced by factors similar to those influencing women's mental health in general, because of social factors, such as stigma and isolation, lesbians may be more vulnerable to common mental illnesses. Wright and Antony (2002) detail some good practice guidelines in working with lesbian women.

WOMEN WHO ARE MOTHERS

The aims of the Women's Strategy in relation to women who are mothers are:

- To enable women service users, particularly those with a serious mental illness, to maintain their parenting role wherever possible. To recognise fully and address women's fear of their children becoming 'looked after' as a result of their mental health problems.
- To ensure that women with a current or previous history (including family history) of serious mental health problems, receive timely and appropriate care and support to minimise the potential for recurrence and/or deterioration of their mental health.
- The early detection of any aspect of mental ill health in women at the ante-natal or post-natal stage, with no personal or family history of such difficulties (e.g. LeCuyer and Maus 2003).

Women's mental health should be carefully monitored at each stage of the perinatal period and workers should:

- Assess mental health need at ante-natal stage
- Assess for early detection of post-natal depression (Beck (2001) in a meta-analysis of studies found four new predictors of postpartum depression: self-esteem, marital status, socioeconomic status, and unplanned/unwanted pregnancy)
- Enable women with serious mental illness to maintain parenting role wherever possible

- Work in partnership with social services children's team
- Foster close links and training with midwifery and maternity services, health visitors and community mental health teams, GPs and community/practice nurses
- Facilitate access to community support e.g. Surestart, Newpin
- Ensure mothers who require in-patient care accommodated with babies
- Promote family-friendly child visiting in in-patient settings
- Ensure discharge planning considers parenting roles and child's well-being
- Provide convenient appointment times
- Respite/crisis support with or without children as needed
- Consider other caring responsibilities – carer grant and plans.

However, there has been a neglect of sociological and ethnographic perspectives in research on perinatal maternal ill health (Thurtle 1995) focusing on the woman's own view of her health and social circumstances.

WOMEN OFFENDERS WITH MENTAL ILL HEALTH

Women offenders are twice as likely to have received mental health help in the 12 months prior to custody. The Women's Mental Health Strategy advocates:

- Early intervention approach and diversion from custody by multi-agency package of care and support for women offenders e.g. drug treatment, parenting support, abuse counselling, supported accommodation, education and training, benefits
- To enable women offenders with mental ill health to remain in the community (unless they are convicted of offences that pose a severe risk to the public)
- To co-ordinate the joining-up of services to develop tailored community packages of care for women offenders with mental ill health
- To ensure the same level of tailored support for women prisoners on resettlement in their originating locality
- To ensure that women prisoners receive the same quality of primary and specialist mental health care as women residing in the community

● To ensure that, on resettlement, continuity of mental health care is provided for women.

WOMEN OFFENDERS IN PRISON

A very high proportion of women in prison suffer from mental ill health (Smith and Borland 1999) and around a quarter of the women in a US maximum security prison were found to have a diagnosable personality disorder (Warren *et al.* 2002). There is a need to ensure mental health prison in-reach services promote assessment and treatment interventions for:

● Women with severe and enduring MH problems
● Acute mental illness
● Survivors of abuse and violence
● Dual diagnosis (substance misuse and MH problems)
● Self-harm
● Eating disorders
● Those diagnosed as having a borderline personality disorder
● Training, support and supervision of prison health care staff
● Aftercare on release.

WOMEN WHO SELF-HARM

Service providers should recognise self-harm as a coping strategy which may often be linked to childhood sexual abuse (Reece 1998). Providers should aim to:

● Develop policies/protocols, training and staff support to assess and manage self-harm effectively
● Focus on alternatives and harm reduction and safe, supportive environment
● Address underlying causes
● Develop policies/protocols, staff training and staff support to assess and manage women who self-harm effectively – primarily as a coping mechanism or survival strategy – in in-patient and community mental health services
● Train staff routinely to assess for self-harm in care planning.

WOMEN WHO RECEIVE A DIAGNOSIS OF BORDERLINE PERSONALITY DISORDER

The policy implementation guidance *Personality Disorder: no longer a diagnosis of exclusion* (NIMHE 2002) requires mental health services to ensure that they mainstream the specific needs of women who receive a diagnosis of borderline personality disorder. They have a complexity of need as their propensity to self-harm, eating disorders, misuse substances, episodes of (or long-term) psychosis, major depression and compulsion to engage in abusive relationships (depending on the severity of their distress) are co-occurring features. They are likely to be survivors of severe and prolonged abuse, notably childhood sexual abuse, suffering from a variant of post-traumatic stress disorder and trauma-based therapeutic approaches are advocated. Suggested actions are:

● Develop community based multi-disciplinary teams for people with personality disorder
● Address stigma often associated with this diagnosis
● Combine psychological therapies and focused drug therapy when needed.

WOMEN WITH DUAL DIAGNOSIS WITH SUBSTANCE MISUSE

The main contention of the recent implementation guidance, the Dual Diagnosis Good Practice Guide (DH 2002), is that substance misuse is usual rather than exceptional amongst people with severe mental health problems and that the relationship between the two is complex. Individuals with these dual problems deserve high-quality, patient-focussed and integrated care that should be delivered within mental health services.

There are significant gender differences in the social context, form of substance misuse and presentation of women and men with dual diagnosis that need to be addressed fully in the development of local service planning. For instance, Green *et al.* (2002) found that women with mental health diagnoses were significantly less likely to initiate treatment of their substance misuse problems.

Van der Walde *et al.* (2002) highlight the invidious position of women with alcohol misuse problems: biologically, women react differently to alcohol ingestion than do men. Women reach higher blood alcohol levels and sustain more somatic and cognitive damage than men when consuming equivalent amounts of alcohol. Psychosocially, women alcoholics face societal rebuke and chastisement of a greater magnitude than do men. Finally, barriers to treatment faced by women, such as the need for child care, cost of treatment, familial opposition, denial of alcoholism, and inadequate diagnostic training of physicians, must be overcome to create successful treatment approaches for the female alcoholic. Liebschutz *et al.* (2002) found that around 80% of the female in-patients at a detoxification unit had past histories of physical and sexual abuse.

WOMEN WITH EATING DISORDERS

Around 60,000 people in UK have eating disorders which may co-occur with other problems e.g. depression, substance misuse. Anorexia has the highest mortality rate of any psychiatric illness. Services for eating disorder should aim:

- Effectively to meet the needs of, predominantly, girls and women with mild to severe eating difficulties
- To develop and establish specialist eating disorder services on a consistent basis countrywide that can provide assessment, consultation, liaison and treatment.

Services for people with eating disorders should develop in accordance with recently published NICE guidelines (2004) and aim to:

- Improve detection and treatment in primary care
- Treat concurrent physical health problems
- Provide education about eating disorders
- Support voluntary sector and self-help
- Provide family therapy – especially for adolescents with anorexia.

MENTAL HEALTH PROMOTION

It is important to ensure that all staff have adequate training to make them mindful of the mental health promotion needs relating to the gender and ethnicity of their clients and to ensure gender (and ethnically) sensitive mental health promotion are included in service planning for the community.

An evidence base exists for a number of mental health promotion activities including:

- **Arts and creativity** e.g. women only art groups which encourage self-expression and emotional processing combined with social support
- **Reducing fear of crime**: community crime reduction partnerships e.g. safer lighting, community policing etc. can contribute to women's overall sense of safety and participation in their communities
- **Stress workshops for the general public**: open access all-day workshops were evaluated as highly successful in reducing symptoms of common mental health problems
- **Home visiting programmes**: support to new mothers can help reduce symptoms of post-natal depression and increase feelings of self-esteem and self-efficacy
- **Parenting skills**: increase a sense of competence in dealing with common childhood behavioural and developmental issues
- **Primary care**: can offer a broad range of easily accessed mental health promotion opportunities including:
  - *Brief interventions (alcohol)* aimed at harm reduction
  - *Social prescribing* e.g. exercise sessions at local gym (Raine *et al.* 2002); arts on referral rather than immediate recourse to psychotropic prescribing for depression or anxiety
  - *Community mothers*: practical and social support to new mothers from other mothers in the community
  - *Self-help/voluntary referrals*: signposting women to appropriate self-help and voluntary sector groups in the community
  - *Managing peri- and post-natal depression*: promoting early assessment and treatment through appropriate health-visitor training and support.

Older people

- *Volunteering*: Opportunities for women to participate in their communities through a range of voluntary work which enhances self-esteem and reduces social isolation. Weber (1999) conducted a naturalistic inquiry into women's experience of 'juggling motherhood and child care' and found seven categories reflective of experiential well-being: mutuality, spirituality, child-centredness, acceptance, happiness, security, and enrichment of the world.

- *Telephone support*: Help and advice lines to improve access to information and support.

People with mental health problems

- *Supported employment*: user-led initiatives offering supported employment to promote recovery and opportunities to participate in services including 'real workplace' settings and the generally beneficial effects of employment on women's mental health (Bogard *et al.* 2001; Killien 2001)
- *Social support*: women-only day services and self-help initiatives reducing social isolation
- *Physical health care*: ensuring that people with mental ill health have regular physical health check-ups and appropriate treatments.

Black and minority ethnic groups

- *Appropriate mental health services*: developing culturally appropriate services for black and minority ethnic groups which are responsive to different religious, linguistic and cultural needs.

MANAGEMENT AND PLANNING TO MAINSTREAM GENDER

Provider organisations in the statutory and voluntary sector need to take a number of actions to mainstream gender appropriate services. It is recommended that Primary Care Trusts and other organisations:

- Appoint a women and mental health lead
- Establish a multi-agency forum to promote implementation
- Establish women's service-user groups
- Undertake resource mapping of women's mental health services in relation to:

  ○ Service structure and function
  ○ Skills
  ○ Staff
  ○ Expenditure.
- Identify gaps and unmet needs for women only services
- Link to service planning and commissioning
- Review existing mixed-sex mental health services (including primary care, community mental health services and in-patient services)
- Ensure that existing service evaluation, monitoring, clinical governance, satisfaction surveys and other audits are routinely analysed by gender and that this information is used to promote action and service development
- Promote gender-awareness training and other appropriate therapies/interventions for women in all services.

Workforce development and training

There are a number of aspects of workforce development and training which support the implementation of better services for women (e.g. gender awareness training cf. Nutt (1979)). There is some evidence that therapists have more positive attitudes to women currently than was the norm thirty years ago (Phillips 1985) which may reflect a positive change within the wider culture and more blurring of gender roles and social definitions of gender-appropriate behaviour and also more enlightened training programmes (Berlin 1987; McKeown *et al.* 2003).

The Department of Health/NIMHE Mental Health Care Group Workforce Team is developing a curriculum and competencies for mental health work with women.

Needs of women in leadership positions e.g. action on harassment, family-friendly policies, promotion opportunities should be considered by all organisations wishing to develop positive practice in this area.

Staff support

Staff support in the workplace including supervision, appraisal, crisis support, and confidential counselling can enhance the effectiveness of women workers, delivered in a gender-sensitive manner. Managers should be sensitive to the emotional sequelae of working with intense psychological distress (e.g. Wasco and Campbell (2002) found high levels of anger and fear in rape victim advocates).

Governance

Most – if not all – service providers are required to undertake audit and evaluation of their services and this is often a requirement for continued funding. Much data is collected but it is not always *routinely* analysed by gender and ethnicity. For instance, audits of clinical risk management may highlight issues around safety or abuse which differentially affect women. Similarly, clinical audits and user surveys may underline the different needs of men and women.

Evidence-based practice studies may draw attention to different service outcomes for men and women from particular interventions and thus may help to shape services in a constructive way.

Involvement of women service users and carers is crucial in ensuring that the content and process of data collection is valid and appropriate.

Best value reviews and other external or internal reviews and inspections (e.g. Commission for Health Improvement reports) can also provide a rich vein of observations and areas for improvement.

Modern service improvement technologies such as process mapping, analysis and service re-design techniques can be powerful in achieving desired service changes.

Further research is needed regarding a whole range of service-delivery issues. For instance:

- Risk and protective factors related to women's mental health
- Causation, prevalence and clinical course of various mental health problems analysed by gender
- Gender response to treatment interventions
- Particularly significant areas for further investigation which predominantly affect women include eating disorders, peri-natal mental ill health, and trauma of abuse and violence
- Involving service users and carers in determining priorities, service planning, development and delivery.

Also needed is research which focuses on:

- Risk and protective factors for women's mental health
- Understanding the causation, prevalence and response to treatment of various interventions for women's mental health
- Issues which predominantly affect women.

Implementing research findings into practice is also challenging (Owen and Milburn 2001) and there is a need to research methods of implementing change.

SERVICE STANDARDS FOR MEETING THE SPECIFIC NEEDS OF WOMEN SERVICE USERS

Findings from governance activities such as service audit, evaluation and research is essential to promote the development of relevant and robust service standards and policies which have a proven impact on women's well-being including:

- Choice of gender of key worker or therapist
- Progressive policies on self-harm
- Ensuring that women's physical health needs are addressed
- Promoting environmental safety
- Sensitive policies on close observation (e.g. in in-patient settings)
- Family friendly areas/child care facilities
- Monitoring medication
- Consideration of caring responsibilities
- Sensitivity to cultural needs of black and minority ethnic women
- Women-only respite and crisis support.

CONCLUSIONS

There is a great deal of literature about women and mental health. However, there is a paucity of high-quality evidence-based research to support various assertions which play an important role in the design and development of services.

The following observations can be made:

- Much of the published research on women's mental health has used methodologies which are less powerful in terms of scientific replicability or predictability such as anecdotal, qualitative and narrative approaches
- Qualitative approaches nonetheless are extremely valuable in defining the 'right questions' and in grounding future theories and hypotheses
- There are some powerful and consistent messages which come from women's individual testimony
- However, qualitative approaches are not seen as 'powerful' in terms of bidding for service development resources
- Qualitative approaches lack replicability and if their conclusions are overstated may perpetuate ineffective interventions
- Much research is confined to the 'less prestigious journals'

- Better funded mainstream research and audits do not routinely analyse powerful data sets by gender and thus there is insufficient attention to gender differences in response to various therapies and interventions
- Gender differences in presentation and response to interventions should be evaluated more systematically and should receive an appropriate share of the 'research revenues' leading to more cost-effective delivery of a range of services.

What is needed is a programme of research that collates and disseminates robust evidence relating to the effectiveness of services, interventions and the views of women as users of the services.

References

Barnes, M., Davis, A., Guru, S., Lewis, L. and Rogers, H. (2002). *Women-only and women-sensitive mental health services: an expert paper.* Report to the Department of Health. See also www.socialresearch.bham.ac.uk

Batcup, D. (1997). The problems of researching mixed-sex wards. *Journal of Advanced Nursing*, **25**, 51018–24.

Beck, C.T. (2001). Predictors of postpartum depression. *Nursing Research*, **50**(5), 275–85.

Berlin, Sharon. (1987). In *The woman client: providing human services in a changing world* (eds. Burden, Dianne S. and Gottlieb, Naomi), pp. 146–61. Tavistock/Routledge, New York.

Bernhard, L.A. and Applegate, J.M. (1999). Comparison of stress and stress management strategies between lesbian and heterosexual women. *Health Care for Women International*, **20**(4), 335–47.

Blehar, Mary C. (2003). Public health context of women's mental health research. *The Psychiatric Clinics of North America*, **26**(3), 781–99.

Bogard, C.J., Trillo, A., Schwartz, M. and Gerstel, N. (2001). Future employment among homeless single mothers: the effects of full-time work experience and depressive symptomatology. *Women's Health*, **32**(1/2), 137–57.

Bunting, S.M. (1997). Applying a feminist analysis model to selected nursing studies of women with HIV. *Issues in Mental Health Nursing*, **18**(5), 523–37.

Burman, E., Gowrisunkur, J. and Walker, K. (2003). Sanjhe Rang/shared colours, shared lives: a multicultural approach to mental health practice. *Journal of Social Work Practice*, **17**(1), 63–76.

Campbell, Rebecca. (2002). *Emotionally involved: the impact of researching rape.* Routledge, New York.

Campbell, J.C. and Lewandowski, L.A. (1997). Mental and physical health effects of intimate partner violence on women and children. *The Psychiatric Clinics of North America*, **20**(2), 353–74.

Collin, B.S., Hollander, R.B., Koffman, D.M., Reeve, R. and Seidler, S. (1997). Women, work and health: issues and implications for worksite health promotion. *Women's Health*, 25(4), 3-38.

Contratto, Susan. (2002). A feminist critique of attachment theory and evolutionary psychology. In *Rethinking mental health and disorder: feminist perspectives*, (eds. Ballou, Mary and Brown, Laura S.), pp. 29-47. Guilford Press, New York.

Creedy, D., Nizette, D. and Henderson, K. (1998). A framework for practice with women survivors of childhood sexual abuse. *Australian and New Zealand Journal of Mental Health Nursing*, 7(2), 67-73.

Davar, Bhargavi V. (2001). *Mental health from a gender perspective.* Sage Publications India, New Delhi.

Davis, R.E. (2000). Refugee experiences and South-east Asian women's mental health. *Western Journal of Nursing Research*, 22(2), 144-62.

Department of Health (DoH). (1999). National Service Framework for Mental Health. Department of Health, London. Available at: www.doh.gov.uk/nsf/mentalhealth.htm

Department of Health (DoH). (2000). The NHS Plan. Department of Health, London. Available at:www.doh.gov.uk/nhsplan/nhsplan.htm Department of Health (DH) 2003.

Eichenbaum, Luise and Orbach, Susie. (1982). *Outside in, inside out: women's psychology: a feminist psychoanalytic approach.* Penguin Books, Harmondsworth, Middlesex, England.

Elliott, M. (2001). Gender differences in causes of depression. *Women's Health*, 33(3/4), 163-77.

Ettorre, Elizabeth and Riska, Elianne. (2001). Long-term users of psychotropic drugs: embodying masculinized stress and feminized nerves. *Substance Use & Misuse, Special Issue: Dependence on psychotropics: A multidimensional perspective*, 36(9), 101187-211.

Finfgeld, D.L. (2001). New directions for feminist therapy based on social constructionism. *Archives of Psychiatric Nursing*, 15(3), 148-54.

Gibbs, J.T. and Fuery, D. (1994). Mental health and well-being of black women: toward strategies of empowerment. *American Journal of Community Psychology*, 22(4), 559-82.

Good Practices in Mental Health (GPMH) (1994). Women and Mental Health: An Information Pack of Mental Health Services for Women in the United Kingdom. GPMH, London.

Green, C.A., Polen, M.R., Dickinson, D.M., Lynch, F.L. and Bennett, M.D. (2002). Gender differences in predictors of initiation, retention, and completion in an HMO-based substance abuse treatment program. *Journal of Substance Abuse Treatment*, 23(4), 285-95.

Gülçür, L. (2000). Evaluating the role of gender inequalities and rights violations in women's mental health. *Health and Human Rights*, 5(1), 46-66.

Hall, L.A, Sachs, B., Rayens, M.K. and Lutenbacher, M. (1993). Childhood physical and sexual abuse: their relationship with depressive symptoms in adulthood. Image of the *Journal of Nursing Scholarship*, 25(4), 317–23.

Helfrich, C.A., Lafata, M.L., MacDonald, S.L., Aviles, A. and Collins, L. (2001). Domestic abuse across the lifespan: definitions, identification and risk factors for occupational therapists. *Occupational Therapy in Mental Health*, 16(3/4), 5–34.

Horwitz, Allan V. (2002). *Creating mental illness*. University of Chicago Press, Chicago.

Humphreys, J., Parker, B. and Campbell, J.C. (2001). Intimate partner violence against women. *Annual Review of Nursing Research*, 19, 275–306.

Jebali, C.A. (1995). Working with women in mental health: a feminist perspective. *British Journal of Nursing*, 4(3), 137–40.

Killien, M.G. (2001). Women and employment: a decade review. *Annual Review of Nursing Research*, 19, 87–123.

Kohen, Dora, Kornstein, Susan G., Clayton, Anita H. (eds.). (2000). *Women and mental health*. Routledge, New York.

Koss, M.P. (1990). The women's mental health research agenda. Violence against women. *The American Psychologist*, 45(3), 374–80.

Kulkarni, J. (1997). Women and schizophrenia: a review. *The Australian and New Zealand Journal of Psychiatry*, 31(1), 46–56.

Lam, A. G. and Stanley, S. (2001). Client diversity. *Psychotherapy: Theory, Research, Practice, Training*, 38(4), 479–86.

LeCuyer, Maus E.A. (2003). Stress and coping in high-risk mothers: difficult life circumstances, psychiatric mental health symptoms, education, and experiences in their families of origin. *Public Health Nursing*, 20(2), 132–45.

Liebschutz, Jane, Savetsky, Jacqueline B., Saitz, Richard, Horton, Nicholas J., Lloyd-Travaglini, Christine and Samet, Jeffrey. (2002). The relationship between sexual and physical abuse and substance abuse consequences. *Journal of Substance Abuse Treatment*, 22(3), 121–8.

Maziak, Wasim, Asfar, Taghrid, Fouad, Fouad M. and Kilzieh, Nael. (2002). Socio-demographic correlates of psychiatric morbidity among low-income women in Aleppo, Syria. *Social Science & Medicine*, 54(9), 1419–27.

McKeown, M., Anderson, J., Bennett, A. and Clayton, P. (2003). Gender politics and secure services for women: reflections on a study of staff understandings of challenging behaviour. *Journal of Psychiatric and Mental Health Nursing*, 10(5), 585–91.

Miers, M. (2002). Developing an understanding of gender sensitive care: exploring concepts and knowledge. *Journal of Advanced Nursing*, 40(1), 69–77.

Mullen, P.E., Romans-Clarkson, S.E., Walton, V.A. and Herbison, G.P. (1988). Impact of sexual and physical abuse on women's mental health. *Lancet*, 1(8590), 841–5.

Nyamathi, A., Wenzel, S.L., Lesser, J., Flaskerud, J. and Leake, B. (2001). Comparison of psychosocial and behavioral profiles of victimized and nonvictimized homeless women and their intimate partners. *Research in Nursing & Health*, 24(4), 324–35.

Orbach, S. (1978). Fat is a feminist issue. Paddington Press, New York.

Owen, S. and Milburn, C. (2001). Implementing research findings into practice: improving and developing services for women with serious and enduring mental health problems. *Journal of Psychiatric and Mental Health Nursing*, 8(3), 221–31.

Padgett, D.K. (1997). Women's mental health: some directions for research. *The American Journal of Orthopsychiatry*, 67(4), 522–34.

Perkins, R., Nadirshaw, Z., Copperman, J. and Andrews, C. (1996). Women in Context: Good Practice in Mental Health Services for Women. GPMH, London.

Perrott, K., Morris, E., Martin, J. and Romans, S. (1998). Cognitive coping styles of women sexually abused in childhood: a qualitative study. *Child Abuse and Neglect*, 22, 1135–49.

Phillips, Roger D. (1985). *Academic Psychology Bulletin*, Special Issue: Gender roles, 7(2), 253–60.

Porter, Robin Young. (2000). Clinical issues and interventions with ethnic minority women. In *Psychological intervention and cultural diversity* (ed. Aponte, Joseph F. and Wohl, Julian), (2nd ed.). Allyn & Bacon, Boston.

Pugliesi, K. (1992). Women and mental health: two traditions of feminist research. *Women and Health*, 19(2/3), 43–68.

Raine, Pamela, Truman, Carole and Southerst, Annie. (2002). The development of a community gym for people with mental health problems: influences on psychological accessibility. *Journal of Mental Health* (UK), 11(1), 43–53.

Reece, J. (1998). Female survivors of abuse attending A&E with self-injury. *Accident and Emergency Nursing*, 6(3), 133–8.

Repper, J., Perkins, R., Owen, S., Deighton, D. and Robinson, J. (1996). Evaluating services for women with serious and ongoing mental health problems: developing an appropriate research method. *Journal of Psychiatric and Mental Health Nursing*, 3(1), 39–46.

Repper, J., Perkins, R. and Owen, S. (1988). 'I wanted to be a nurse ... but I didn't get that far': women with serious ongoing mental health problems speak about their lives. *Journal of Psychiatric and Mental Health Nursing*, 5(6), 505–13.

Robinson, G.E. (2001). Psychotic and mood disorders associated with the perimenopausal period: epidemiology, aetiology and management. *CNS Drugs*, 15(3), 175–84.

Romito, Patrizia and Gerin, Daniela. (2002). Asking patients about violence: a survey of 510 women attending social and health services in Trieste, Italy. *Social Science & Medicine*, 54(12), 1813–24.

Smith, C. and Borland, J. (1999). Minor psychiatric disturbance in women serving a prison sentence: The use of the General Health Questionnaire in the estimation of the prevalence of non-psychotic disturbance in women prisoners. *Legal and Criminological Psychology*, 4(2), 273–84.

Showalter, E. (1985). *The female malady*. Virago, London.

Sramek, John J. and Frackiewicz, Edyta J. (2002). Effect of sex on psychopharmacology of antidepressants. In *Psychiatric illness in women: emerging treatments and research* (eds. Lewis-Hall, F., Panetta, J.A., Williams, T.S., Herrera, J.M.) American Psychiatric Publishing Inc., Washington.

Thurtle, V. (1995). Post-natal depression: the relevance of sociological approaches. *Journal of Advanced Nursing*, 22(3), 416–24.

Trotman, Frances K. and Brody, Claire M. (eds.). (2002). *Mental health and older women. Springer series, focus on women, psychotherapy and counselling with older women: cross-cultural, family, and end-of-life issues.* Springer Publishing Co, New York.

Trotman, Frances K. (2000). Psychotherapy with African American women: innovations in psychodynamic perspectives and practice. In *Annals of the American Psychotherapy Association*, pp. 33–61 (eds. Jackson, Leslie C. and Greene, Beverly), Guilford Press, New York.

Van der Walde, Heidi, Urgenson, Francine T., Weltz, Sharon H., and Hanna, Fred J. (2002). Women and alcoholism: a biopsychosocial perspective and treatment approaches. *Journal of Counseling & Development*, 80(2), 145–53.

Van Hook, M.P. (1999). Women's help – seeking patterns for depression. *Social Work in Health Care*, 29(1), 15–34.

Warren, Janet I., Burnette, Mandi, South, Susan Carol, Chauhan, Preeti, Bale, Risha and Friend, Roxanne. (2002). Personality disorders and violence among female prison inmates. *Journal of the American Academy of Psychiatry & the Law*, 30(4), 502–9.

Wasco, Sharon M. and Campbell, Rebecca. (2002). Emotional reactions of rape victim advocates: a multiple case study of anger and fear. *Psychology of Women Quarterly*, 26(2), 120–30.

Webb, C. (2002). Feminism and clinical nursing. *Journal of Clinical Nursing*, 11(5), 557–9.

Weber, G.J. (1999). The experiential meaning of well-being for employed mothers. *Western Journal of Nursing Research*, 21(6), 785–95.

Weintraub, T.A., Paine, L.L. and Weintraub, D.H. (1996). Primary care for women: comprehensive assessment and management of common mental health problems. *Journal of Nurse Midwifery*, 41(2), 125–38.

Welch, S., Collings, S.C. and Howden-Chapman, P. (2000). Lesbians in New Zealand: their mental health and satisfaction with mental health services. *The Australian and New Zealand Journal of Psychiatry*, 34(2), 256–63.

Williams, J., Watson, G., Smith, H., Copperman, J. and Wood, D. (1993). *Purchasing effective mental health services for women: a framework for action.* MIND Publications, London.

Women's Mental Health: Into the Mainstream. Department of Health, London. Available at: www.doh.gov.uk/mentalhealth/women.htm

Wright, N. and Owen, S. (2001). Feminist conceptualizations of women's madness: a review of the literature. *Journal of Advanced Nursing*, **36**(1), 143–50.

Wright, R. and Anthony, P. (2002). Lesbians and mental health: are we helping or hindering? *Mental Health Practice*, **5**(8), 12–15.

7

Service user involvement in mental health research and development

Ann Davis

... the involvement of consumers will lead to research which is more *relevant* to the needs of consumers (and therefore to the NHS as a whole), more *reliable* and more *likely to be used*. If research reflects the needs and views of consumers, it is likely to produce results that can be implemented.

Involvement works: the second report of the Standing Group on Consumers in NHS Research, 1999

INTRODUCTION

This chapter outlines why mental health service user involvement has emerged as an important concern in the research and development (R&D) field, what issues it raises for those involved in R&D and the implications of this development for the service user and the R&D communities. In considering these implications it describes and draws on lessons learnt by a Midlands-based, service-user-led network in mental health research and education: Suresearch.

WHY INVOLVE SERVICE USERS IN R&D?

In developing mental health R&D that plays an active part in improving services for the one out of six citizens likely to experience mental distress during their lives, the involvement of service users, as well as carers, has been identified by government as vital. (SAGCI 1998; DoH 1999; NIMHE 2002). This aspiration is being pursued by government funding bodies who have made it a requirement that those designing and submitting research bids provide evidence that they have involved service users in their work. This development calls into question the established traditions of mental health R&D, which has positioned service users as objects of study rather than active participants in the research process (Townend and Braithwaite 2001; Repper and Perkins 2003). It therefore raises a number of timely challenges for the approaches and processes of mental health R&D.

These challenges are being faced across the range of National Health Service (NHS) R&D and there is much to be learnt from exchanges between specialist areas in the health field. But there are also some important differences about user involvement in the mental health field that need to be acknowledged and worked with in working to make service user involvement a reality in mental health R&D.

To understand and work productively with the current service user involvement agenda in R&D it is important to understand the context in which it has evolved. The focus on service user involvement in this sphere has its roots in several approaches that have characterised health and welfare policy and practice since the 1980s in the UK (Braye 2000; Barnes and Bowl 2001).

The first, and currently the most dominant approach reflects the way in which public services in the UK have been increasingly viewed by government as key players in a market of health and welfare provision. As such they have been exhorted to place the interests of those on the receiving end at the heart of their endeavours. As the NHS Plan states that,

> ... *patients are the most important people in the health service.*
> ... *Too many patients feel talked at rather than listened to. This has to change. NHS care has to be shaped around the convenience and concerns of patients. To bring this about, patients must have more say in their own treatment and more influence over the way the NHS works.*

> (DoH 2000, p. 88)

This approach positions people using services as customers or consumers rather than as citizens with recognised rights to public service support. As Barnes and others have noted (Barnes 1997) there are demonstrable problems in realising this consumerist approach. In Barnes' view consumerism depends on a number of preconditions, including:

- The existence of a range of alternatives to existing services
- Accessing service users to information about alternatives and also the characteristics of alternatives that might suggest that they would not only overcome dissatisfaction with existing services but would also not substitute new problems for current problems
- The practicality of moving from one option to another
- The guarantee that moving from one option to another would not of itself generate damaging disruption.

It is Barnes' contention that for most people using health and social care services, 'it is clear that all these circumstances will rarely apply' (Barnes 1997, p. 34). As a result consumerism is constrained by the realities not only of service provision but the values and practices of health and welfare professionals.

A second approach that has characterised this period has been the growth of a number of service-user-led organisations who have focussed their concerns on the abuse of power in health and social care systems (Barker and Peck 1997; Barnes and Bowl 2001). In pursuing these concerns service-user organisations have campaigned against the discrimination and neglect experienced by those using health and welfare services. A number of these organisations, including some in the mental health field, are also concerned with challenging the stigma, social exclusion and discrimination experienced by service users who are denied their full membership of society because of their use of health and welfare services (Brandon 1991; Campbell 1996b; Sayce 2000).

In focussing on the civil, political and economic and social rights of service users, these organisations have raised questions about the practice and the impact on service users of the paternalism of politicians and professionals delivering policy and provision. In doing so they have argued that it is important to view service users not as passive recipients of services but as active, knowledgeable agents with considerable expertise based on what they have learnt from using and surviving mental health services (Bowl 1996; Barnes and Shardlow 1997). Working for the empowerment and inclusion of service users, these organisations have directed their energies mainly in the direction of societal and service change. A small number have also pursued their concerns for service change by entering the marketplace of health and welfare provision as providers, developing user-led alternatives to community-based services (Lindow 1994; Barker and Peck 1997).

As Perkins and Repper have highlighted, there are two distinct trends that can be distinguished in the mental health service-user movement in the UK: radical and reformist. The former, characterised by an antipsychiatry stance, rejects mainstream psychiatric services and seeks to provide user-controlled alternatives outside of the service mainstream (Curtis *et al.* 2000). The latter embraces consumerism and directs its energies towards improving mainstream services in ways that increase user involvement and control (Perkins and Repper 1998).

The modernisation agenda for public services that was launched in the late 1990s by the government reflects an uncritical fusion of the range of these competing positions. In claiming to place service-user interests at the heart of modernisation and seeking to ensure that public service organisations involve service users in the planning, delivery and evaluation of services, government statements have drawn on consumerism as well as notions of empowerment to justify their stance. Under the banners of involving stakeholders and developing partnerships between policy makers, professionals and service users, they have promoted the vision of service users, as well as carers, having an active involvement in the planning, delivery and evaluation of services (Simpson *et al.* 2002). At the same time, the modernisation agenda has developed targets, performance indicators, monitoring and auditing procedures to keep service providers and professionals on track (Secretary of State 1998; DoH 1999). This approach makes continual reference to the importance of researching and evaluating services in striving to ensure that services are positively responsive to the needs of service users.

An initiative which exemplifies this approach was the establishment in 1996 of Consumers in NHS Research – now known as INVOLVE. This government-funded organisation was established to promote the involvement of consumers in R&D in the NHS. With a working definition of consumers as:

> *patients, potential patients, carers, organisations representing consumers' interests, members of the public who are the targets of health promotion programmes and groups asking for research because they believe they have been exposed to potentially harmful circumstances, products or services.*
>
> (SGCNHS 1999, p. 1)

INVOLVE seeks to work across the National Health Service to increase the activity of consumers in all aspects of R&D. In doing so they have, through their work and its associated publications, highlighted both the barriers to service-user involvement in the NHS as well as the gains to all involved in service provision and research if these barriers are identified and dismantled (Consumers in NHSRUSU 2000).

INVOLVING SERVICE USERS IN MENTAL HEALTH R&D

In relating these debates within the service-user involvement agenda to the mental health field it has to be recognised that there are both similarities and differences in considering people who acquire a diagnosis of mental illness and use mental health services as being the same as other groups of patients/consumers/users (Rogers *et al.* 1993).

A critical difference that has been highlighted in the service-user literature is that people who use mental health services, unlike citizens seeking treatment for other forms of health care, can be subject to legal compulsion to be assessed and treated. The powers to detain and treat individuals under the Mental Health Act 1983, introduces a distinctive element to the experience of mental health service use. This impacts not only on the small but increasing numbers of people subject to compulsory detention, but also frames the experience of all those experiencing mental distress.

As Campbell argues:

> *The psychiatric system is founded on inequality. By and large, the user is at the bottom of the pile. Our unequal position is symbolised by the compulsory element in psychiatric care. I do not intend to argue either for or against the use of legal compulsion in treatment. But the fact of its existence has repercussions for all service users and these must be recognised. That an individual can be compelled to receive psychiatric treatment affects each in-patient regardless of whether his stay is formal or informal.*
>
> (Campbell 1996a, p. 59)

Recognising this reality for mental health service users has important implications for models of service user involvement in service planning and delivery as well as R&D (Bowl 1996). In particular, it raises questions about claims that are made to user involvement that are rooted in notions of equality, choice and partnership (Repper and Perkins 2003).

Another important difference that needs to be noted are the range of services that are important to the mental well-being and recovery of those individuals experiencing mental health difficulties. Responses to mental distress and diagnosed mental illness are much wider than those offered by the health services alone. Mental health professionals and researchers have traditionally viewed the reduction of symptoms and psychiatric service use as the prime measures of the success of psychiatric interventions. However, user literature suggests that many service users

> *... see these as but side issues to their 'real' problems which they locate as being able to participate in society, support themselves and to enjoy feelings of well-being. Hence many users of mental health services see their principal needs much as others do – they would value employment, a decent income, decent housing and a chance to make and sustain social relationships. These and symptom reduction are not always mutually exclusive but they may conflict.*

> (Barnes and Bowl 2002, p. 95)

User-based research relating to what is helpful to people in recovering from mental health crisis and distress lists income, employment, decent housing and personal relationships as top priorities alongside information about medication and other forms of treatment (Rose 1996; Hannigan *et al.* 1997; Mental Health Foundation 1997; Beresford 2000). This suggests that in developing an approach to user involvement in mental health R&D, it needs to be acknowledged that the established psychiatrically driven research priorities need to be widened to accommodate a focus on the totality and complexity of individual's lives, rather than just symptomatology and psychiatric service use.

What these issues of difference highlight is that in working with the current range of understandings of the nature and purpose of user involvement in mental health R&D, continuous attention needs to be given to issues regarding constraint and scope. People using services experience constraint in exercising choice and making full use of services. This experience of constraint is likely to influence the ways in which service users respond to any requests made to them to become involved in researching mental health provision. At the same time, a failure to recognise the full scope of the services and experiences that service users have reported make a difference to their recovery and well-being will limit the contribution that service users can make to developing the focus and research methodologies of mental health R&D (Rose 2001).

Whether people using mental health services are seen to be constrained consumers, a marginalised and excluded community, or equal partners in the planning, delivery and evaluation of those health and welfare services relevant to their needs, current government initiatives have underlined the importance of their active involvement in mental health R&D. The National Service Framework for Mental Health, in its consideration of R&D, states that it is the government's aim 'to develop the knowledge base for mental health services, making the knowledge accessible to clinicians, practitioners, managers, service users and carers' (DoH 1999, p. 113). In pursuing this aim, it is suggested that it is important to promote service users influence on the research agenda and develop research tools with service users in order to gather their views on how services can best meet their needs.

The National Institute for Mental Health in England (NIMHE)'s standing research programme – the Mental Health Research Network (MHRN) – in its review of mental health research concludes that in the past it has not provided support or leadership for practice development, has been too reliant on small localised studies and has not actively involved 'those on the front line – service users and carers. As a result, research has failed to inform policy, lacking coherence, relevance and, critically, credibility for service users and professionals' (MHRN website: www.mhrninfo). In developing its response to redressing this situation through the MHRN, criteria have been developed for future research that will be developed through the network. Their criteria include evidence of service user input to research proposal development. At the same time the MHRN has launched the Service User Research Group in England (SURGE). This service user research support network is responsible for encouraging collaborative efforts between service users and clinical academic partners, developing the capacity of service users to be involved in research and encouraging service-user-led research.

In embracing service user as well as carer involvement as an essential component of improving the quality and focus of mental health R&D, the mental health policy and practice community will be committing themselves to a step which cannot but involve them in questioning and transforming the status quo. The mental health R&D agenda has been, to date, shaped in its knowledge, concerns and methodologies by established mental health clinicians and academics (Barnes and Shardlow 1997). Delivering fully on the current service-user-involvement aspirations is not a question of 'bolting on' user views to what already exists. If, as INVOLVE maintains, user involvement is to deliver increased reliance, reliability and influence on practice and service delivery, the R&D community needs to reflect on how it is going to maximise this opportunity. Such reflection requires engagement with the ideas, interests and concerns of user activists, researchers and educators. It also requires an acknowledgement that this user community has knowledge and expertise that needs to be understood and incorporated in all aspects of mental health R&D in the future (Rose 2001).

This is difficult work. Mental health service-user activists and researchers have developed a sustained critique over a number of decades of the status quo in mental health practice and R&D. (Beresford 2000; Thornicroft *et al.* 2002). Some have questioned whether mental distress can be fully understood as an illness. Others, accepting the designation of distress as mental illness, have developed sustained critiques of the medicalised approaches to working with it as well as researching it (Mental Health Foundation 1997). Those service users who have become involved in R&D have not always been convinced, on the basis of their own experience, that their work has been used to make a positive difference to policy and provision (Nettle 1996) and have questioned whether research should be considered as a priority by service users and their organisations.

Exchanges on these issues need to start with furthering mutual understanding of the nature and terrain of mental health R&D, the frameworks that are used to select topics and develop research designs and tools, and clarifying the basis on which collaboration can be developed as a foundation on which user involvement in R&D can be progressed. Without this work, it is likely that attempts to develop service user involvement in the R&D agenda will falter and fail or at best be tokenistic gestures from an entrenched and traditional mental health R&D community.

In its published briefing notes for service user involvement in research the Consumers in NHS Research and Support Unit suggest that there are three types of consumer involvement which need to be viewed as part of a continuum:

- Consultation – asking consumers/service users for their views and using those views in making decisions about research priorities and proposals
- Collaboration – building active and ongoing partnership with consumers/service users in all or some aspects of the research and development process
- User control – providing opportunities for consumers/service users to design and undertake research and disseminate the findings.

(Consumers in NHS Research SU 2000)

While this framework is helpful for researchers in thinking through the implications of service-user involvement in R&D, it has been developed from the perspective of the established R&D community. To engage fully with the processes required to build meaningful user involvement it also needs to be informed by the viewpoints of service users. As Campbell has suggested, the service-user community has discovered that the term 'user involvement' has been used to refer to a spectrum of activities, which include:

- Activities where service users have real power to choose and initiate what they do
- Activities where service users are involved at the invitation of service providers
- Activities where service users do not want to be involved but are cajoled or persuaded by mental health professionals.

(Campbell 2001)

The importance of relating these two approaches in thinking through the development of user involvement in R&D is that the relevance, reliability and usefulness of research in which users have been involved, at whatever level, is related to the terms on which they have been engaged to take part.

SURESEARCH: ONE APPROACH TO SERVICE USER INVOLVEMENT IN R&D

Suresearch is a Midlands-based user-led network that has been developing its contribution to mental health research and education for over four years. Members of Suresearch have a common commitment to work for the improvement of mental health services through research and education. Whilst the network is user-led, it welcomes allies from the academic and clinical fields who share this commitment and wish to provide support to service users. The membership of a hundred comprises over eighty individuals whose expertise lies in their experience of service use. The network offers its services to users, practitioners and policy makers interested in developing user involvement in research, education and service provision (Davis and Braithwaite 2001).

Suresearch was formed in 2000 as the result of a day's workshop, at the University of Birmingham, attended by service users and academics already involved in making a contribution to mental health research and education. At this workshop two presentations were made by service users and academics who had undertaken small research projects in collaboration. The approach of these projects was to work in ways that ensured that the expertise of service users was valued at all stages of the research process. In addition, the projects used interviewers who had experience of service use to interview service users connected with the services being researched. The discussions about what had been learnt by service users and research academics during these projects led to an identification of some common concerns and issues.

Everyone taking part in the workshop was convinced that there was a need to harness more fully the experience and expertise of service users in research designed to discover what service responses were valued by service users and to disseminate the findings to those planning and providing those services. However, it was acknowledged that service users who became involved in this kind of endeavour could find themselves isolated and lacking support as research partners. When this occurred, people felt discouraged and disinclined to develop their skills and interests as researchers. This experience was not, however, inevitable. In the two research projects presented on the day, ways had been found of providing the kind of mutual respect and support that had given service users a sense of being valued and had built up their self-esteem and confidence. As a result they had increased their interest and appetite for further involvement in mental health research.

From this day's workshop the idea evolved of creating a user-led network in partnership with mental health clinicians and academics that would provide ways of developing mutual support and learning as well as growing opportunities for user-led, as well as collaborative, research. The workshop resulted in participants agreeing to try to establish such a network, with stated aims and regular opportunities to meet and exchange ideas and interests.

The aims of Suresearch which emerged from this workshop were to:

- Increase the involvement of mental health service users in research and education
- Provide opportunities for its members to work in partnership with each other to share and develop skills and knowledge
- Develop and provide programmes of education and training for its members
- Respond to, and take up opportunities for, research, consultancy and education
- Influence the quality, ethics and values of mental health research and education
- Link with other local, regional and national partnerships in mental health.

Four years later, the Suresearch membership has grown to 100 (80 of whom are service users) and is involved in an expanding range of research and education activities. The network runs monthly meetings open to members and other interested individuals. Members of the network are not obliged to attend meetings, they can maintain contact through mailings, by phone or email. The regular Suresearch meetings provide opportunities for information exchange and networking. Some Suresearch members are actively involved in other local and national user-led organisations and networks, some are making their first connection with a user-led network, sometimes they have decided to work with Suresearch as a result of being interviewed by a user researcher from Suresearch who told them about the network.

In between meetings, members involved in research or education projects meet to progress their work and take part in training and skills development. Suresearch have an office base in the Institute of Applied Social Studies, the University of Birmingham, and a presence on the executive management group of the Heart of England MHRN Hub (MHRN website: www.mhrninfo). The research portfolio of Suresearch covers a range of commissioned research projects which are undertaken by teams of Suresearch researchers. At the same time, Suresearch members make use of their experience and expertise by contributing as researchers or advisors to research projects run by other organisations or academic departments, in teams or on their own.

The portfolio of Suresearch research projects includes work on users experience of compulsory admission under the 1983 Mental Health Act; poverty and mental health; personal finances, social exclusion and mental health; employment and mental health; social security benefits and mental health; mental health training needs; user views of mental health services; women and mental health and user contributions to clinical governance in the mental health services. All of this work has been characterised by collaborative, user-focussed and user-led approaches. In addition, members are involved in training initiatives with a wide range of professional and user organisations and presentations at major research and professional conferences.

In 2003, twenty Suresearch members (three of whom were clinicians/academics) took part in a user-led, one-day review of the network. Using evidence from Suresearch research projects as well as exchanges of personal experiences from elsewhere, this review highlighted that there were three positive features of the network that were contributing to its growth and research productivity:

- The establishment of positive working relationships
- The development of research capacity
- The maintenance of user involvement in research.

Positive working relationships

Suresearch is valued by its members because it has adopted a consistently positive approach to service users expertise, potential and skills. It has succeeded in instilling confidence in service users about their worth and abilities. Service user members have found that they can become involved at their own pace, making their own decisions about when and how they want to join research projects. As a result, members have valued not feeling pressured about the commitment they make to the network. As members of research project teams they have received ongoing support and mentoring from peers and associated academics that have sustained them in developing their expertise and skills. They have also valued the monetary rewards they have received for their work. Despite the constraints of the benefit system, finance departments restrictive procedures and the attitudes of research funders, Suresearch has sought to make equal payment for equal work amongst its members.

Developing research capacity

Suresearch has a commitment to involving service users in all aspects of research – design, delivery, analysis, report writing and dissemination. This means that members can take part in as many or as few aspects of research work as they feel ready to engage with. Focussed training has been provided for the tasks required in each aspect of each project so that those with no previous experience, as well as the experienced, can play a full part.

Suresearch has sought to develop the research capacity of members over time. It has never sought core funding for this work but has used the expertise of service user and academic/clinician members to devise and deliver the kind of training that members have identified as being important to developing their skills in this area. Alongside the focussed training for specific projects the network has delivered a research training programme for interested members that has not been project related but has drawn on material generated by ongoing Suresearch projects. This programme has covered topics such as:

- Turning ideas into research proposals
- How research is done
- Research ethics – do's and don'ts
- Looking at data

- Producing reports
- Getting listened to – locally and nationally.

Whilst this programme was devised to meet the expressed needs of Suresearch members, it has welcomed participation from members of local user-led organisations who are interested in receiving research training.

Other initiatives have evolved which make a contribution to developing skills relevant to research. In 2003, for example a writing group was formed to provide support and guidance for members wanting to develop their written communication skills. This group writes a bi-monthly column for MIND's Openmind magazine. It has also been asked to take on the guest editorship of a user-led edition of the *Journal of Social Work Education.*

Maintaining service user involvement in research

Suresearch has had considerable success in sustaining user involvement as evidenced by the growth in both their membership and in their research portfolio. In reflecting on why this has happened, our review suggested that the following characteristics of the network had been critical to this success:

- The relationships developed by members has meant that a safe environment in which mutual respect and mutual valuing of a diversity of expertise has been established
- New friendships as well as research-related opportunities have evolved over time to the mutual benefit of all concerned
- The networking that Suresearch encourages ensures that people have opportunities to meet new people from different walks of life, learn new things and enjoy themselves in stimulating exchanges that has led to new friendships and interests.

This environment of mutual learning has been enhanced by an unwavering commitment to meetings being user led and the development and achievements of members being recognised and celebrated. Several members have built on the skills and confidence they have acquired and opened up new areas in their lives through employment, consultancy and returning to education. This has meant that the success of Suresearch has been measured by what members have themselves decided to do with their lives rather than being narrowly tied to the research outcomes of the network. Our experience has been that members whose lives have taken another course have remained in touch with the network and made information and contacts developed in their new situations available to the Suresearch membership. This has enriched the network to the benefit of all.

CONCLUSIONS

The current focus by government and other research-funding bodies on user involvement in mental health R&D represents a recognition of the importance of service-user contributions in working to develop high-quality and relevant research in the mental health field that can positively impact on practice and policy. To make the most of this opportunity to build vibrant and sustainable rather than tokenistic user involvement requires all those involved to re-examine the basis on which R&D has developed in the past and build approaches that maximise the expertise and talents of all. Without this work future R&D will not make the impact on services that government is promoting. In engaging in this work, attention has to be paid to changing the ways in which service users and those involved in research relate to each other. As the Suresearch network has discovered, its not just what you do, it's the way that you do it.

References

Barker, I. and Peck, E. (1996). User empowerment – a decade of experience. *The Mental Health Review*, 1(4), 5–13.

Barnes, M. (1997). *Care, communities and citizenship*. Longman, London.

Barnes, M. and Bowl, R. (2001). *Taking over the asylum: empowerment and mental health*. Palgrave, Basingstoke.

Barnes, M. and Shardlow, P. (1997). From passive recipients to active citizens: participation in mental health user groups. *Journal of Mental Health*, 6(3), 289–300.

Becker, S. (1997). Research for change: form theory to influence. *Social Services Research*, 4, 1–12.

Beresford, P. (2000). *Our voice in our future: mental health issues*. Shaping Our Lives/National Institute for Social Work, London.

Braye, S. (2000). Participation and involvement in social care: an overview. In *User involvement and participation in social care: research informing practice*. Kemshall, H. and Littlechild, R. (eds). Jessica Kingsley, London.

Bowl, R. (1996). Involving service users in mental health services: Social Services Departments and the National Health Service and Community Care Act 1990. *Journal of Mental Health*, 5(3), 287–303.

Brandon, D. (1991). *Innovation without change? Consumer power in psychiatric services.* Macmillan, Basingstoke.

Campbell, P. (1996a). Challenging loss of power. In Read, J. and Reynolds, Jill (eds) *Speaking our minds: an anthology.* Macmillan, Basingstoke.

Campbell, P. (1996b). The history of the user movement. In Heller, T., Reynolds, J. and Gomm, J.R. (eds) *Mental health matters.* Macmillan, London.

Campbell, P. (2001). The role of users of psychiatric development – influence not power. *Psychiatric Bulletin*, 25(3), 87–8.

Consumers in NHS Research Support Unit. (2000). *Involving consumers in research and development in the NHS: briefing notes for researchers.*

Davis, A. and Braithwaite, T. (2001). In our own hands. *Mental Health Care*, 41, 413–14.

Department of Health. (1999). *National Service Framework for Mental Health.* Department of Health, London.

Department of Health. (2000). *The NHS national plan.* Department of Health, London.

Hannigan, B., Bartlett, H. and Cilverd, A. (1997). Improving health and social functioning: perspectives of mental health service users. *Journal of Mental Health* 6(6), 613–19.

Hickey, G. and Kipping, C. (1998). Exploring the concept of user involvement in mental health through a participation continuum. *Journal of Clinical Nursing* 7(1), 83–8.

Lindow, V. (1994). *Purchasing mental health services; purchasing alternatives.* MIND, London.

Mental Health Foundation. (1997). *Knowing our own minds: a survey of how people in emotional distress take control of their own lives.* Mental Health Foundation, London.

National Institute of Mental Health England website www.nimhe.org.uk

Nettle, M. (1996). Listening in the asylum. In Read, J. and Reynolds, Jill (eds) *Speaking our minds: an anthology.* Macmillan, Basingstoke.

Perkins, R. and Repper, J. (1998). *Dilemmas in community mental health practice. Choice or control.* Radcliffe Medical Press, Oxford.

Repper, J. and Perkins, R. (2003). *Social inclusion and recovery: a model for mental health practice.* Elsevier Science.

Sayce, L. (2000). *From psychiatric patient to citizen: overcoming discrimination and social exclusion.* Macmillan, Basingstoke.

Secretary of State for Health. (1998). *Fit for the future: modernising social services.* Cmd. 3805. Stationery Office, London.

Simpson, E.L., House, A.O. and Barkham, M. (2002). *A guide to involving users, ex-users and carers in mental health service planning, delivery or research: a health technology approach.* Academic Unit of Psychiatry and Behavioural Sciences, University of Leeds, Leeds.

Standing Advisory Group on Consumer Involvement in the NHS R&D programme to the Central Research and Development Committee

1996/7. (1998). Research: *What's in it for consumers?* NHS Executive, London.

Standing Group on Consumers in NHS Research. (1999). *Involvement works: the second report of the Standing Group on Consumers in NHS research.* NHS Executive, London.

Thornicroft, G., Rose, D., Huxley, P., Dale, G. and Wykes, T. (2002). What are the research priorities of mental health service users? *Journal of Mental Health,* 11, 1–5.

Townend, M. and Braithwaite, T. (2002). Mental health research – the value of user involvement. (Editorial). *Journal of Mental Health,* 11, 2, 117–19.

Part II

Policy and its implications for mental health research in the NHS

8

Higher education policy and its implications for mental health research in the NHS

David Sallah and Judy Whitmarsh

The pace of change within both Higher Education Institutions (HEIs) and the health care economy has created a challenging environment for research and development and, in particular, for mental health services. The full impact of the implementation of Research Governance in the NHS (DoH 2002) has brought added pressures on researchers in terms of its structures, often managed by individuals with very little knowledge of the process of research and the need to innovate, together with very elongated and tiresome approval systems. Some of these hurdles could take over three months to surmount even before the start of a research project. The Higher Education White Paper, published in January 2003, has also added to these pressures by creating a vision that is challenging both in terms of widening participation for student admissions, and the decision to concentrate research in just a few universities (DfES 2003). Other main drivers of the research agenda within the HEI sector are the Robert's Review of Research Assessment (Roberts 2003), the dual support system which recommends that the full economic cost of research projects must be specified in grant applications, and the Higher Education Funding Council for England's (HEFCE) consultation on establishing threshold standards for postgraduate degree standards. This chapter will discuss the key intentions of the Higher Education White Paper (DfES 2003) with particular emphasis on research and development and its potential impact on the NHS mental health services. In attempting to do this, we will firstly outline the issues that can contribute to changing or hindering the closure of the gap that exists between research and development, and conclude by advocating a pluralistic approach to research and development activity and its use in mental health care.

INTRODUCTION

Health research can be divided into three main categories: firstly, research that relates to policy which is central to driving the research and development agenda in the health service; secondly, research that is initiated by professionals; and finally, research that seeks to draw comparisons in terms of effectiveness with various existing benchmarks. The focus on community care and the development of care trusts (HMSO 1990, DoH 2001a) has provided the opportunity for health professionals to extend their roles, resulting in government insistence on the importance of finding the evidence on what works, in order to provide national institutions such as the National Institute for Clinical Excellence (NICE), the Healthcare Commission and the National Institute for Mental Health in England (NIMHE) with the means to develop their modernising change programmes. The centrality of evidence in government policy has evolved as a result of modernising the mental health services through the implementation of the National Service Framework (NSF) for mental health (DoH 1999) and increasing the resources available to improve services and practice.

However, the modernisation programme has exposed and created past and current gaps between the demand for, and the supply of, research in many areas. For example, NICE requires research evidence in order to inform the development of clinical guidelines for practitioners and NIMHE needs evidence in order to deliver the objectives as set out in the National Service Frameworks. The NHS cannot deliver this goal of providing the evidence on its own and needs to form partnerships, particularly with higher education institutions, in terms of forming research groups and of implementing the findings into practice to drive the development plan for the service.

The higher education white paper

In the autumn of 2003, the Higher Education White Paper, which set out the Government's position on higher education as a whole, was published (DfES 2003), and taking into account the earlier Widening Participation in Higher Education White Paper, published in April 2003, it details proposals to reform higher education in England and Wales and to create an Office for Fair Access to higher education.

The White Paper itself was well signposted by leaks and official releases in advance of publication. Its key proposals are for increased flexibility in fee-setting; the UK Government evidently has embraced the prevailing rhetoric worldwide that those who benefit most from higher education should pay for it. The White Paper draws attention to the fact that average earnings over the past decade have grown faster than academic salaries, leading, in part, to recruitment and retention problems and deteriorating staff–student ratios. The state of universities in the UK, as acknowledged in the White Paper is partly due to Government policy failures that have resulted in declining core funding, creating a system where collaboration and partnership working is frowned upon. Consequently, the Government's acknowledgement in the White Paper that it has a role to play in balancing competing interests, as well as a responsibility to intervene under some circumstances, is timely.

The White Paper addresses other main issues; key amongst them is a stronger focus on university teaching with informed student choice as a driver to driving institutional quality. To enable this, universities are being asked to develop and adopt human resource strategies that explicitly value teaching, and reward and promote good teachers (DfES 2003).

Another main issue of note and relevance to the direction of the discourse in this chapter is that the right to use the title of 'university' may be made dependent on undergraduate degree-awarding power – and therefore on the quality of teaching – rather than research degree awarding as it is at present.

RESEARCH

The government's own spending review of funding for universities confirms an infrastructure 'backlog' of some £8 billion with a further need for doubling maintenance costs. As a result of the spending review, expenditure in science and research is to increase by 30% between 2002 and 2005. The White Paper identifies a dedicated capital stream (£500 m per annum by 2004/5) for the development of the infrastructure, funding for research councils is to be increased to enable them to meet the full cost of research and a further £50 m per annum to support collaborative research has been identified. Overall, the Paper advocates that research funding is to be targeted even more to existing 'research-intensive' universities – while still providing resources for other institutions to develop and improve their research. Universities are now expected to demonstrate that their research is 'financially sustainable' (neither definition nor criteria are given).

Furthermore, the Government and the Higher Education Funding Council for England (HEFCE) are to develop new standards for postgraduate places which may lead to some institutions losing PhD places, or even postgraduate-degree-awarding status – a situation that could lead into a model where postgraduate-degree-awarding powers are restricted to successful research consortia. Other research specific changes proposed by the White Paper are:

- The PhD stipend is to be increased, with higher rates in some fields
- The Arts and Humanities Research Board is to be elevated to the status of research funding council by 2005
- A review of the Research Assessment with a focus on 'different approaches to the definition and evaluation of quality research' which will lead to the development of expanded assessment criteria
- A review of governance and management
- Incentives for high-quality researchers
- More research-only posts
- Postdoctoral salaries to be increased by £4000
- 1000 new academic fellowships
- A new fellowship scheme to provide secondments to high-rating research institutions for staff from non-research-intensive institutions.

The publication of the White Paper received a torrent of strong reactions on all fronts. Unions and students are clearly against it, some of the staff particularly at managerial level welcome its proposals and parliamentarians, particularly from the ruling Labour Party, revolted and voted against its introduction. The Government won the resultant vote with a very narrow margin and the measures proposed in the White Paper are currently going through the parliamentary process to becoming law as the Higher Education Bill.

The Government's intention, as outlined in the White Paper, is to expand on many existing measures to improve cross-sector linkages with higher education, including incentives for so called less research-intensive universities to develop links with local businesses. The need to work closer with the NHS is therefore strengthened with the encouragement, for example, of increasing the Higher Education Innovation Fund, to stimulate regional exploitation of university research and community, cultural and social roles for universities. Another key proposal in the White Paper is the development of 'employer-focussed' two-year foundation degrees which are to become 'the standard two-year qualification', with Further Education (FE) colleges, as well as universities, fully involved in its development; and in the case of FE colleges, to become awarding institutions.

The Higher Education Bill, introduced in the House of Commons on 8 January 2004, is intended to assist in the implementation of a number of policies set out in the White Paper (DfES 2003). In addition to this, the Bill also contains provisions relating to two other areas not covered by the White Paper: the provision of new powers to share information relating to student support, and the devolution of the tuition fee regime and student support in relation to Wales to the National Assembly for Wales. The Bill itself is divided into 5 Parts. Part 1 makes provision relating to a new Arts and Humanities Research Council, which is to be set up by Royal Charter, and the funding of arts and humanities research. Part 2 deals with the review of student complaints. Part 3 permits institutions to charge variable fees and, providing they have an approved plan, fees above a basic rate. Part 4 includes provisions to transfer functions to the National Assembly for Wales, provisions to prevent student loans being written off on discharge from bankruptcy, amendments to allow loans in respect of money owed by students to universities to be paid to the latter so as to facilitate deferral of fee payments by students and provisions about the disclosure of information. Finally, Part 5 contains miscellaneous and general provisions. The territorial coverage of the Bill varies in each of the countries of the United Kingdom but it is overall a nation-wide legislation. Part 3 of the Bill provided the most divisive debates within the higher-education sector, the UK legislature and the country as a whole, leading to revolt in parliament amongst the ruling Labour Party parliamentarians to support their Government.

STUDENT FEES IN HIGHER EDUCATION

Section 26 of the Teaching and Higher Education Act 1998, makes provision for the fees which Higher Education Institutions (HEIs) charge for full-time undergraduate students in a given year, to be determined by the maximum fee remission grant for that year. The current Bill enables HEIs to set their own fees, up to a basic amount specified in regulations, which would no longer be linked to the level of grant for fees. Institutions that wish to charge fees above this rate will only be able to do so if they have in force a plan under this part of the Bill, approved by the relevant authority; in England, the new Director of Fair Access to Higher Education. The intention is that loans will be made available, on an income-contingent basis and with no real rate of interest, to allow students to defer payment of fees until they have completed their studies and are earning enough before they are required to make payments. Under this new arrangement, higher education institutions will receive loan payments directly from the Government, so that they can receive fee payments up front and students can repay later.

NEW ARRANGEMENTS FOR RESEARCH FUNDING

Research in the arts and humanities is at present partly funded by the Arts and Humanities Research Board (AHRB). This is a company limited by guarantee, which has charitable status, and receives its funding through the Higher Education Funding Council for England (HEFCE), the Higher Education Funding Council for Wales, the Scottish Higher Education Funding Council, and the Department for Employment and Learning in Northern Ireland. Research in the sciences and social sciences is at present partly funded by seven research councils established by Royal Charter. These research councils receive money from the Office of Science and Technology under the Science and Technology Act 1965. That Act also contains various other provisions relating to the existing research councils, including requirements to keep accounts and records, and to provide reports to the Secretary of State. The creation of a new Arts and Humanities Research Council (AHRC), to be established by Royal Charter, is said to put arts and humanities research on the same footing as research in the sciences and social sciences. How does all this affect the evolving research and development policy and its implementation in the NHS?

THE LANDSCAPE FOR RESEARCH AND DEVELOPMENT IN THE NHS

The empirical basis for theories regarding how to improve appropriate use of research evidence in policy and clinical decisions, particularly in mental health, is still unclear. Weiss and Weiss (1996) argue that, both decision-makers and social scientists behave as though social science research makes a genuine contribution to public policy; the contribution that the scientific approach makes to defining what works in mental health is questionable as well. This point of view provides various dimensions for debate; on one hand, many researchers are sceptical about the extent to which research is used, and on the other, many policy-makers are sceptical about the usefulness of research. This is explained better by developing the assertions of Lindbolm and Cohen (1979) who argued that suppliers and users of social research are dissatisfied; the former because they are not listened to, the latter because they do not hear much they want to listen to. One of the ways that this divergence of emphasis, which consequently translates into research funding and its application in practice, can be bridged is to engage the two camps (suppliers and users) of health service research to work towards agreeing the priorities for research. Elsewhere in this book (see Introduction, Chapters 1, 7, and 8), the various ways that the Department of Health is managing this gap by involving stakeholders of mental health research has been articulated.

For decades now, policy makers have repeated the mantra that economic competitiveness and national well-being depend crucially on the skills, adaptability and motivation of the workforce. By the same token, even a cursory glance through the relevant policy documents reveals that what policy makers actually have in mind when they talk about 'skill' is considerably broader now than in the past, when it tended to be equated with the manual craft worker and technologist. There is an emphasis now on 'multi-skilling' the workforce based on a pathway through an imaginary 'skills escalator'. The success of this approach depends on an abundant, flexible and highly skilled workforce, which the NHS could not guarantee.

The shortage of health service researchers is considered by some to be a threat to the NHS's R&D programme as a whole, and research in primary care is a particular concern because of the apparent vicious circle of disadvantage, in which, because there are few well-qualified researchers (and little sustained investment in developing this capacity), the research outcomes are limited in number and quality. There is an acknowledgement that the conduct of research in the health sector is multi-disciplinary and involves various multi-professional groups within the health service itself and other related outside disciplines and services, HEIs being a major partner in teaching and learning and in research. In short, the NHS alone cannot address the issues that relate to improving the care and treatment of patients and deliver improved systems of care provision. As a result of this, research into health and health services leading to development would invariably employ an array of knowledge, skills and methods to assess the effectiveness of interventions. The policies shaping the continuing modernisation of the NHS, some of which are outlined in this book, are a testimony to the desire on the part of the Government and the NHS to foster partnership and collaborative working. The consequences of these multi-disciplinary activities mean that there is a great deal of potential for enriching the quality of health and health care research by involving universities. In developing these partnerships, the research capacity and capability within the NHS needs to be improved in order to work in collaboration with the universities on a programme of research that underpins and shapes development of care and treatment.

Even though key NHS policy papers set out the context for developing the NHS (DoH 1997; 1999; 1999b) the change that is necessary to drive the modernisation programme is only being recognised since the introduction performance measures, such as Clinical Governance. The importance of research to delivering this agenda has been strengthened by the launch of the NHS research funding policy in support of the modernising NHS. In the mental health services, the National Service Framework (DoH 1999) provides a challenge for the service and researchers to find the evidence to drive the quality of service, treatment and care to users of the service and for staff who work within it.

However, the contribution of nurses, midwives, health visitors and allied health professions to research has neither flourished nor matched the extent to which they impact on practice. In the case of some of these professions, nursing, for example, there is a view that nursing should both be the subject of research and development and also a contributor at every stage of the research and development cycle. The Department of Health has recognised this as a concern that needs improvement.

There is evidence that nursing, midwifery and Allied Health Professional (AHP) departments are generating increasing research income, (an increase from £3 m in 1996/7 to £9.7 m in 1999/2000), better submission rates to the Research Assessment Exercise of 2001, and an increase in category A staff; however, the principal funders have been the Department of Health, NHS regional offices and trusts, and not the research councils. The Higher Education Funding Council for England (HEFCE) support for research has been £3 m a year of QR funding to 11 departments in Unit of Assessment (UOA) 10 which covers nursing and midwifery. The survey commissioned by HEFCE further speculates that some of the £7 m a year, which went to UOA 11, will have reached AHP departments.

Despite continuous lobbying of both government and research funders, including the Health Technology Assessment programme, the research capacity and capability within nursing, midwifery and allied health professionals (AHP) remains very low compared to that which is available to doctors. In a recent study to assess the evidence for the extent to which research is being promoted amongst these professions, it was found that these departments are generating increasing research income with a corresponding increase in capacity (HEFCE, DoH 2003), providing the evidence for continuing capacity and capability building.

RESEARCH AND DEVELOPMENT FUNDING

In the case of medical research, the distribution of research and development funds (public and charitable) is appallingly unjust. For example, Hacking (2004) revealed that about £1.5 billion is spent annually on a not-for-profit medical R&D in England with the NHS contributing about £450 million. Of this amount, over two-thirds goes to just three cities (London, Oxford and Cambridge), often referred to as the 'Golden Triangle'. The situation relating to NHS R&D is even worse as 68% of the total allocation of £437 million allocated went to trusts in London (Hacking 2004). Hacking ascribed this disparity in funding medical research to historical accident; explaining that as research funds normally follow teaching funds, the cities of London and Oxford, as teaching centres, did attract most of the funding. This of course happened before the expansion of universities and the development of health services in industrial cities. Hacking (2004) called for a redistribution of research funding based on a geographical basis, concentrating on value for money, equity of health service linked with improved health outcomes for populations, the burden of disease and implementation of the Government economic policy of reducing disparities. Reducing these disparities is a mammoth task, not least due to the vested interests of these teaching hospitals which are arguing that a geographical redistribution of funding could result in extra costs that could impinge upon both resources and people and an unimaginable change management programme to deliver the goal. In either case, it is inconceivable that there might be a gradual phasing-in of the redistribution programme over time, and, as suggested, by some twinning arrangements between hospitals within the Golden Triangle and others outside it.

ETHICS IN MENTAL HEALTH RESEARCH

To say that research is essential to the successful promotion of health and well-being is hardly a new fact. In mental health a considerable number of key advances in the last century have depended on research; however, health and social care professionals and the public they serve are increasingly looking to research for further improvements. Unfortunately, recent events in health research have increased the anxieties of the public, particularly when research causes real distress when things go wrong (Kennedy 2002). Resultantly the Labour Government of the UK decided to set up a framework for research to ensure that the public can have confidence in, and benefit from, health and social care research. This framework is known as Research Governance (DoH 2001).

The standards in this framework apply to all research which relates to the responsibilities of the Secretary of State for Health – that is, research concerned with the protection and promotion of public health, research undertaken in or by the Department of Health, its non-Departmental Public Bodies and the NHS, and research undertaken by or within social care services that might have an impact on the quality of those services. This includes clinical and non-clinical research, research undertaken by NHS staff using NHS resources, and research undertaken by industry, the charities, the research councils and universities within the health and social care systems. With the advent of clinical governance and the duties under the research governance arrangements, health professionals are being increasingly called upon to examine the ethics that lie behind treatment or research decisions.

Ensign (2003) advances the notion that research is neither a basic right nor a necessity for society or for individuals. Ensign further insists that this viewpoint should guide and inform the practice of research and stimulate awareness of the changes we may impose upon participants' lives by the fact of the research process. Whilst this position could be questioned from the point of view that there is a value for both the individual and society through research, the point being made is clear: research and researchers need a code of practice that should shape their thinking and serve as their guiding principle during the research process; ethical codes. Historically, ethical codes and guidelines arose from a need to safeguard participants in quantitative, mainly biomedical, research. As qualitative research methods gained popularity and credence, traditional ethical principles appear to have been transferred to the qualitative methodology, sometimes without the necessary consideration of their pertinence and suitability (see also Murphy and Dingwall 2001).

The role of the research and ethics committees as a provider of independent advice to researchers and to ensure that the research conforms to appropriate ethical standards is central to protecting the dignity, rights, safety and well-being of all actual or potential research participants (Corec 2004). This responsibility is, however, shared with the researchers, research sponsors, universities and all those involved with the research.

As a further safeguard to patient confidentiality, the Caldicott Guardian (DoH 2001) ensures that patient information relating to patients, travels within the NHS guided by the following principles:

- Every proposed use or transfer of patient-identifiable information should be clearly defined and reviewed
- Personal-identifiable information should only be used if there is no alternative
- Personal-identifiable information should only be accessed on a 'need-to-know' basis
- All staff must be aware of their responsibilities to respect patient confidentiality.

The process of assuring ethical approval acts as signposts, some of which are easily read and understood, others lead researchers up tangential paths. Research ethics committees are the gatekeepers (Homan 2001) of health and social care research because of their very unique position of giving access to the research field. However, while most research ethics committees offer constructive help to researchers about their applications, some produce numerous obstacles to access; this raises issues around the power held by research and ethics committees and the way in which they may potentially manipulate the direction of research (some members are themselves researchers).

It is suggested by Hood *et al.* (1999) that the socially disadvantaged are subject to more research since they are not protected by powerful interests. Few would deny that the research in mental health specifically targets the socially disadvantaged and anecdotal evidence suggests that many of those to be researched are suffering from 'research fatigue'. Some researchers with acknowledgement from funders do offer inducements, such as money, gifts or tokens for certain products as an incentive to participate in research. Coady (2001) argues that a risk/benefit equation must be part of ethical research design. The researcher should calculate the risks to the subject, whether physical, mental or psychological, and balance these against the benefit the research may provide for the participants and the community. This adoption of a consequentialist principle may perhaps be more appropriate to a quantitative research methodology where, arguably, the outcomes of the research may be more reliably linked to the intervention and the variables may be manipulated. However, the outcome, or even harm, resulting from the ethnographic interview may not be so readily calculated and balanced against the benefits of the research (Murphy and Dingwall 2001). Perhaps because qualitative research, including the feminist perspective, and the ethnographic type interview, is seen as 'soft' research (Denzin and Lincoln 1998) and commonly studies marginalised or oppressed groups, the potential for harm is not often articulated. It is argued variously that potential harm to participants could result from:

- Participant anxiety, guilt, stress
- Damage to self-esteem
- Loss of close relationship with researcher on completion of study
- Embarrassment in interviews about opinions held or not held
- Dissatisfaction with everyday life following consciousness-raising
- Challenge to status quo.

Harmful participant outcomes may not become apparent until some time after the interviews, thus creating a distance from the intervention and possibly confusion about the origins of the damage. Harm may also be caused to participants by the writing and dissemination of the research findings. Published findings may allow authorities detailed information of groups, which can be used to control and manipulate them. Participants may be hurt or offended by the inclusion or exclusion of details of their stories. The mass media may sensationalise reports, leading to a result that is very different to the aim of the researcher. In conclusion, the researcher's perspective on the findings may be very different to that of the participants and, with the current move towards offering participants a research summary, this may lead to feelings of having been duped by the researcher for their own purposes (Murphy and Dingwall 2001). The place that ethics plays in mental health research is crucial both in terms of content, context, nature of the research methodology and dissemination and implementation of outcomes.

CONCLUSION

The UK Government is now stressing that greater weight should be given to evidence in all aspects of health and social care, placing the onus on the service and the academic community to deliver such evidence. Investment in research varies hugely, the size of the R&D communities is different and the number of specialist journals available for publication differs from specialty to specialty. Whatever is known about the capacity and capability for mental health research, it is unlikely that the same critical mass and number of collaborations would be reached as in areas such as cancer or coronary heart disease, which are both national priorities alongside mental health.

The shortage of health service researchers is considered by some to be a threat to the NHS's R&D programme as a whole, and research in primary care is a particular concern. The focus on evidence in clinical practice is an opportunity to develop health care professionals with knowledge, skills and competencies in research and evidence-based practice; the higher education institutions should be partners and collaborators. It is time to shift the focus slightly from social research, which the universities mainly concentrate on, to clinical research. The recognition for clinical research should concentrate research education for health care professionals in many higher education settings with emphasis on doing research rather than *using* research.

References

Ainley, P. (1993). *Class and skill: changing divisions of knowledge and labour.* Cassell, London.

Bridges, D. (2001). The ethics of outsider research. *Journal of Philosophy of Education.* 35(3), 371–86.

Coady, M. (2001). Ethics in early childhood research. In MacNaughton, G., Rolfe, S.A. and Siraj-Blatchford, (eds.), pp. 64–75. *Doing early childhood research: international perspectives on theory and practice.* Open University Press, Buckingham & Philadelphia.

COREC (Central Office for Research Ethics Committees). (2003). Update: Changes Affecting Procedures for Applications to NHS Research Ethics Committees (04/03/03). www.corec.org.uk/interim.htm(hash)newhas accessed 27.1.04

Department of Health. (2001). *Research governance framework for health and social care.* DH Publications, London.

Department of Health. (2001a). Health and Social Care Act. DH Publications.

Department of Health. (2001b). Caldicott Guardians: Summary of responses to consultation. www.doh.gov.uk/ipu/confiden/implemen/calresp1.htm accessed 27.1.04

Department of Health. (1999). National Service Framework for Mental Health: Modern Standards and Service Models. DH Publications.

Department of Health. (2000). NHS Plan. A Plan for Investment. A Plan for Reform. DH Publications.

Department of Health. (1999a). *Modernising mental health services.* DH Publications.

Denzin, N.K. and Lincoln, Y.S. (eds.) (1998). *The landscape of qualitative research: theories and issues.* Sage Publications, Thousand Oaks, London, New Delhi.

DfES (2003) White Paper. *The future of higher education* (Cm 5735). Stationery Office, London.

Ensign, J. (2003). Ethical issues in qualitative health research with homeless youths. *Journal of Advanced Nursing, 43*(1), 43–50.

Hacking, J. (2004). Medical research fools' gold'. *Health Service Journal,* 114(5899), 32–3.

HEFCE. (2003). Research Report 01/64. *Promoting research in nursing and the allied health professions.* A report to Task Group 3 by the CPNR, CHEMS Consulting, the Higher Education Consultancy Group and the Research Forum for Allied Health Professions. **November 2003.**

Hood, S. Mayall, B. and Oliver, S. (eds). (1999). *Critical issues in social research.* Open University Press, Buckingham & Philadelphia.

Homan, R. (2001). The principle of assumed consent. *Journal of Philosophy of Education, 35*(3), 329–44.

HMSO. (1990). Health and service and Community Care Act. Stationery Office, London.

Kennedy. (2002). The report of the public inquiry into children's heart surgery at Bristol Infirmary 1984–95.

Murphy, E. and Dingwall, R. (2001). The ethics of ethnography. In Atkinson, P., Coffey, A., Delamont, S., Lofland, J. and Lofland, L. *Handbook of ethnography,* pp. 339–52. Sage Publications, London, Thousand Oaks, New Delhi.

Keep, E. and Mayhew, K. (1999). The assessment: knowledge, skills and competitiveness. *Oxford Review of Economic Policy, 15*(1), 1–15.

Lindblom, C.E. and Cohen, D.K. (1979). *Usable knowledge: social science and social problem solving.* Yale University Press, New Haven, CT.

Roberts, G. (2003). *Review of research assessment.* Report by Sir Gareth Roberts to the UK Funding Bodies. http://www.ra-review.ac.uk/

Weiss, J.A. and Weiss, C.H. (1996). Social scientists and decision makers look at the usefulness of mental health research. In Lorion, R.P., Iscoe, I., Deleon, P.H., and Vandenbo, G.R. (eds.) *Psychology and public policy: balancing public service and professional need*, pp. 165–181. American Psychological Association, Washington, DC.

9

NHS research and development in mental health

Clair Chilvers, Sue Spiers and Susan Barnes

BACKGROUND

The identification of mental health as a ministerial priority reflects not only the burden of mental ill health and its devastating social consequences, but also the low priority that has been given to improving health and social care services for people suffering from mental distress. The stigma associated with a diagnosis of severe mental illness, or indeed of suffering from a common mental health problem, has undoubtedly contributed to the inadequate attention paid to mental health services in the past. This has had a number of consequences for mental health research.

Firstly, the funding from charitable sources for mental health research is small: there are none of the wealthy charities associated with other common conditions such as cancer and heart disease. Yet, mental illness is a common condition; one in six people are suffering from a mental health problem at any one time. Secondly, the research base for mental health is not strong. Mental health research has been regarded as being particularly difficult to do: for common mental illnesses, research needs to be done in a primary care setting where the research culture is less well embedded than in secondary care, and for severe mental illness, the often chaotic lives led by people suffering the distress of mental illness leads to problems of keeping contact with research participants, and with treatment compliance. Nevertheless, a number of randomised trials in both settings have been successfully conducted.

In this chapter a perspective is taken of how the National Research Plan for mental health, promised in the *National service framework for mental health* (DoH 1999a), is being developed and of how recent government policy has acknowledged and supported the need for research. A brief summary is then given of current policy on research and development (R&D) within the National Health Service (NHS), followed by a description of the state of mental health R&D in the NHS. This covers the Strategic Review carried out in 2001/02 (DoH 2002a) updated with information from the most recent reports from research active NHS hospitals and primary and community care. Finally, current priorities for mental health research are discussed in the context of recent policy documents, findings from a service-user panel, and the mechanism for priority setting is described.

To set the scene, the burden of mental ill health from *Our healthier nation* (DoH 1999b) is shown in Table 9.1.

RESEARCH AND DEVELOPMENT IN THE NATIONAL HEALTH SERVICE

In March 2000 the Government announced plans to modernise the funding of research within the NHS (DoH 2000a). This identified two complementary funding streams:

- NHS *Support for science*, to provide the NHS contribution to the science base, and
- NHS *Priorities and needs R&D funding*, to support the development of the knowledge base required by the NHS.

R&D for a first class service (DoH 2000a) described the purposes of NHS R&D funding. The NHS needs access to reliable knowledge relevant to its business. This knowledge is generated by national and international research. NHS *Support for science* pays for the costs to the NHS of supporting research carried out within the NHS. Much of the research is carried out in partnership with universities.

The NHS also requires specific knowledge directly relevant to improving health and delivering high-quality health and social care. It relies on an evidence base to support its practice and NHS *Priorities and needs funding* contributes to the R&D needed to provide that evidence base. It does this through Department of Health national R&D programmes, through research capacity building, and through funding allocated to NHS R&D providers (mainly hospitals and primary care

Table 9.1 The burden of mental ill health

Years of life lost

- Suicide and undetermined injury cause 4,500 deaths every year
- Suicide accounts for 400,000 years of life lost before age 75 years
- Suicide is the leading cause of death among men aged 15–24 years and the second most common cause of death among people aged under 35 years
- Over 95% of those who commit suicide had been suffering from mental illness before their death
- 10–15% of people with severe mental illness kill themselves
- People with mental illness are also at increased risk of dying early from respiratory disease, cancer and coronary heart disease

Years of health lost

- 16% of the adult population suffers from a common mental disorder such as depression or anxiety
- 12% of children and adolescents suffer from a conduct or emotional disorder
- 30% of people over 85 years suffer from dementia
- Four people in every 1000 suffer from a psychotic disorder such as schizophrenia

Health disadvantage

- Women are more likely than men to seek help for a mental health problem
- Suicide is three times more common in men than in women
- Women living in England born in India and East Africa have 40% higher suicide rates than those born here
- Men in unskilled occupations are four times more likely to commit suicide than those in professional work

Counting the cost

- Treating mental illness costs the NHS and social services an estimated £7.5 billion each year
- People with mental illness have increased sickness absence, change jobs more often and are more likely to be unemployed

Source: Our Healthier Nation (DoH 1999b).

organisations working in collaboration with universities). Currently, the national programmes are: the Health Technology Assessment Programme, the Service Delivery and Organisation Programme, the Policy Research Programme, the Methodology Programme, the New and Emerging Aspects of Technology Programme and the Forensic Mental Health Programme. Although each operates somewhat differently, the key point is that they fund research and development of direct relevance to the NHS. Most of the research is commissioned by setting research priorities after wide consultation and inviting applications for funding. Key principles for these national programmes are their rigorous peer review systems, the appropriate involvement of service users and carers and their value to the NHS.

Research capacity is built by means of research fellowships and research infrastructure units. Funding allocated to NHS R&D providers to support direct research costs is problematic in that the basis for the awards is largely historical and does not necessarily reflect the current volume of research activity. For example, much of this funding may be tied up in research sessions for NHS clinical posts which were based on past research activity. Disentangling R&D funding to ensure that it is spent on research rather than patient care, or the obverse of discovering research that is supported by patient care monies has become a preoccupation of research managers within the NHS and the Department of Health. Research funding has for some years been a declining proportion of the overall NHS budget, and it has not kept pace with the expansion of the biomedical research base. Between 1997/8 and 2001/2 the NHS R&D budget increased by 11.5% but fell from 1.2% to less than 1% of the total NHS budget. Over the same period, Medical Research Council funding increased by 20% and medical research charity funding by 10% per year. The difficulty in resolving current anomalies in research funding is therefore unsurprising.

With the introduction of the Research Governance Framework for Health and Social Care (DoH 2001a) there is general awareness of best research practice and full implementation is expected by April 2004. The Human Rights Act (1998) and the EU Directive on Clinical Trials (2001) are also having a fundamental impact on clinical research, and there is a perception that barriers will be erected which may have a negative impact on non-commercial research in the future in terms of feasibility, cost and reliability.

The reform of the research ethics committee system with the introduction of Multicentre Research Ethics Committees and more uniformity of operation of Local Research Ethics Committees overseen by the Central Office for Research Ethics Committees lays the foundation for a more standardised system. Further work will be needed to demonstrate the advantages of the new systems.

Although the principle of service user and carer involvement in research is now well accepted, and organisations such as INVOLVE (formerly Consumers in NHS Research) are well established, there has been a shift in attitude in the general public away from participating in research. There is less willingness to take part in research studies with a consequent decline in response rates and the introduction of potential biases and a lack of generalisability of research findings.

Mental health research is among the most forward-looking in terms of user and carer involvement, and in terms of the notion of service-user led emancipatory research. This needs to be built on so that service users appreciate the benefits to them of taking part in research studies: benefits both in terms of ensuring that the research measures outcomes that are important to them, and in terms of a more immediate beneficial effect of being treated according to a well-defined protocol.

Two other immediate issues related to equality and research in the NHS are ethnicity and gender. These are particularly important in mental health and are described in more detail in Chapters 5 and 6. There are good reasons for ensuring that research is appropriately inclusive. For example, there may be differential outcomes for men and women (perhaps due to differing rates of metabolism of pharmaceuticals, or to different attitudes to psychological treatments). Imposing age limits in a research study needs careful consideration, both in terms of the interface between adolescent and adult services and whether in most instances an upper age limit is needed at all.

Ethnicity is being addressed within the Department of Health through pilot work on commissioning by the Policy Research Programme. The National Institute for Mental Health in England (NIMHE) initiative on black and ethnic minority research issues is also taking forward this agenda. The need for culturally sensitive services is already being reflected in research.

THE STATE OF MENTAL HEALTH RESEARCH AND DEVELOPMENT IN THE NHS

Mental health research and development has been assessed by a strategic review carried out in 2001/02 and by an analysis of annual R&D reports from NHS organisations carrying out research.

The strategic review of mental health research & development in the NHS (DoH 2002a)

Strategic reviews of NHS R&D in the Government priority areas of cancer, coronary heart disease and mental health were carried out in 2001/02 by the Research and Development Directorate at the

Department of Health. The Mental Health Review (DoH 2002a) was carried out over a seven month period and steered by an advisory group of experts including academics, policy advisors and mental health service users.

The objectives of the Strategic Review were:

- To assess current NHS R&D activity; to identify overlaps and gaps
- To consider the capacity and organisation of R&D in the NHS in terms of bridging these gaps and the possible need for further infrastructure development
- To contribute to the development of a longer-term strategy for research and development in mental health.

Although the Strategic Review was predominantly of research on 'adults of working age', data were collected on research relating to children and older people.

The Strategic Review comprised a number of related elements:

- An assessment of mental health research in the NHS, mapping research against the priorities set out in the *National service framework for mental health* and *NHS plan*
- A review of priorities from a service-user perspective by means of a panel
- A survey of research in social services departments across the country
- An overview of international mental health research using bibliometrics.

Key findings from the assessment of mental health research activity:

- Although there was evidence of some large-scale activity with more than 30 major externally funded research units, centres and programmes, there were relatively few large-scale projects in progress
- There was significant evidence of partnership working between NHS R&D providers, and with UK and international universities
- Randomised controlled trials were few (just over 30 at that time)
- Almost half the projects registered on the National Research Register (a register of current research funded by the Department of Health and voluntarily by some other funders) had no external funding and were very small in scale
- There was a lack of systematic reviews of research evidence
- There was a lack of critical mass of expertise in many R&D providers carrying out mental health research

- In terms of potential, more than 3000 NHS staff were active in mental health research, and of these 1000 were working towards a higher degree (mostly at masters level)
- There was little research carried out within social services departments
- There was a lack of funding sources for mental health research. The main funders were the Department of Health, the Medical Research Council, and the Wellcome Trust
- There were a number of significant gaps relating to the *National service framework for mental health*: substantive and focused work on mental health promotion, research on access to care, and on the types of services needed to support carers.

Mental health research outputs from 15 countries

This work was commissioned from the City University School of Informatics and consisted of an analysis of research papers in mental health in the Science Citation Index and the Social Sciences Citation Index from 1996 to 2000. It concentrated on 15 OECD countries, of which 12 were in Europe (Lewison and Wilcox-Jay 2002). Over 63,000 papers were included in the analysis.

Key findings
- Mental health research has grown by 2% per year, more slowly than biomedical research in general. The USA accounts for 47% of the output and the UK for 12%.
- In terms of potential impact, UK outputs were above the world average in terms of citations, and more clinically orientated than the outputs from the USA and most other countries.
- For the UK the strongest areas were primary health care, learning disability, evidence-based practice and forensic mental health. The UK was weakest in outputs on substance misuse, user involvement and dual diagnosis.
- A correlation of outputs on suicide prevention with suicide rates in each of the countries included in the analysis indicated that the UK outputs reflected the rates of suicide in the UK.

The development of NHS R&D programmes in mental health

NHS Trusts and other NHS organisations carrying out research are now required to describe their research in terms of programmes. Each programme consists of linked projects around a coherent theme. It is expected that programmes would have a mixed economy of funding from external sources as well as from the Department of Health. Programmes are assessed for their strength and relevance to national priorities.

Of the 1522 R&D programmes described in the Annual Reports for 2002/03, 154 were related to mental health. These came from 49 NHS R&D providers; an average of 3 programmes per provider. The largest number of mental health programmes was 21 from one specialist mental health trust. Sixty eight per cent of programmes were rated as strong. In comparison with the previous year, there is clear improvement in the quality of the programmes of work but still a need for organisations involved in small scale research to develop critical mass by collaboration. Programmes were mapped against the seven standards of the *National service framework for mental health*, and demonstrated a clear need for more high quality research relevant to mental health promotion, primary care, access to services, services to support carers and suicide. More focused research is needed on issues relating to black and ethnic minority groups, and to women's service needs. Future research should include social care and involve service users and carers at all stages in the research process.

CURRENT PRIORITIES FOR MENTAL HEALTH RESEARCH

Two policy documents are the starting point for setting mental health research priorities: the *National service framework for mental health* (DoH 1999a) and the *NHS plan* (DoH 2000b).

The *National Service Framework for Mental Health* makes a number of commitments to research:

> *'Department of Health investment in mental health R&D will focus on the knowledge base required to implement the National Service Framework.'*

Priorities for research into the organisation and delivery of services include:

- The individual and collective performance of the component parts of the National Service Framework
- Investigating variations in the use of in-patient beds, and their implications
- The management of co-morbidity, and the interface between primary care, specialist mental health services and substance abuse services

- Ways to enhance staff morale, retention, recruitment and performance.

In terms of clinical interventions, the following are all given high priority:

- Evaluating the effectiveness and cost-effectiveness under usual service conditions of psychological and psychosocial interventions
- Comparing the outcomes for self-harm between different types of services
- Assessing relative cost-effectiveness, service-user satisfaction and concordance rates of atypical antipsychotic drugs, newer antidepressants, and complementary therapies, compared to standard management.

Service-user satisfaction is regarded as an important outcome measure. The management of severe personality disorder is also highlighted as a research topic.

Service-user involvement in research is a theme that cross cuts the research priorities. In particular, importance is attached to the need to use outcome measures that are meaningful to service users, such as occupational activities, enhancement of self-esteem and views on the services that they use.

The *NHS plan* (DoH 2000b) presented as 'a plan for investment, a plan for reform', included a number of objectives to change the delivery of health services in England. A commitment was given in the NHS Plan to developing a strong set of national research and development programmes.

In the *NHS plan*, mental health was identified as one of the clinical priorities and modernising mental health services as one of a number of Government priorities. Particular recommendations for mental health within the *NHS plan* included:

- A proposal for 1000 new graduate primary care mental health workers
- Additional early intervention teams to reduce the period of untreated psychosis
- New crisis resolution teams
- More aggressive outreach services
- Redesign of services for women
- Improved support for carers
- Further investment in secure psychiatric and prison services.

There was also an undertaking that this significant agenda would be supported by a coherent research and development programme. Since then a number of other policy documents have been published relevant to the development of the mental health research agenda. These are summarised in Table 9.2.

Early work on the research agenda

The Mental Health National Service Framework (DoH 1999a) referenced the output of a series of working groups set up to support its development. The report of these groups in June 1999 outlined a number of research priorities, which were reflected in the Framework (see Table 9.3).

Some concern had been expressed about the strength of the evidence base for both the *National service framework for mental health* and *NHS plan*. It was important to commission work as early as possible to examine how available research findings could contribute to the evidence base and to highlight robust emerging themes which would assist in the implementation of the NSF.

A series of workshops were held during 2000/02 with key experts to explore the evidence base in specific areas: assertive outreach, suicide prevention, severe personality disorders and the management of sex offenders. These workshops identified issues for future research.

Early work commissioned included the *Scoping review of the effectiveness of mental health services* (Jepson *et al.* 2000) which linked the aims, recommendations and milestones of the *National service framework in mental health* with the results and conclusions of relevant systematic reviews. The focus of the review was on types and locations of care and care processes rather than therapeutic interventions.

Forty-two good-quality systematic reviews had been undertaken or were in preparation at that time, most reporting that the quality of the primary research was poor. The majority of the reviews related to people with severe mental illness and evaluated community-based interventions such as assertive community treatment and case management. The reviewers recommended that outcome measures such as users' social networks, user and carer satisfaction with services, social relationships and quality of life should be incorporated into future systematic reviews and primary research.

The reviewers found that many health service interventions had not been addressed in published systematic reviews; in particular, reduction of social stigma associated with mental illness, more accurate diagnosis

Table 9.2   Mental health policy documents with references to research priorities

The mental health policy implementation guide (DoH 2001b) supports the implementation and delivery of the three principal new service models – early intervention in psychosis, assertive outreach and crisis resolution. Supplementary documentation aimed at providing a framework for staff to develop services in partnership with service users has been subsequently produced, some of which highlight the lack of research in particular areas and the urgent need for research to be commissioned or the improvement in research in a particular area through dedicated funding (DoH 2002b).

Standard 7 of the *National service framework for older people* (DoH 2001c) incorporates a research strategy for older people including targeted research funding to identify gaps in knowledge about health and social care services for mental health problems concerning older people.

Changing the outlook: a strategy for developing and modernising mental health services in prison (DoH 2001d) sets out a joint Department of Health and Prison Service approach to modernisation and reform achieved through mental health in-reach services requiring monitoring and evaluation at a national level. As many as 90% of prisoners have a mental illness, substance abuse or both which can contribute to re-offending and social exclusion (Brooker *et al.* 2003).

A sign of the times: modernising mental health services for people who are deaf (DoH 2002c) considers the needs of an estimated 50,000 to 75,000 people in England and highlights the need for research in areas of effectiveness of early diagnosis in preventing mental illness in deaf children, risk assessment and management, incidence of suicide, service-user involvement and advocacy. It also recommends research to identify the number of prisoners who are deaf and their mental health needs in order to ascertain the best ways of providing in-reach services.

The national suicide prevention strategy for England (DoH 2002d) supports the target of reducing the death rate by suicide by at least 20% by 2010 through six goals including the promotion of research (DoH 1999b). The National Institute for Mental Health in England is now taking the strategy forward and the first annual report demonstrates good progress in commissioning the necessary research.

There are clear gender differences in mental illness with anxiety, depression and eating disorders more common in women. The report *Women's mental health: into the mainstream* (DoH 2002e) forms part of the Government's strategic development of mental health care for women. The report outlines mental health provision for specific groups of women suffering from mental illness including women offenders and highlights gender as an essential dimension in research to develop a better understanding of the difference in the mental ill health of women and men.

Table 9.2   Continued

Mental illness can have a major impact on carers, families and friends as well as the person affected by the illness. Despite a lack of evidence to support the effectiveness of any carer support service, positive outcomes have been associated with the provision of these services. *Developing services for carers and families of people with mental illness* (DoH 2002f) provides guidance on the development and maintenance of mental health carer support services. The need to have measures to assess the impact and effectiveness of services and the involvement of carers in the evaluation process is fundamental, and a programme of research was commissioned during 2002.

Mental health problems are common in primary care with about 40% of people attending a primary care practitioner having a significant mental health issue. *Primary care mental health programme* (National Institute for Mental Health in England 2003) sets out a programme for primary care mental health which will help practitioners improve the fundamentals of care and facilitate innovative practices in line with primary care standards 1 and 2 of the *National service framework for mental health*. The collation, development and prioritisation of emerging research themes from within the programme is seen as necessary to develop the potential of primary care mental health research fully and this will be done within the infrastructure of NIMHE's Mental Health Research Network.

Personality disorder: no longer a diagnosis of exclusion (DoH 2003a) highlights the need for more research into therapeutic interventions for this client group. In forensic services the development of pilot personality disorder centres will provide a focus for research into effective interventions.

Research on service evaluation and organisational change in mental health has, by and large, ignored ethnic and cultural dimensions and the report *Inside outside: improving mental health services for black and minority ethnic communities in England* (DoH 2003b) highlights a need to enhance the cultural relevance of research and development. This will be done by the development of appropriate research methodology for use with black and ethnic minority groups and improvement in research governance in relation to ethnicity and cultural diversity. The inclusion of an ethnic or cultural component in all future mental health research will be vital to make outcomes relevant to a multicultural society.

---

and assessment of common mental health problems, interventions within hospital settings, 24-hour staffed accommodation, more accurate assessment of risk of harm (to self or others) and interventions to support carers.

Since the Department of Health NHS R&D programme was started in 1991, a large number of mental health related studies have been commissioned. In a series of reports from the PRiSM Group at the

Table 9.3   Research priorities identified in the National service framework for mental health based on the work of the mental health topic working groups

Service delivery and organisation

- Evaluating the individual and collective performance of the component parts of the NSF
- Investigating variations in the use of in-patient beds and their implications
- Investigating ways to enhance staff morale, retention, recruitment and performance, and improve service-user engagement and outcomes

Clinical and practice interventions

- Evaluating the effectiveness and cost-effectiveness under usual service conditions of psychological and psycho-social interventions
- Comparing the outcomes of self-harm between different types of services
- Assessing relative cost-effectiveness, service-user satisfaction and concordance rates of
  - Atypical antipsychotic drugs
  - New antidepressants
  - Complementary therapies compared to standard management
- Evaluating the better management of antisocial attitudes and behaviour which attract the definition of severe personality disorder

Service user involvement

- Developing and evaluating a range of occupational activities to maximise social participation, enhance self-esteem and improve clinical outcomes
- Developing research tools with service users to assess their view on how services can best meet their needs

Source: National Service Framework for Mental Health (DoH 1999a).

Institute of Psychiatry, this work was analysed and summarised and the content reviewed in relation to the *National service framework for mental health*. Gaps in research coverage were identified and translated into researchable questions (Thornicroft *et al.* 2002).

An area of particular concern was in-patient care. The available literature demonstrated a lack of clarity about the purpose of psychiatric admission, the process of admission, therapeutic interventions in the in-patient setting and thresholds for using psychiatric intensive care services. The report *In-patient care for mental health problems; a review of research and identification of researchable questions* (Gournay 2001) highlighted the paucity of even reasonable quality research into in-patient care. Researchable questions were identified under a number of themes:

- Race, culture and ethnicity
- Supplements and alternatives to in-patient care
- Costs of in-patient care
- Therapeutic interventions
- Psychiatric intensive care
- Suicide
- Violence
- Dual diagnosis.

The Department of Health Policy Research Programme commissioned five scoping reviews to report on the current state of research and to identify the most urgent gaps with respect to the NSF and NHS Plan. Expert briefings based on the reviews were launched at the NIMHE conference in 2003 (DoH Policy Research Programme and National Institute for Mental Health in England, 2003):

- Early intervention for people with psychosis
- Employment for people with mental health problems
- Post-qualification mental health training
- Self-help interventions for mental health problems
- Women-only and women-sensitive mental health services.

The Department of Health Service Delivery and Organisation Programme responded to the research recommendations in the *National service framework for mental health* by commissioning reviews on services to support carers of people with mental health problems (Arksey *et al.* 2002) and continuity of care for people with severe mental illness' (Freeman *et al.* 2001).

Recommendations from service users
As part of the Strategic Review, a panel of service users with experience of mental health research (either as academic researchers or as participants) considered current mental health research priorities and made recommendations about future priorities.

The panel commented on the current research agenda and made suggestions for new research areas (DoH 2002a). These are summarised next.

The current research agenda:

- The panel challenged the setting of research priorities wholly on the basis of existing government policy. This was seen as unduly restrictive.

- Discussion of research priorities by service users should not be confined to defining topics for study but ought to include the research process and the role of users in it. Service users should be empowered to participate fully in the research process and carry out their own research.
- Issues of race and culture were inadequately addressed.
- Approaches to research should be more holistic in scope, researching the overall well-being of service users, and outcome measures capturing social, economic, cultural, financial and housing issues should be incorporated.
- Research should extend beyond the NHS to social care and have a focus on the joining up of different policy areas.
- Much good research is not published in mainstream academic journals, but in the so-called 'grey literature'. This literature should be included in reviewing evidence from mental health research.
- Current mental health research is predominantly based on a 'medical' model of mental health problems. This distracts from the broader social, economic, political and cultural issues in understanding madness and distress.
- The existing research identifies self-help as a priority; it would be appropriate to recast this in terms of self-management emphasising the importance of mental health service users having control over the support that they receive.
- There was a strong challenge to the assumption 'that sexual offences were a form of, or expression of, mental illness or distress'.

Service user priorities:

- A developmental approach to research funding and priority setting so that service users and their organisations could be fully involved and be able to participate on equal terms with researchers in all stages of the research process. Research into the blockers and drivers for user involvement should also be included.
- Funding and development of user-controlled and emancipatory research.
- Issues of discrimination and bias in relation to culture and race.
- Research into social inclusion rather than a focus on symptoms and symptom management.
- Routine use of user-defined outcome measures.
- Research on broader public policy which impacts on people with mental health problems and which may increase or reduce the risk of

people developing mental health problems. Examples included the effects of social security benefits policies.

- Research on positive risk management and how this may promote more holistic approaches to the well-being of people suffering from mental distress; a shift of focus from the delivery of services to the interests of service users.
- Research on user-controlled or user-led services exploring non-medicalised, complementary forms of support and assistance.
- Research to identify the scale of the problem of abuse of mental health service users: this includes race issues and issues relating to the inappropriate prescribing of drugs.
- Research to explore the assumption that violence is a consequence of madness and mental distress.
- Research that learns from positive initiatives to support other groups of service users such as people with learning disabilities or disabled people.

An action plan for mental health research

Previous sections have indicated the need for an 'action plan' for mental health research as promised in the *National service framework for mental health*. One thing is clear: there is no shortage of ideas and topics. To date the action plan has been developed, as described above, by analysis of policy documents, commissioning early reviews and scoping reports and following through the research needs identified. The current action plan is summarised in Table 9.4, and the full list of projects completed, in progress and being planned is regularly updated on the Department of Health website.

The future

An 'action plan' cannot be static. Two pieces of work are planned to develop the mental health research landscape further. The first is an analysis of current mental health research in the UK based on a similar exercise undertaken for cancer (National Cancer Research Institute 2002). A dynamic database is being developed to capture mental health and social care research funded by the Medical Research Council, the Economic and Social Research Council, the Wellcome Trust, charitable sources and the various Department of Health programmes. The database will be available to the funders themselves, the research community and policy makers. It will assist with identifying gaps in research coverage to inform future research, and common and

Table 9.4   Action plan for mental health research 2003

Research priorities

Evaluation of clinical initiatives from the *NHS plan*
- Access into the mental health system
- Primary care mental health workers
- Early intervention in psychosis
- Assertive outreach
- Crisis resolution and home treatment for severe mental illness
- Support for carers of people with mental health problems

Other clinical priorities
- Evaluation of self-help initiatives
- Suicide prevention measures including mental health promotion in young men
- Use of nurse prescribing
- Management of personality disorders
  - Psychological therapies in borderline personality disorder
  - Child and adolescent precursors of personality disorder
- Management of dual diagnosis (substance misuse and mental health problems)
- Delivery of in-patient care
- Forensic mental health services
  - Pathways into forensic services
  - Treatment of sex offenders
- Mental health services for prisoners
- Mental health services for homeless people

Cross cutting themes
- Incorporating the views and priorities of service users and their carers in the research process
- Black and ethnic minority issues
- Gender issues
- Incorporation of occupational and other social outcome measures in research
- Intervention trials

Infrastructure

- Development and expansion of the Mental Health Research Network
- Development of research interest groups
- Mental Health Research Funders Group
- Mental Health Research Advisory Group of the NIMHE

complementary interests of research funders and researchers, to help avoid duplication of effort and enable partners to be identified. Research will be classified on a number of dimensions: from basic biology through aetiology to applied research, by specific mental health problems based on the DSM IV (American Psychiatric Association 1994), and by research setting (population-based, in-patient care, forensic etc).

The second piece of work being undertaken to develop the mental health R&D landscape is a forward look at priorities over the next five to ten years, to identify emerging themes. A number of recent workshops have begun this, but wider consultation is necessary to confirm themes and prioritise. As well as academics and policy makers, a key part of this consultation will be engaging with mental health service users, with carers of people with mental health problems, and with front-line staff. The topic-specific research groups of NIMHE's Mental Health Research Network (www.mhrn.info) will contribute to the process. The NIMHE Research Advisory Group, comprising many of those constituents in mental health R&D just mentioned, will take the lead in overseeing the conduct of this process. The output will be a plan of research priorities for the medium term which can be updated with emerging priorities. The objective is to build a solid base for mental health policy development in the future. In parallel with research development in the UK, systematic searches and reviews of research undertaken elsewhere will be needed to synthesise findings as they emerge.

Research commissioning

Having identified research priorities, commissioning is undertaken through the most appropriate Department of Health programmes described earlier. The Policy Research Programme commissions work of Government priority, but there is strong competition for funds. The Service Delivery and Organisation Programme has a fast track procedure for issues of high priority to the NHS. The Health Technology Assessment Programme has a process for setting priorities from the many research ideas suggested to it by its stakeholders. This can lead to a substantial delay in commissioning research, and a fast track procedure is being developed.

The Department of Health depends on other research funders to contribute to the development of the evidence base, and continued dialogue between funding bodies and the Department is important in bringing research priorities to the notice of funders. Although generally

Table 9.5 The Mental Health Research Network

The Mental Health Research Network

The National Institute of Mental Health in England (NIMHE, see Chapter 10) has, as one of its standing programmes, the Mental Health Research Network. The overall purpose of the network is:

To provide the infrastructure to support high-quality mental health and social care research, including randomised trials of interventions in mental health, large-scale effectiveness trials, studies of service organisation and delivery, and studies led by users of services and their carers.

The Network is led by a managing partnership from the Institute of Psychiatry in London and the University of Manchester. It started with five research hubs, based in South London, the North West, the West of England, the Midlands, and Eastern England. The intention is to add a further two hubs during 2004.

By improving the co-ordination of mental health research, it will be more timely, of better overall quality, and better integrated with social care. By widening participation in research, a more direct interest in research findings will be generated with direct knock-on effects on the quality of treatment and patient care.

The involvement of service users in research will be systematised in the network placing their needs firmly at the centre of the research agenda. A service-user hub (SURGE) is part of the network structure.

operating in response mode, continuing advocacy for the need for mental health research can help to improve the chances of successful applications in difficult areas of research. The Mental Health Research Network is particularly helpful in this regard as a platform for large-scale research (Table 9.5).

Disseminating the results of research

The process of scientific enquiry is non-linear and the process of getting research results into practice far from straightforward. Research moves through a process of accumulating results until there is sufficient evidence to be confident of a research finding. Thus, a single study is rarely sufficient to justify a change in treatment or service organisation. Syntheses of research findings are critical to identifying a sufficient weight of evidence and development of the Cochrane Collaboration was a milestone in this regard. Likewise, the National Institute for Clinical

Table 9.6 NICE and mental health

Technology appraisals – completed

No.	Title	Publication date
19	Alzheimer's disease – donepezil, rivastigmine and galantamine	January 2001
13	Attention deficit hyperactivity disorder (ADHD) – methylphenidate	October 2000
66	Bi-polar disorder – new drugs	September 2003
51	Depression and anxiety – computerised cognitive behaviour therapy	October 2002
59	ECT – Electroconvulsive therapy	April 2003
43	Schizophrenia – atypical antipsychotics	June 2002

Technology appraisals – in progress

Title	Anticipated publication date
Alzheimer's disease (mild to moderate) – donepezil, rivastigmine and galantamine	May 2005
Alzheimer's disease (moderate to severe) – memantine	May 2005
Conduct disorder in children, parent - training/ education programmes	To be confirmed
Dementia (non-Alzheimer) – New pharmaceutical treatments	May 2005

Excellence (NICE) set up to ensure equality of standards of care across the country both in terms of technology assessments and guidelines has had a major impact on getting research results into practice.

Other developments such as the National Electronic Library for Health and the discipline of knowledge management will also make an impact but there is some way to go. NIMHE's regional development centres have a central role to play in bridging the worlds of research and development in mental health.

Table 9.6 Continued	
Guidelines – completed	
Ref Title	Publication (or issue) date
CG1 Schizophrenia: core interventions in the treatment and management of schizophrenia in primary and secondary care	December 2002
CG9 Eating disorders	January 2004
CG16 Self Harm	July 2004
CG22 Anxiety (generalised)	December 2004
CG23 Depression	December 2004
Guidelines – in progress	
Title	Anticipated publication date
Bipolar disorder	June 2006
Dementia	February 2007
Depression in children	August 2005
Disturbed (violent) behaviour	February 2005
Obsessive compulsive disorder (OCD)	September 2005
Post-traumatic Stress Disorder (PTSD)	March 2005

CONCLUSIONS

The increase in the quantum of mental health research of direct relevance to policy has happened relatively quickly in Britain. The priority given by the Government to improving services for people with mental health problems has led directly to the need for timely and focused research. By facilitating a regular dialogue between policy makers, bodies that fund research, academics, front-line staff and service users and their carers, together with important developments in infrastructure, it is proving possible to bring to bear the ideas of the research community on the management of these difficult and sometimes intractable problems.

A more co-operative and less competitive relationship between researchers in what is a relatively small field is proving advantageous in developing more timely and larger scale mental health research. There is still much to do; there is no shortage of ideas for the future, and there are some immediate priorities that have not yet been addressed. Taking a longer view of research priorities, and particularly addressing issues that are important to sufferers from mental health problems, will help to inform future policy. Success will be measurable by seeing research reflected in good practice through the development and implementation of guidelines and the improvement of services across the spectrum of settings. Prevention of mental health problems is the ultimate aim, and this will involve co-operation and close working between all the relevant agencies. In research terms this is particularly difficult and requires cross-disciplinary collaboration. That is the next challenge.

References

American Psychiatric Association. (1994). *Diagnostic and statistical manual of mental disorders* (4th edition). American Psychiatric Association, Washington DC.

Arksey, H., O'Malley, L., Baldwin, S. *et al.* (2002). Overview report: services to support carers of people with mental health problems. Report to Service Delivery and Organisation Programme, London. Online. Available: www.sdo.lshtm.ac.uk/

Arksey, H., O'Malley, L., Baldwin, S. and Harris, J. (2002). Literature review: services to support carers of people with mental health problems. Report to Service Delivery and Organisation Programme. Online. Available: www.sdo.lshtm.ac.uk/mentalhealthcarers.htm

Bailey, S., Carpenter, J., Dickinson, C. and Rogers, H. (2002). Expert Paper on Post-qualifying mental health training. Report to Policy Research Programme. Online. Available: www.socialresearch.bham.ac.uk

Barnes, M., Davis, A., Guru, S. *et al.* (2002). Women-only and women-sensitive mental health services: an expert paper. Report to Policy Research Programme. Online. Available: www.socialresearch.bham.ac.uk

Brooker, C., Repper, J., Beverley, C. *et al.* (2003). *Mental health services and prisoners: a review.* Online. Available www.dh.gov.uk/PublicationsAndStatistics

Croudace, T., Jones, P., Kritzinger, R. *et al.* (2003). *Early diagnosis of schizophrenia and other psychoses: an assembly of evidence (to year end 2002) in support of indicated prevention research.* Report to Policy Research Programme. Department of Health, London.

Department of Health. (1999a). *National service framework for mental health: modern standards and service models.* Online. Available: www.doh.gov.uk/nsf/mentalhealth.htm

Department of Health. (1999b). *Saving lives: Our healthier nation.* HMSO. Online. Available: www.doh.gov.uk/ohn.htm

Department of Health. (1999c). Mental Health Topic Working Group. Final Report. Online. Available: www.doh.gov.uk/research/re3/clarkereport/srsg.htm

Department of Health. (2000a). *Research and development for a first class service: R&D in the new NHS.* Online. Available: www.doh.gov.uk/research/rd3/nhsrandd/newfunding.

Department of Health. (2000b). *The NHS plan. A plan for investment, a plan for reform.* The Stationary Office. Online. Available: www.doh.gov.uk/nhsplan

Department of Health. (2001a) *Research governance framework for health and social care.* Online. Available: www.doh.gov.uk/

Department of Health. (2001b). *The mental health policy implementation guide.* Online. Available: www.doh.gov.uk/mentalhealth/implementationguide.htm

Department of Health. (2001c). *The national service framework for older people.* Online. Available: www.doh.gov.uk/nsf/olderpeople/docs.htm

Department of Health. (2001d). *Changing the outlook: a strategy for developing and modernising mental health services in prison.* Online. Available: www.doh.gov.uk/prisonhealth/mhstrategy.htm

Department of Health. (2002a). *Strategic review of mental health research and development in the NHS.* Online. Available: www.doh.gov.uk/research/documents/mhfinalreportc.pdf

Department of Health. (2002b). *Mental health policy implementation guide: adult acute in-patient care provision and dual diagnosis.* Online. Available: www.doh.gov.uk/mentalhealth/dualdiagnosis.htm

Department of Health. (2002c). *A sign of the times: modernising mental health services for people who are deaf.* Online. Available: www.doh.gov.uk/mentalhealth/signofthetimes.htm

Department of Health. (2002d). *National suicide prevention strategy for England.* Online. Available: www.doh.gov.uk/mentalhealth/suicideprevention.htm

Department of Health. (2002e). *Women's mental health: into the mainstream.* Online. Available: www.doh.gov.uk/mentalhealth/women.htm

Department of Health. (2002f). *Developing services for carers and families of people with mental illness.* Online. Available: www.doh.gov.uk/mentalhealth/devservcarers.htm

Department of Health Policy Research Programme & National Institute for Mental Health in England. (2003). *Expert briefings in mental health.* Online. Available: www.nimhe.org.uk/expertbriefings

Department of Health. (2003a). *Personality disorder: no longer a diagnosis of exclusion.* Online. Available: www.doh.gov.uk/mentalhealth/personalitydisorder.htm

Department of Health. (2003b). *Inside outside: improving mental health services for black and minority ethnic communities in England.* Online. Available: www.doh.gov.uk/mentalhealth/improvingmh.htm

Freeman, G., Crawford, M., Weaver, T., Low, J. and de Jonge, E. (2001). *Promoting continuity of care for people with severe mental illness whose needs span primary, secondary and social care. A multi-method investigation of relevant mechanisms and contexts.* Report to Service Delivery and Organisation Programme, www.sdo.lshtm.ac.uk/continuityofcare.htm

Gournay, K. (2001). Inpatient care for mental health problems: a review of research and identification of researchable questions. Report to the Department of Health, London.

Jepson, R. *et al.* Scoping Review of the Effectiveness of Mental Health Services. NHS Centre for Reviews and Dissemination, University of York. Report No 21.ISBN 1 900640 19 8.

Lewis, G., Anderson, L., Araya, R., Elgie, R., Harrison, G., Proudfoot, J., Schmidt, U., Sharp, D., Weightman, A. and Williams, C. (2003). *Self-help interventions for mental health problems.* Report to Policy Research Programme.

Lewison, G. and Wilcox-Jay, K. (2002). *Research outputs of mental health from 15 countries.* www.doh.gov.uk/research/documents/mhfinalappendicesc.pdf

Marshall, M., Lewis, S., Lockwood, A., Drake, R., Jones, P. and Croudace, T. (2003). *Systematic review of the relationship between duration of untreated psychosis and outcome.* Report to Policy Research Programme.

Marshall, M. and Lockwood, A. (2003). *A systematic review of the effectiveness of early intervention in psychosis.* Report to Policy Research Programme.

Marshall, M., Lockwood, L., Lewis, S. and Fiander, M. (2003). *Essential elements of an early intervention service – the opinion of expert clinicians.* Report to Policy Research Programme.

National Institute for Mental Health in England. (2003). Primary Care Mental Health Programme – Consultation document. Online. Available: www.nimhe.org.uk/priorities/primarycare.asp

National Cancer Research Institute. (2002). *Strategic analysis of cancer research.* Online. Available: www.ncri.org.uk

NHS Service Delivery and Organisation Programme. Continuity of care for people with severe mental illness. SDO Briefing paper 2002. www.sdo.lshtm.ac.uk/continuityofcare.htm

NHS Service Delivery and Organisation Programme. Services to support carers of people with mental health problems. SDO Briefing paper. 2002. www.sdo.lshtm.ac.uk/mentalhealthcarers.htm

Newbronner, E., Hare, P. and Acton-Shapiro. (2002). *Consultation report: services to support carers of people with mental health problems.* Report to

Service Delivery and Organisation Programme, www.sdo.lshtm.ac.uk/
mentalhealthcarers.htm

Schneider, J., Heyman, A. and Turton, N. (2002). *Occupational outcomes: from evidence to implementation.* Report to Policy Research Programme. (Abridged version at www.dur.ac.uk/CASS/Research/papers/ET%20abridged.pdf)

Thornicroft, G., Bindman, J., Goldberg, K., Gournay, K. and Huxley, P. (2002). Researchable questions to support evidence-based mental health policy concerning adult mental illness. *Psychiatric Bulletin*, **26**, 364–7.

10

Mental health in the mainstream: a localised implementation strategy in development

Antony Sheehan and Ingrid Steele

INTRODUCTION

The present government has placed mental health as one of its top three clinical priorities; alongside cancer and coronary heart disease (DoH 2002). A major modernisation agenda was heralded by the White Paper, *Safe, sound and supportive – modernising mental health services* in 1998, followed up by a long-awaited *National service framework for mental health* (DoH 1999a). The *National service framework for mental health* described the nature of services that should be delivered through a series of seven standards to be achieved over a ten year timescale. The *NHS plan* (DoH 2000a) then set out a number of specific targets promising, for example, 220 assertive outreach teams and 335 crisis resolution teams by 2004. Implementation guidance designed to provide leadership and direction, which was issued in 2001, described in some detail what the new teams and services should look like.

This very specific – and prescriptive – policy framework was accompanied by implementation arrangements at local level which were designed to facilitate collaboration, by the many players whose involvement would be required to turn the national vision into local reality. The chosen vehicle, Local Implementation Teams (LITs) were each faced with an enormous programme of similar tasks, for which they had little relevant experience and no external support. In describing the purpose of the National Institute for Mental Health in England (NIMHE), we will outline the structures and the thinking that underpin its establishment and function.

REASONS FOR NIMHE

During the first half of 2001, discussions took place within the Department of Health about the need for a robust structure to deliver policy into practice. The vehicle through which this aspiration was to be delivered was though a national institute.

The establishment of a National Institute of Mental Health for England (NIMHE), it was suggested, would provide a unique opportunity to implement positive change in mental health and mental health services in line with the evidence base. In the quest for the search for the evidence, NIMHE's role was to bring together the research, development and dissemination functions, and develop effective partnerships between agencies, service users, carers, professionals and managers. NIMHE would be a focal point for driving through the changes for mental health across primary and secondary care services set out in the *National Service Framework for mental health* and the *NHS plan*. NIMHE was born.

John Hutton, then Minister of State for Health, agreed in early May 2001 to the establishment of NIMHE, following which a project team was established, including health and social care staff, service users and communications expertise, in order to consult on NIMHE's priorities and how it would be organised. The group also project managed the establishment of NIMHE.

It was agreed that NIMHE should cover the whole field of mental health in primary, secondary and tertiary care, and of services for people of all ages. Bringing the whole of mental health under one umbrella would, it was contended, result in greater collaboration and challenge some of the boundaries which limit the provision of effective care (for example, exploring boundary and transition issues between adolescent and adult mental health services). It was envisaged that this would also provide an impetus to research and development in under-developed areas, such as forensic services, dangerous and severe personality disorder and prison mental health services.

During the early summer of 2001, work proceeded to establish NIMHE, including agreement of a budget, management structure and initial work programme, as well as the role of NIMHE in relation to other organisations. In May, a stakeholder conference was held to develop the consensus on the role and structure of the new organisation further.

VALUES AND PRINCIPLES

The values and principles to guide the work of NIMHE set out to challenge negative public attitudes and behaviour and to involve service users, their family members and carers, and professionals.
NIMHE values services which:

- Promote a better quality of life for people who experience mental distress, service users, their families, and the whole community
- Involve service users and their carers in the planning and delivery of their work
- Draw on both service-user experience and existing good practice
- Recognise the diversity of the communities they serve including race, culture and gender values
- Are accessible so that help can be obtained when and where it is needed
- Promote the safety of service users and carers, staff and the wider public
- Support the development of services and research that offer choices
- In turn value, empower and support mental health service staff.

NIMHE will seek to ensure that:

- Mental health services improve outcomes for service users and their families and carers
- The Institute's work learns from all perspectives, both inside and outside the current mental health service system
- The Institute's work is well co-ordinated between all staff and agencies
- Research is of high priority, co-ordinated and timely to inform both policy and practice development
- The Institute makes best use of research findings
- The Institute promotes the delivery of continuity of care for as long as this is needed
- The Institute is properly accountable to the public, service users and carers.

SETTING UP THE INSTITUTE

The project team focused on the establishment of a small central hub and the eight regional development centres, with government office co-terminous boundaries. Initial tasks included a programme of detailed consultation with potential partners and consumers of the services of NIMHE.

NIMHE was launched at a time when services were taking stock and preparing to implement the proposals in the *NHS plan*. Most new investment was not due until the following financial year, and professionals in the field, service users and their carers were anticipating not only significant development and the resources to deliver the change required, but also development support in order that implementation could be taken forward. The announcement of NIMHE was seen as a significant aspect of this preparatory year, and was intended as a clear statement of the priority ministers were affording to mental health.

Between November 2001 and January 2002, the NIMHE project team consulted on what should be the precise role and purpose of the Institute.

As a result of the consultation, a first series of national programmes were chosen, and a final set of work programme ideas were worked up by the project team and agreed by NIMHE Chief Executive, Antony Sheehan; National Director, Louis Appleby; and then Health Minister, Jacqui Smith.

PLACE IN MODERNISATION AGENCY

As part of the Modernisation Agency, NIMHE is accountable to the Department of Health and to ministers. Within the agency, NIMHE takes lead responsibility for mental health programmes and thus has a key role in the future development of mental health services. NIMHE works in close collaboration with the overall programme of the Modernisation Agency – for example, its clinical governance and leadership programmes.

NIMHE'S MISSION

The Institute's mission is:

> ... *to improve the quality of life for people of all ages who experience mental distress.*

Supplementary description

Working beyond the NHS, we help all those involved in mental health to implement change, providing a gateway to learning and development, offering new opportunities to share experiences and one place to find information. Through NIMHE's development centres and programmes of work, we will support staff to put policy into practice and offer help to resolve local challenges in developing mental health.

To achieve these aims, service users, families and communities will be at the heart of all our work. We will embrace diversity, champion achievements, help to break down bureaucracy and promote flexible ways of working. NIMHE is forging new partnerships at a national and international level. We will take a lead in connecting mental health research, development, delivery, monitoring and review.

CONNECTING POLICY, DELIVERY AND IMPLEMENTATION

A unique situation for mental health vis-à-vis other condition areas has been achieved through linking together mental health policy and performance, legislation and NIMHE. This has enabled a coherent way of working across policy development to implementation support.

NIMHE AREAS OF ACTIVITY

Within NMHE there are four key areas of activity:

- Eight development centres, the 'engine rooms' of NIMHE, provide the main point of contact with people who provide and use mental health services, to share experiences and find effective solutions that work in practice.
- A mental health research network, led by the University of Manchester and Institute of Psychiatry as the managing partnership, classified as a standing programme of NIMHE to support high-quality mental health and social care research studies.
- A wide range of other work programmes, to create new collaborative partnerships and action at national level, which will help staff in local services to deliver change such as improving access and choice,

acute in-patient care, primary care, suicide prevention, equalities and the mental health workforce.
- A small central hub, based in Leeds, with responsibility for a number of core work programmes, central business management functions, national liaison, communications (including positive practice) and knowledge management.

THE DEVELOPMENT CENTRES

By 2003, eight development centres had been established to support strategic health authorities, local authorities, NHS trusts and local implementation teams with their NHS Plan and NSF implementation responsibilities. The development centres do this in a number of ways.

Learning sets and networks bring together groups of people with a common interest to share experience, support positive practice and explore innovative approaches to service development and how the wider community is engaged in improving mental health. Information about positive practice, research evidence, policy issues and local opinion is gathered and disseminated. Training and education priorities are influenced on the basis of aggregated information, and some small-scale training programmes are provided.

Local stakeholders are involved in the conception, prioritisation, delivery and monitoring of programmes, through networks and communications systems. Local leadership is developed through leadership programmes, through facilitating fellowships and through secondments.

Most development centres have a broadly representative 'stakeholder' group – these are relatively large and tend to meet quarterly. Some also have a smaller 'management' group made up of a subset of the membership of the larger group. These arrangements for local governance have been found to work quite well, and the lack of formal prescription from the centre about how they should be established has helped to secure local ownership.

There is some ambiguity about the personal accountability of the development centre directors. Typically, they answer in varying degrees to the chair of the 'stakeholder' (and/or 'management' group), the Chief Executive of their 'host' organisation and the Chief Executive of NIMHE.

There are some potential tensions about the balance of time that development centres spend on local work (which keeps local stakeholders on board and helps raise NIMHE's profile locally) and NIMHE's national work.

NIMHE AND RESEARCH

The Mental health research network

Concern about a lack of capacity in mental health research was a key driver in the gestation of NIMHE. It was argued that mental health service-based research had been relatively poorly co-ordinated, lacked coherence and had often failed to inform policy or practice in a timely or effective manner. Problems facing clinical services had only been slowly translated into research priorities, studies were often too small to produce generalisable results, and rival institutions could be reluctant to collaborate on major studies.

Even when a clinical problem led to useful research findings, dissemination and the development of good practice and training resources had been inconsistent, with the result that policy was sometimes poorly implemented and clinical services lacked coherence and consistency.

NIMHE, it was argued, would address these problems, and by working in conjunction with organisations such as the Workforce Action Team and Modernisation Agency, bring a co-ordinated approach. NIMHE would inform priority setting for relevant research, and would support dissemination and the growth of best practice through training programmes and the recruitment of respected clinicians to provide strong leadership.

The creation of NIMHE, with its strong research focus, confirms the priority that the government places on research in the reform of mental health services. Research has a central place in supporting the strategy set out in *Modernising mental health services* (Department of Health 1998), which initiated a radical programme to improve access to effective treatment and care, reduce unfair variation, raise standards, and provide quicker and more convenient services.

The Mental Health Research Network is a standing programme and the research arm of NIMHE. It is developing a managed network that brings together researchers and providers of mental health and social care services.

It is co-ordinated by a managing partnership comprising two leading academic centres – the Institute of Psychiatry and the University of

Manchester. They have responsibility, over time, to establish and maintain a network of research hubs, the first being North West and London, The Heart of England, Cambridgeshire and Norfolk, and a West Hub (covering part of the South West of England). The network will provide the infrastructure to support high-quality mental health and social care research, including randomised trials of interventions in mental health, large-scale effectiveness trials, studies of service organisation and delivery, and studies led by users of services and carers. The Network is led by a research director from one of the academic centres. Working within a framework set by NIMHE, the strategy of the Network is overseen by an advisory group which has service user, carer, professional, managerial and academic involvement as well as members from the constituent organisations of the network. A prioritised programme of research is shaped by NHS policy and is in line with the strategy set out by NIMHE.

The Mental Health Research Network has three key functions:

- To organise and deliver large-scale relevant research projects which inform policy or contribute to implementation strategies (and to contribute to an effective dissemination programme in partnership with NIMHE's regional development centres).
- To identify the research needs of the NHS and social care, working with users of the service and their carers.
- To develop research capacity, by service users and carers undertaking research programmes, and through the promotion of areas which have been neglected historically, such as social care, recovery, service-user-led and longitudinal research, and mental health promotion.

The Mental Health Research Network is also establishing a central role for service users and carers in the development and implementation of its programme, in which their personal experiences and use of services will shape and inform the work of the network. As well as ensuring high-quality, high-impact research the Network will promote the development of novel research methodologies (including both qualitative and quantitative methods). These methods will reflect the many contexts in which mental health care is provided and will address the diverse cultural needs of service users and carers.

NIMHE will liaise with the Department of Health research funding programmes (the Policy Research Programme, the Health Technology Assessment Programme and the Service Delivery and Organisation Programme) through the NHS Research & Development Portfolio

Director for Mental Health. The Director of the Managing Partnership of the network is also seeking support for research programmes and projects from the Medical Research Council the Wellcome Trust and other funders. The Mental Health Research Network should provide an attractive infrastructure that could attract substantial funding from the major research funders, both in the UK and internationally.

NIMHE'S NATIONAL PROGRAMMES

Health Minister, Jacqui Smith, launched NIMHE's first series of national programmes on 25 June 2002.

Primary care

To support the delivery of *NHS plan* commitments in primary care and mental health, is a joint NIMHE/Natpact programme, led by NIMHE West Midlands and London Development Centres. It is an ambitious programme of work, which has been widely consulted on, covering staff development, commissioning and developing effective partnerships, developing a primary care user perspective, integrated care and services, and R&D. A Primary Care Programme Board, chaired by Professor Andre Tylee, has been established and a CD-Rom to raise awareness about mental health has been circulated to 40,000 people. Trailblazers, a well-established leadership and change methodology, is already being delivered through some of NIMHE's development centres.

Community teams

To support the development of new community teams, such as assertive outreach, early intervention and home treatment programmes.

In addition to work led by NIMHE's development centres, the Sainsbury Centre for Mental Health national training programme is focusing on assertive outreach and crisis resolution and has four work streams:

- Team leaders
- Psychiatrist programme
- Regionally based training for whole team development
- 'Train the trainer' programme to help develop capacity locally and regionally.

Acute in-patient care

This programme was launched in April 2002 to implement acute in-patient care guidance. Over half of all adult acute wards in England now have a trust forum and lead consultant psychiatrist in place. Acute in-patient care targets have been incorporated into National Service Framework monitoring and service mapping, and a themed review of in-patient services has been completed and published. The Sainsbury Centre for Mental Health has been commissioned to undertake a benchmarking exercise of staffing levels in adult acute wards.

Practical guidelines on therapeutic working in acute wards are in development, led by Stephen Pereira, consultant psychiatrist at North East London Mental Health NHS Trust and honorary fellow of NIMHE.

Commissioned by NIMHE, Mentality have drafted *Not all in the mind*, a physical health needs resource for publication in 2003.

Substance misuse

A joint programme with the National Treatment Agency, the Opening Doors Programme began in October 2002 and has delivered improvements in priority areas of booking and choice, equalities, service-user experience and waiting times.

Thirty teams have taken part in the first wave of the programme, implementing improvements such as assessment procedures which reduce duplication, slicker referral and discharge protocols, better quality information for service users and carers, more flexible opening hours and more user-friendly shared care with GPs.

Suicide prevention

The suicide prevention strategy was implemented to meet the *Saving lives – our healthier nation* targets of reducing the number of suicides by one fifth by 2010 (Department of Health 1999b). Following the strategy's launch, the early focus has been on a few early deliverables to support implementation:

- Developing a toolkit to support standard seven of the National Service Framework (the prevention of suicides)
- Planning a new pilot aimed at reaching young men at risk of suicide
- Initial work to develop a support pack for people in contact with bereaved families
- Continued work, as part of the 'mind out' mental health promotion work, to promote responsible reporting of suicide in the media.

Equalities

This programme embraces mental health promotion, social inclusion and emerging work on black and minority ethnic mental health and women's mental health.

NIMHE has worked jointly with communications and public health in the Department of Health on the 'Mind Out' mental health promotion campaign. Joint plans for future sustained programmes of work are being developed using development centres and building further national collaboration.

NIMHE has also worked in partnership with the Social Exclusion Unit to support their work in mental health, and pilots to improve access, together with development sessions on social inclusion, have been provided to a number of development centres. The first phase of an action research and support programme for young people was completed in Liverpool.

Inside outside has been published, setting out the reform of mental health care for people from black and minority ethnic communities (NIMHE 2003a). Strong links with other initiatives, such as the 'Circles of Fear' project are being made and implementation programmes on black and minority ethnic communities and women have been developed.

Workforce

Workforce is an implementation-focused programme, working with the Changing Workforce Programme in the Modernisation Agency, human resources in the Department of Health, workforce development confederations, the NHS University and the Sainsbury Centre for Mental Health.

The Workforce Programme is developing its work and support under core priorities including:

- Strategic planning and workforce development
- Developing effective communications and knowledge management
- Supporting new roles into practice
- Recruitment and retention.

The Department of Health has commissioned training programmes on primary care and graduate workers.

National occupational standards for mental health were developed during 2002/03 and published in June 2003.

Intelligence in progress

This programme brings together performance management data into a meaningful picture of progress happening at a local level. Pennine NHS Trust is the programme lead and works closely with local services, NIMHE's development centres, organisations involved in dataset development and the new Commission for Health Audit and Inspection. They began their work formally this financial year (2003/04).

The work programmes use different approaches to create a dynamic to support change. The access, booking and choice, and substance misuse programmes, for example, have produced generic process design methodologies of process mapping and the 'PDSA cycle' (Plan Do Study Act). By contrast, the acute in-patient care programme has used the learning from a collaborative approach to create regional and local development networks.

The aim has been to develop a well-co-ordinated programme of work in each of the areas, which will promote consistency in improvement, share learning and reduce duplication. The programme should have a balance of 'bread and butter' and innovative, forward-looking activity, be both proactive and responsive, but have an early impact. It should also help to create an infrastructure for sustainable change and development support.

Shortly after the launch of these national programmes, an additional programme was added through liaison with the Modernisation Agency to give mental health access to the same support that acute care had received in recent years to support the re-engineering of local services.

Access, booking and choice (ABC)

This is a joint initiative with the Modernisation Agency's Booking Programme. One hundred and forty project teams (84% of Mental Health Trusts) from across the country participated in the first phase of the ABC programme and all NIMHE development centres are now skilled in process redesign tools and techniques. The second phase is continuing to support the 140 teams already taking part in the programme and is also working with new teams.

A *Redesigning mental health – access and choice service improvement guide*, to summarise progress to date, was published in June 2003 (NIMHE 2003b).

DEVOLVED AND UNITED

NIMHE has sought to become a federal organisation, 'devolved and united'. Each development centre is governed by local stakeholder arrangements and approaches its work with sensitivity to the local community's needs and expectations. NIMHE is governed by a national strategic partnership, with representation from all development centres (directors and chairs), service users and carers, and NIMHE Central.

NIMHE's central team is a group of peripatetic staff with a small base in Leeds, providing support across the organisation, including knowledge development and communications, cross cutting liaison and whole systems service redesign and development, plus corporate business and performance management.

The central team arrange national events to promote specific policy initiatives, consultations, or NIMHE programme areas. There is one annual national event CONNECTIONS, a two- to three-day event in June to report on progress in the delivery of mental health and share positive practice as widely as possible. About 400 people involved in mental health attend each day.

NIMHE PUBLICATIONS AND ONLINE KNOWLEDGE SHARING

Development centres and national programmes publish their own thematic and locally focused publications.

In addition, NIMHE publishes an annual review (published in June), positive practice, research and other evidence-based materials, and work programme materials (published via hard copy and electronic media).

NIMHE (www.nimhe.org.uk), helps to raise awareness and share the learning from regions and work programmes. A delivery stories database shares examples of local positive practice. A new knowledge community has also been built which offers people an evidence-based, online, interactive facility to share and collaborate on mental health issues.

RELATIONSHIPS

Among the organisations with which NIMHE is making connections at national level in the Modernisation Agency are the clinical governance team, changing workforce team, leadership programme, redesign team, NATPACT and the primary care development team; NIMHE facilitates a mental health inter-agency network where these and other colleagues meet regularly. NIMHE has also prioritised establishing and developing relationships with other national organisations with an interest in mental health, such as SCIE (Social Care Institute for Excellence), CHI (Commission for Health Improvement) now developing into CHAI (Commission for Audit and Inspection), and voluntary organisations.

NIMHE has recruited a wide range of people in a variety of ways, including fellowships, secondments and project workers. Many posts have been created as partnerships with others and all have been designed to enable people to remain involved with another organisation, or field of activity, whilst bringing time, skills and experience to the work of the Institute.

As the organisation grows and consolidates over the next two to three years, there will be a need to continue to attract able people, but also to 'recycle' their skills back into the mental health service. This will be achieved through associate, part-time and fellowship arrangements, which enable people to contribute to NIMHE whilst retaining service responsibilities.

NIMHE'S STRATEGIC PRIORITIES

NIMHE has selected some strategic priorities for the next three years:

- System transformation – to ensure that the overall system of mental health care enables the provision of efficient and effective care and treatment
- Workforce development – to ensure that there are sufficient staff, with the right skills, experience and leadership to provide the services needed
- Changing practice – to ensure people have rapid access to the best possible care.

These will be developed through the development centres and through national programmes in the context of priorities.

Transformation of the system that plans and delivers treatment and care is essential to create a mental health service that is built around the individual needs of the people who use it. This is a theme that runs through Government policy, both for the NHS and for other public services – it is not sufficient just to do more of the same.

For mental health, NIMHE will concentrate on a number of key areas, from supporting implementation of the service models set out in the *National service framework for mental health* (such as crisis resolution and early intervention) and new mental health legislation (as and when approved by Parliament), to working directly with communities to improve mental health support. The latter will include a substantial programme to recruit community development workers for minority ethnic people. The reform of mental health care in prisons will also be supported.

Research will form an important activity in support of this priority, with a significant programme to be established through the Mental Health Research Network.

Among the instruments to be developed are models for commissioning and providing mental health services within primary care, and supporting their implementation, mechanisms for capturing and sharing knowledge about mental health and mental health services, and outcomes measures which embrace morbidity, mortality, quality of life and user experiences.

An important part of this priority is to mainstream mental health, so that provision is fully integrated with other programmes and services. To further this aim, NIMHE will promote the recognition of mental health within generic health and social care, and support local work to include mental health in strategies for neighbourhood renewal.

Workforce development is essential for people-intensive mental health services. As with other aspects of health and social care, mental health services must attract more people – from a diversity of backgrounds – to increase capacity to deliver the *NHS plan* and *National service framework for mental health.*

NIMHE will work alongside agencies already engaged in similar activity, including the Modernisation Agency's changing workforce programme, the Leadership Centre and the workforce development confederations.

Areas of work will include developing shared capabilities, which include cultural, gender and other competencies, supporting initiatives for new ways of working, and promoting effective leadership. Both pre- and post-registration training must meet the needs of the new patterns of services.

The work on system reform will help to provide the framework for effective care and fundamentally different ways of supporting people. The work on workforce will help to provide the staff and skills required. The third priority is work designed directly to change and improve the individual experience of service users and their families, through changing practice.

Key activities will include improving access and choice across the whole range of mental health services, including substance misuse services and pathways into care for women and people from minority ethnic communities.

The engagement of groups, communities and individuals who are disadvantaged will be promoted, and services helped to change in order to meet their needs. This can be done by supporting the social inclusion and citizenships of people with mental health problems, with a particular emphasis on access to education, employment and meaningful occupation.

In addition, NIMHE will continue to support improvements in acute in-patient care, promote approaches which are known to reduce the risk of suicide and work with NICE and SCIE to ensure guidelines are disseminated and supported in implementation.

CHALLENGES FOR THE FUTURE

The fast pace of the reform of health and social care may result in NIMHE's location changing in the medium term. As the Modernisation Agency considers how it will move to become localised itself, this is likely to have an impact on NIMHE's positioning.

NIMHE is also working through the organisational challenge of implementing the principle of 'subsidiarity' – that activity has led to the development centres unless there are persuasive reasons to keep it central or work collaboratively across NIMHE. The current split is about 75% devolved locally to development centres, 25% held centrally for NIMHE central and national programmes.

THE ACID TEST

The kinds of reforms described here will help to make NIMHE a sustainable body, able both to command respect as a source of advice nationally, whilst remaining relevant to people working in the field and, even more crucially, to those who use mental health services and their families.

NIMHE is nothing if it cannot make a difference – to what service users and their families say and feel, to the experiences they report of the support and space they are given. That is the acid test of progress, which NIMHE has set itself.

References

Department of Health. (1998). *Modernising mental health services: Safe, sound and Supportive.* HMSO, London.

Department of Health. (1999a). *National service framework for mental health: modern standards and service models.* Available Online: www.doh.gov.uk/nsf/mentalhealth.htm

Department of Health. (1999b). *Saving Lives: our healthier nation.* HSC 1999/152; LAC(99)26, HMSO, London.

Department of Health. (2000a). *The NHS plan.* HMSO, London.

Department of Health. (2000b). *NHS priorities and planning guidance 2003–2006.* The Stationery Office, London.

NIMHE. (2003a). National Institute for Mental Health in England. *Inside Outside Improving mental health services for black and minority ethnic communities in England.* Department of Health, London.

NIMHE. (2003b). National Institute for Mental Health in England. *Redesigning mental health. Access and choice service improvement guide.* Department of Health, London.

11

A critical introduction to clinical governance

Tim Freeman and Michael Clark

> *. . . a history respectful of contingency, mistrustful of inevitability, indifferent to any predetermined route or destination; a history refusing to take for granted (as the victors' texts always want) that the way things turned out was the way they were always meant to be . . .*
>
> (Schama 2000, p. 17)

> *A consideration of clinical governance involves engaging with issues of autonomy and control in the context of the complex relationships that exist between clinicians and managers and between policy makers and service providers. It also involves unpacking the vague, or contested, idea of governance itself . . .*
>
> (Walsh and Small 2001, p. 110)

> *It includes all of the favoured approaches to performance measurement (the approach that one of my colleagues referred to as 'hitting the donkey with the carrot') . . .*
>
> (Broadbent 2003, p. 5)

INTRODUCTION

Part of the terrain upon which it may be expected that research and development will come together in health care in England is that of 'clinical governance'. We should not, though, blithely presume that just because clinical governance policy contains references to 'research' and 'evidence-based', research and development will find common ground to meet within it in individual Trusts. Indeed, as 'evidence-based practice' is itself a contested concept (see the discussions in Trinder and Reynolds (2000)), it is far from being a given that clinical governance will automatically result in research being taken up into clinical practice in mental health or any other area of health care.

Nor should we simply accept 'official' accounts that this policy is an inevitable government response to wide variations in clinical practice and the loss of public confidence in health care quality (Scally and Donaldson 1998; Nicholls *et al.* 2000). Whilst these undoubtedly made health care quality a political imperative requiring a response, the official view does little to explain the specific form of the policy prescription. Rather, we should critically review the policy of clinical governance. In this chapter we shall do this by placing clinical governance within the context of broader shifts in modes of governance between the state, citizens and professional groups. This allows us better to explore continuities and discontinuities with previous governance arrangements in the UK NHS, the difficulties posed by its internal tensions, and the scope for research and development to come together. In doing this, we shall articulate the highly contested nature of clinical governance.

As increased decentralisation and use of regulated markets in service delivery has exponentially increased across Western Europe, there has occurred a consequential greater emphasis on oversight methods of accountability (Power 1997; Hood *et al.* 1999). Debates over models of external review are ultimately concerned with professional control i.e. judgements concerning the appropriate balance between professional self-regulation and accountability. The use of new models strikes new balances of trust and control between patients, professionals and government.

Within the UK, the role of central government in health care quality improvement has become increasingly prescriptive. In 1997, the government outlined a programme of NHS quality reforms in an ambitious agenda reflecting broader governance trends towards the performance management of devolved organisations against national standards (Newman 2000; Geddes and Martin 2000; Ball *et al.* 2002; Freeman 2002; Broadbent 2003). There were new national structures to set and monitor standards, including the National Institute for Clinical Excellence (NICE), and enhanced systems of performance assessment, inspections and ratings. A new statutory duty imposed on Trusts for quality required structures of clinical governance within local health care provider units to ensure local delivery of the national agenda. For the first time, individuals and organisations were accountable for achieving central quality targets (Ferguson and Lim 2001). These requirements were also explicitly linked to performance assessment mechanisms:

> *Although the emphasis on controlling, guiding, influencing, managing or regulating may differ according to who is doing the 'governing', the underlying rationale is clear: individuals and/or organisations need to be made more accountable in order to achieve outcomes that are deemed desirable.*
>
> (Ferguson and Lim 2001, p. 464)

We shall look more critically at clinical governance, particularly in the wider context of models of governance, but first we shall examine it in its own terms.

CLINICAL GOVERNANCE, ITS ORIGINS AND STATUS

Definitions

Clinical governance has been officially defined as:

> *... a framework through which NHS organisations are accountable for continuously improving the quality of their services and safeguarding high standards of care by creating an environment in which excellence in clinical care will flourish.*
>
> (DoH 1998, p. 33)

It has been characterised as both a controls assurance framework (Martin 2001; Emsley 2002) and a whole-system approach to continuous quality improvement (Hackett *et al.* 1999; Cullen *et al.* 2000; Latham *et al.* 2000; Nicholls *et al.* 2000; Halligan and Donaldson 2001; Wallace *et al.* 2001).

How are such divergent readings possible? Support for both may be found within the White Paper *The new NHS: modern, dependable* (DoH 1997). Short-term targets relate to development of assurance committee structures, whilst the long-term vision is fixed on cultural change, away from a climate of blame and fear towards open reporting of incidents, reflective learning and service development. This is reinforced by the five-year vision for clinical governance outlined in *Clinical governance: quality in the new NHS* (1999), supporting the development of open, participative cultures, active user involvement, multidisciplinary team-working and quality improvement. Yet, the language of continuous quality improvement contrasts sharply with the assurance-focused style of performance management exhibited by the Department of Health and many of its agencies, and there is a danger that the long-term quality improvement agenda is being diluted.

Published responses to the policy of clinical governance cover the spectrum from rejection (Goodman 1998) via cautious approval (Davies and Mannion 1999; Walshe et al. 2000; Davies et al. 2001), to enthusiastic endorsement (Donaldson and Muir-Gray 1998; Scally and Donaldson 1998). Such divergences of opinion are in part due to contested understandings of the 'nature of the beast'. The contrast between the definition provided by *The new NHS: modern, dependable* (DoH 1997) and *The national service framework for diabetes: delivery strategy* (DoH 2002b) on one hand and *Clinical governance: quality in the new NHS* (NHSE 1999) on the other (Table 11.1) encapsulate the tensions between competing claims made on behalf of clinical governance. While the former definitions locate the essence of clinical governance within local structures and processes backed by a statutory duty, the latter locates it within a change in organisational culture towards greater openness, learning and service improvement. We are offered (DoH 1998) significantly different visions of the best approach to health care. To the extent that clinical governance provides an accountability framework of standards against which organisations and/or individuals may be assessed by external agencies, it constitutes a performance management system. On the other hand, to the extent that it relies on development and support to encourage continuous quality improvement it constitutes a whole-system approach to Continuous Quality Improvement (CQI).

While both assurance and improvement approaches rely on indicators, they use them to different ends: the former to make summative judgements on care quality, the latter to foster learning and improvement within clinical teams (Freeman 2001). The dual emphasis on assurance and improvement may be an attempt to bridge the gap between managerial and clinical approaches to quality (Buetow and Roland 1999). The difficulty, though, is that there is no attempt to resolve the tensions between the two dialectically:

> *The performance focus contrasts sharply with the language of continuous quality improvement, and the interplay of these two discourses informs activity at the sharp end of service delivery.*
> (Newman 2000, p. 55)

There is a resulting struggle for the soul of clinical governance (Miles et al. 2000). While quality improvement and central control are

Table 11.1 Clinical governance: definitions	
DoH (1997, 3.6)	A new system of clinical governance in NHS Trusts and primary care to ensure that clinical standards are met, and that processes are in place to ensure continuous improvement, backed by a new statutory duty for quality in the NHS.
DoH (1998, p. 33)	. . . a framework through which all National Health Service (NHS) organisations are accountable for continuously improving the quality of services and safeguarding high standards of care by creating an environment in which excellence in clinical care will flourish.
NHSE (1999, p. 5)	Above all clinical governance is about changing organisational culture in a systematic and demonstrable way, moving away from a culture of blame to one of learning so that quality infuses all aspects of the organisation's work.
Scally and Donaldson (1998, p. 62)	Clinical governance is a system through which NHS organisations are accountable for continuously improving the quality of their services and safeguarding high standards of care by creating an environment in which excellence in clinical care will flourish.
Goodman (1998, pp. 1726–7)	. . . a rolling unpunctuated tangle of prepositional and adverbial phrases similar to the many that have appeared in the past few years on the walls of our hospital wards and clinics . . . a small idea, a rehash of all sorts of 'management speak' and poorly thought through generalisations that can depress and dishearten.
Onions (2000, p. 405)	. . . a new NHS concept that seeks, through clinical guidelines and national service frameworks, to encourage and enforce compliance with nationally-devised evidence-based clinical policies.
DoH (2002b, p. 20)	. . . the local delivery mechanism for ensuring safe and high quality care. Clinical governance will ensure that NHS organisations have in place systems to assure the quality of their services and processes to ensure continuous improvement year-on-year.

conceptually distinct and are not strictly antonyms (Harrison and Dowswell 2000), the fear is that performance management may undermine the conditions of trust, honesty and innovation required for quality improvement (Davies and Mannion 1999a).

Clinical governance lacks methodological innovation, in that it includes previous policy initiatives such as risk management, clinical audit and evidence-based practice (Walshe 2000). Yet, it is not simply an exercise in 're-badging' or re-branding. The central newness of this governance is that it imposes a statutory responsibility for quality on individuals and organisations. Clinical governance fits into the context of a range of new external institutions and relationships constituting a strengthening of performance management arrangements. These were explicitly designed to ensure optimal performance of the NHS in line with UK policy directives, implying both the primacy of managerial as opposed to clinical or patient actions and involvement, and the 'given' status of policy objectives (Smith 2002).

This understanding requires us to examine in more depth the concept of governance, and of broader shifts in governance modes. Such an examination of clinical governance in the context of wider governance trends (Newman 2000; Power 2000) offers a powerful revisionist critique of the official history of clinical governance as an inevitable response to variations and failures in care quality and falling public confidence (Nicholls *et al.* 2000). Rather, clinical governance is located within a broader historical and conceptual context to explain its specific form, internal tensions and similarities with parallel developments in other policy arenas (Geddes and Martin 2000; Springings 2002).

Governance and modes of governance

Rhodes (1996) identifies two broad strands of 'governance' literature. Both are sceptical of the ability of a central state to plan economic and social organisation directly. However, they differ fundamentally in their perspective on public management and the role of government in society. The first is associated with reducing the role of the state and employing new public management techniques in order to do more with less (Osborne and Gaebler 1992), and the second with theories of the interdependence of public, private and semi-private actors, such as self-organising networks. In short, while the former is an attempt to translate managerial ideas such as contracting out and client orientation from the private sector to public services, the latter focuses on co-ordinating inter-organisational policy-making (Klijn and Koppenjan

2000). While partnership working between health and social care agencies has been an important part of New Labour's governance strategy, the emphasis has been on an inclusive managerialism rather than community activism (Walsh and Small 2001).

Governance, the emerging pattern that arises from governing (Kooiman 1993), is a form of social co-ordination (Mayntz 1993), of which many patterns, or modes, are available. Starting from Williamson's (1985) analysis of markets and hierarchies as governance structures, Lowndes and Skelcher (1998) identify a number of triads in the literature on governance. They include markets, hierarchies and networks (Thompson *et al.* 1991); markets, bureaucracies and clans (Ouchi 1979; 1991); and community, market and state (Streek and Schmitter 1985). Hood *et al.* (1999) propose four patterns: oversight (bureaucracy), mutuality (clan), competition (market), and contrived randomness. While there are differences of emphasis in these analyses, four ideal types of governance emerge: competition, oversight, network and mutuality (Fig. 11.1). We shall discuss each in turn, and relate them to the context being discussed in this chapter.

Competition/market modes of governance

Market modes of governance deploy contractual relationships between parties, mediated through price mechanisms. While they provide flexibility to actors in terms of their willingness to form alliances, the competitive environment means that parties will generally only collaborate where there are clear mutual benefits, given underlying suspicion between parties. Co-ordination and collaboration are thus

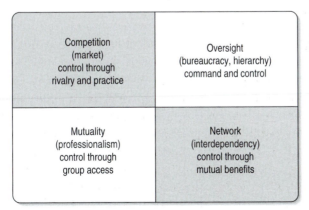

Figure 11.1   Modes of governance, adapted and extended from Hood *et al.* (1999)

difficult. In the NHS, this mode of governance is most closely associated with the internal market reforms of the early 1990s. The distinction between purchasers and providers was intended to produce market incentives to contain costs and increase service quality. While competition in the NHS was severely constrained, the purchaser/provider split was retained in the New Labour reforms. Indeed, *Shifting the balance of power* (2001) further extends the purchasing power of Primary Care Trusts (PCTs) to purchase care from the secondary acute sector.

Oversight/bureaucracy/hierarchical modes of governance

Oversight modes of governance rely on an authoritative supervisory structure to overcome the difficulties of co-ordination and collaboration found in the market. It relies on rules and targets enforced by systems of hierarchical surveillance. The cost can be a stifling of flexibility and innovation, given the formality and routine nature of hierarchical relationships. Performance is assessed in terms of compliance with rules and meeting targets. While oversight has been used extensively in the NHS, historically the focus has been on activity and finance, with clinical quality largely left to clinical professionals (Davies and Mannion 1999b).

Mutuality/clan/professional modes of governance

Mutuality or clan control relies on trusting group norms to control individual behaviour. Such methods of control are seen as particularly effective in circumstances where individuals are bound by strong professional norms, success is difficult to measure, and where the relationship between inputs, processes and outcomes is unclear (Ouchi 1979). Indeed, neither self-interested contracting (market) nor hierarchical enforcement can be relied upon when it is not possible to specify in detail what constitutes as 'good job'. Thus, health care relies on validation by clinical professions, especially medicine. Professions are themselves organisational forms, and mutuality dominated the approach to the control of clinical quality within the NHS until the 1997 reforms. The clinical autonomy of the medical profession to assess performance via peer review is a founding principle of the NHS.

Network governance

Based on the 'governing without government' thesis of Rhodes (1996; 1997; 1999), network governance contends that governing increasingly depends on interactions between public and private sector actors which are relatively autonomous of central states. Consequently, central states can steer only indirectly and imperfectly. Actors are seen as capable of identifying complementary interests, and developing interdependent partnerships based on trust, reciprocity and a sense of common purpose (Lowndes and Skelcher 1998). While partnerships have themselves been characterised as a mode of governance (Davies 2002), Lowndes and Skelcher (1998) contend that partnership arrangements draw on hierarchy, network and market modes of governance at different stages of development.

The typologies above are best viewed as Weberian 'ideal types'; in practice they are not mutually exclusive and tend to function in parallel as hybrids. In the context of clinical governance, the inclusion of clinical, managerial and patient representatives on Commission for Health Improvement review teams could be viewed as an oversight/mutuality hybrid. The use of league tables to assess provider institutions, as in the Performance Assessment Framework, could be seen as an example of an oversight/competition hybrid. On this analysis, clinical governance is not itself a mode of governance – a means by which social co-ordination is achieved. It is less a new 'post-bureaucratic' form (Hoggett 1996) than a shifting blend of different forms of social co-ordination, including market, hierarchy, clan and network modes of governance. The absence in guidance documents of detailed prescription concerning the form of clinical governance arrangements provided some latitude for local interpretation in implementation and varying mixes of local governance.

Principal–agent theory

The dilemmas facing those charged with influencing the behaviour of autonomous professional groups may usefully be explored from the economic perspective of principal–agent theory (Davies & Mannion 1999a; 2000). Here, 'principals' are those individuals or agencies who want things done and 'agents' are those who are engaged in accomplishing tasks for the principals. While such relationships may be contractual or informal, a key feature of all principal–agent relationships is the presence of asymmetries between the parties, leading to the potential for agent opportunism.

Clinicians are in multiple principal–agent relationships with patients, managers and commissioners (Smith *et al.* 1997; Shortell *et al.* 1998). It is illuminating to consider local clinical governance in terms of health service managers with responsibility for health care quality as principals, and the clinicians through whom care quality may be either achieved or lacking as the agents of managers. Davies and Mannion (2000) identify two important differences between such principals and agents: objective functions, and knowledge and information. The former refers to ambiguity over the objectives of health care that may lead to divergence between managers and clinicians. A good example here is the primacy of balanced budgets for health care managers, whereas clinicians may be seeking to maximise health benefits for the patients in their care. The latter refers to the different technical knowledge and situation-specific information available to principals and agents, which may lead to differences in understandings and judgements of appropriate action. Such differences provide scope for divergence between what principals want and what agents deliver:

> *Agents may for example make undesirable trade-offs between multiple competing objectives, or worse, they may exploit their powerful position to indulge in opportunistic behaviour to maximise their own gain at the expense of the principal.*
> (Davies and Mannion 2000, p. 252)

While the opportunistic behaviour of professional agents is likely to be curtailed by self-community and client-control (Sharma 1997), two major approaches are available to principals to reduce the potential for dysfunctional agent behaviour. The first is to check and modify behaviour using hierarchical control structures in an attempt to redress asymmetries of information. This requires the accurate measurement of that agent behaviour deemed important, plus the ability to exert influence over agent behaviour that does not conform to the measurement ideals. In contrast, the second approach is formative, seeking the negotiated realignment of objectives and beliefs that might give rise to agent waywardness. This approach seeks to develop agents' intrinsic professional motivations through the development of trust, in order to realign agent objectives with those of principals.

Managers charged with service improvement may be drawn to coercive methods of behaviour change. Yet, a focus on data to drive improvement suffers from difficulties of collection, interpretation, and perverse incentives (Smith 1995). Given the difficulty of measuring clinical outcomes and difficulties in attribution between clinician behaviour and clinical outcomes, Davies and Mannion (1999a) caution against the over-reliance on oversight to redress information asymmetry between principals and agents:

> *The concern is that insufficient attention will be paid to the sometimes nebulous concepts of trust and culture in a headlong rush for the more tangible appeals of measurement, monitoring and coercive control mechanisms.*
>
> (Davies and Mannion 1999a, p. 15)

Historical development of modes of governance in the UK NHS

While the number of ideal types of governance modes is limited, the relative balance between these approaches and their hybrids is much more variable. Since the UK NHS's inception, the balance between different forms of governance has shifted over time reflecting broader governance trends. Three periods may be distinguished: the 1948 settlement (command and control and clan); New Public Management under the 1991 reforms (market and oversight); and New Labour's 'third way' set out in the 1997 White Paper *The new NHS: modern, dependable* (eclecticism).

The 1948 Settlement

At its inception, the NHS relied on a blend of hierarchy and clan modes of governance. For major decisions about priorities and provision, the NHS relied on a hierarchical system of command and control with strong line management and upward accountability (Robinson 2002). This was tempered by clan modes of governance by the medical profession (Bourne and Ezzamel 1986), in which the professional training and specialised knowledge of clinicians was perceived to make them best placed to judge clinical performance and the quality of clinical care (Goddard *et al.* 2000).

New Public Management (NPM) under the 1991 reforms

In the 1980s, New Right political theory questioned state public services' efficiency and service quality and proposed the application of 'entrepreneurial governance' (Osborne and Gaebeler 1992). This set policy on the course of the internal market, established in the NHS in 1991. The main feature of this was to separate the responsibility for purchasing services from their provision. Potential service providers were encouraged to compete against each other to win contracts. While the system was intended to introduce market forces into public provision, the demands of political accountability quickly led to close regulation and management of the health care internal market via systems of inspection, accounting, regulation and review (Clarke *et al.* 2000).

The approach of semi-autonomous, decentralised provider units subject to 'hands-off' central performance management is explored in the social policy literature under the concepts of New Public Management (NPM) and the regulatory state. Hoggett (1996) identified three defining interlocking strategies of NPM. Firstly, a drive towards operationally decentralised units, with a simultaneous drive for increased central control over strategy and policy. Secondly, the activities of decentralised units were co-ordinated via competition and/or market incentives. Finally, increased performance management and monitoring of the activity of the decentralised units via audits, inspections and reviews. The simultaneous use of both centralisation and decentralisation are a central paradox of the approach (Clarke and Newman 1997), and the need for regulatory mechanisms arises due to the need to 'steer' the behaviour of semi-autonomous organisations. Consequently, NPM is best seen as a combination of competition and oversight modes of governance:

> *The picture that therefore emerges is one of an operationally decentralised organisation with a strong but distant centre engaging in performance monitoring and shaping activity by concentrating on a few indicators which give emphasis to results rather than inputs or processes.*
>
> (Hoggett 1996, p. 21)

Hood *et al.* (1999) contend that NPM in the 1980s and 1990s led to an increase in formality, complexity intensity and specialisation in regulation:

> *New Public Management stressed the importance of [performance accountability], emphasising a change from tactical to strategic prescription, direct to indirect command, detailed instruction to freedom within constraints. Even on that characterisation, new regimes of performance regulation can be expected to emerge in parallel with new management freedoms, and 'compliance' regulation [over procedures, for instance on merit-hiring or complaint handling] can take new, often enhanced, forms in a more managerial service.'*
>
> (Hood *et al.* 1999, p. 6)

The term 'regulatory state' suggests the increasing use of standards, rules and monitoring, under the auspices of public authority.

'Modernisation' – New Labour's third way

At the heart of the modernisation project lie tensions between central prescription, local innovation and upward accountability

1 Political management: Manage the message, ride out the crisis, and corral the media	3 Upward accountability: Set values, targets, objectives, oversight, 'evidence-based'

Rationalism:
Set objectives, evaluate results,
learn and improve

2 Exploration and innovation: Experiment, take risks, pilots, trusts manager's pragmatism	4 Downward accountability: Consult and involve local stakeholders, listen to service users

Figure 11.2 Meanings of modernisation, in Peck (2000)

(Peck 2001; 6 2000). 6's analysis is particularly helpful (Fig. 11.2) in drawing a distinction between local exploration and innovation sanctioned by the centre (item 2), and a pluralist downward accountability routinely seeking local innovation (item 4). The former is consistent with earned autonomy under a performance management framework, the latter with network modes of governance.

Two distinct phases of New Labour's third way may be discerned, suggestive of an emergent strategy seeking to balance the above tensions, rather than an ideological commitment. The first phase is codified in the 1997 White Paper, *The new NHS: modern, dependable* (DoH 1997), and the second in the subsequent *NHS plan* (DoH 2000).

Phase I: The new NHS: modern, dependable *(1997)*
'Modern Public Management'
New Labour vehemently opposed the internal market while in opposition, and instead offered a vision of partnership working and collaborating between health and social care providers. However, New Labour's third way retained and extended the emphasis on decentralisation and performance management, with additional elements of central direction (Fig. 11.3). Commentators have satirised its continuities with New Public Management by coining the term 'Modern Public Management' (Newman 2000).

The role of clinical governance within the reforms was to ensure the local delivery of the national agenda, through internal committee systems and by engaging clinical professionals in quality improvement

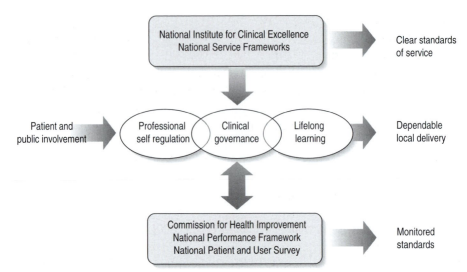

Figure 11.3 The UK health care quality strategy, as outlined in 'A first class service: quality in the new NHS' (DoH 1998)

activities; the dual strategy of internal quality improvement and external quality assurance.

While self-regulation remains in name (Fig. 11.3), it is 'modernised' to be open to scrutiny and publicly accountable for nationally set professional standards (DoH 1998, para 3.44). Hence, oversight modes of governance in connection have dramatically increased. Oversight and clan modes of governance in the context of professional standards make potentially uneasy bedfellows:

> . . . *if necessary clinical governance will provide a systematic framework that can be extended into the clinical community at all levels. Here we have the rationalistic bureaucratic discourse of regulation, which reveals itself through increasingly extensive rule systems, the 'scientific' measurement of objective standards, and the minimisation of the scope for human error. Behind it lies a faith in the efficacy of surveillance as a directive force in human affairs. As such, in terms of its understanding of the principal dynamic in the maintenance of clinical standards, it is the ideological opposite of the belief in the self-sustaining individual professional (or group of professionals) who is motivated by the sense of self-respect that flows from doctors' ownership of professional standards.*
>
> (Salter 2001, p. 874)

The governance eclecticism of the 'third way' may be an attempt to strike a balance between oversight, clan, market and network modes of governance (Goddard *et al.* 2000). The developments signal a significant step away from market modes of governance, towards new forms of regulatory oversight associated with guidance and monitoring. They constitute a strong system of performance improvement, with an underlying emphasis on the increased accountability of professionals to government, drawing on a comprehensive set of high-level performance indicators and central targets (McLaughlin *et al.* 2001).

Phase II: The NHS plan *(2000)* 'earned autonomy'

Smith (2002) considers developments in the emergent performance management framework contained within the *NHS plan* (2000) under three headings: guidance, monitoring and response. These are respectively concerned with transmission of policy objectives; collection of information on the extent to which the guidance has been followed and targets met; and stimulation of remedial action and/or continuous improvement. While the guidance mechanisms of NICE and NSFs remained unchanged, there were additions to both monitoring and response systems designed to develop leadership capacity and introduce incentives for improved performance: a new Modernisation Agency; a performance fund; the notion of 'earned autonomy'; and performance rating ('stars') (Fig. 11.4).

Alongside national institutions to set, monitor and deliver improved quality, and devolved decision making subject to earned autonomy, Robinson (2002) identifies the selective use of market incentives as a spur to improved efficiency. The 1999 Health Act (DoH 1999) promised greater flexibility to NHS and local authorities in planning partnership arrangements by sanctioning pooled budgets, lead commissioning and integrated provision, all designed to allow greater emphasis on client groups in service design across health and social care boundaries. However:

> *Despite claims to the contrary, the emphasis on national standards and accountability set out in 'delivering the NHS Plan' suggest that central direction is still an important part of the ministerial mindset. This is likely to place major limitations on the local autonomy elements of the third way-plus model.*
>
> (Robinson 2002, p. 24)

The end point of earned autonomy, foundation trusts, has highlighted an ideological split within the New Labour government. Supporters

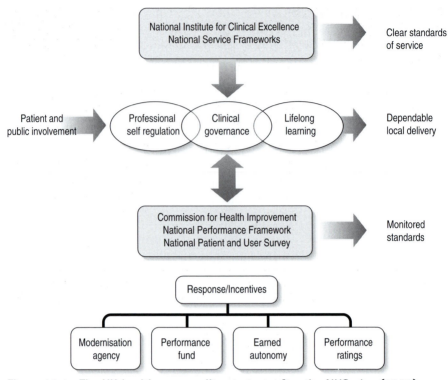

Figure 11.4 The UK health care quality strategy after the NHS plan (2000)

claim it will result in increased choice for local people which will boost performance through increased competition. Critics are wary, concerned about fragmentation and disparities in care quality (Jobanputra and Buchan 2003). Either way, the policy seems likely to increase the role of market modes of governance within the UK NHS.

The continued rise of the regulatory state?

Walshe (2002) summarises the scope and reach of 'second generation' national regulatory agencies associated with the 1997 reforms and the later *NHS plan* (2000) in the English NHS (Table 11.2). These agencies differ from pre-existent bodies such as the Audit Commission or the National Audit Office in their primary focus on regulation, breadth of coverage, and emphasis on clinical quality. As Walshe's emphasis is on regulatory *agencies* he omits three additional regulatory mechanisms: the Performance Assessment Framework (PAF); 'star' ratings; and National Service Frameworks (NSFs), providing information on specific

Table 11.2 'Second generation' NHS regulatory mechanisms: adapted and extended from Walshe (2002)			
Name	Date	Purpose	Methods
National Institute for Clinical Excellence (NICE)	Apr 1999	Provide authoritative guidance on current best practice	Expert review of health technologies, to produce and disseminate guidance
National Service Frameworks	Apr 1999	Provide authoritative advice of the level and type of service provision that patients should expect from specific services, to standardise service provision	Set national standards of care for specific conditions or services. Publish frameworks and audit assessment tools
Performance Assessment Framework	Apr 1999	To monitor the progress of health care organisations in six performance domains: health improvements, efficiency, fair access, care outcomes, patient experience and effective delivery. Ties service priorities to Treasury Service Agreements	Collection, assessment and publication of indicator data
Commission for Health Improvement (CHI)	Nov 1999	Assist in addressing unacceptable variations in care	Review all NHS organisations every 4 years; monitor implementation of NICE guidelines and NSFs; investigate systems failures
Modernisation Agency	Apr 2001	To assist in improving service quality and contribute to meeting performance targets	Provision of training and support services to encourage service redesign initiatives targeted on those areas of service requiring development
National Clinical Assessment Authority	Apr 2001	To support health authorities and trusts faced with concerns over the performance of an individual doctor	Provide advice, take referrals and undertake assessments

Name	Date	Purpose	Methods
National Patient Safety Agency	July 2001	Collate and analyse adverse events in NHS; learn lessons and feed them back; produce solutions, set goals and track progress	Operate a mandatory reporting system and provide national guidance/leadership on safety
Performance Ratings ('Stars')	Sept 2001	Introduce financial incentives to the PAF through development funding and potential to apply for foundation status – 'earned autonomy'	Summary measure of achievement against key targets. Assessment affect access to service development monies
Commission for Health care Audit and Inspection (CHAI)	Apr 2004	To help improve the quality of patient care by assisting to address variations and ensure high standards of patient care	Reviewing NHS organisations on a rolling visit programme; overseeing Performance Ratings and indicators under the PAF; Monitoring NSFs and NICE guideline implementation

Table 11.2 Continued

performance indicators, summaries of organisational performance, and expected models of service respectively.

The need for a balance between trusting professionals to develop high-quality services and checking up on them to ensure that they do so is widely accepted (Davies *et al.* 2001). The evolution of the Commission for Health Improvement (CHI) to the Commission for Health Care Audit and Inspection (CHAI) could be seen as an attempt to rationalise the agencies involved in promoting clinical governance. Under these new arrangements, the modernisation agency has the lead on building trust and capacity for improvement, with CHAI taking the lead on checking via performance ratings and visits. However, the tensions and resultant pressures on those delivering services remain.

Opinions on the desirability of the growth of regulation within the UK NHS differ. Davies and Mannion (2001) are broadly supportive of the balancing of mutuality, oversight and competition in the NHS Plan reforms, and Walshe (2002) summarises the managerialist perspective well:

> *The rise of regulation in the NHS seems, at first sight, to represent a long-term strengthening of central government's control of managerial practice. . . . Their creation could allow a kind of centralised micromanagement, in which there is less and less scope for local variation to develop. However, if the politicians can be persuaded to let go, the new regulators of the NHS could provide a genuinely new approach to improving performance and management, [providing] a more indirect and distanced relationship, in which managed regulation by intermediate and quasi-independent organisations would play a large part. In that environment, the new regulatory agencies could adopt a more responsive approach to regulation.*
>
> (Walshe 2002, p. 969)

Yet, such optimism is not universally shared and the conditional statements in the fourth and fifth lines may well prove to be telling. More fundamentally, critics of New Labour's conception of policy implementation point to a dramatic expansion of treasury control over policy outputs, in terms of performance criteria for service delivery enshrined in the PAF (Lee and Woodward 2002). They characterise the third way approach to policy implementation as increased central policy prescription through treasury resource allocation tied to service agreements. In this context, earned autonomy as introduced under the NHS Plan (DoH 2000) means the delegation of responsibility for administering national priorities – it is administrative rather than political devolution. Together, treasury service agreements and administrative responsibility for delivery have effectively 'nationalised' policy implementation:

> *By attempting to both steer and row through greater central prescription by the core executive, the Third Way of implementation has denied inter-organisational networks at sub-national levels of governance the necessary autonomy to innovate or show foresight.*
>
> (Lee and Woodward 2002, p. 53)

Thus, those emphasising network modes of governance within the clinical governance project see clinical governance as an opportunity (Walsh and Small 2001). In contrast, those concentrating their attention on oversight mechanisms such as the PAF characterise clinical governance as creeping central control (Harrison and Lim 2000; Lee and Woodward 2000; Miles *et al.* 2000). While Ham (1999b) is correct to chide those who characterise the New Labour reforms as simply increased central control, critics do make a strong case. Each reveals a partial truth: clinical governance is not itself a mode of governance, but draws on hierarchical, network and clan modes of governance. The concern is that while there is some scope for administrative autonomy in service delivery, there is arguably an overemphasis on external summative approaches to the extent that the internal, formative, improvement agenda is overshadowed.

CONCLUSIONS

Internally, NHS organisations are obliged to develop systems of clinical governance to ensure that they are delivering high-quality clinical care, consistent with standards established nationally through the National Institute of Clinical Excellence (NICE) and National Service Frameworks (NSFs). Internal mechanisms include clear lines of accountability to the board and a committee structure, and statutory responsibilities for CEOs. NHS organisations are externally supported by the Commission for Health Improvement (CHI), who intend to visit every health care organisation on a rolling four-year visit programme to see that clinical governance arrangements are robust. Organisations scoring well on indicators contained in the Performance Assessment Framework (PAF) will be subject to less scrutiny and receive money for service development, the notion of 'earned autonomy'.

The New Labour NHS reforms address accountability by increasing levels of internal and external scrutiny, while simultaneously reducing and reformulating the role of professionalism within the context of safeguarding clinical quality. The new central agencies, concerned with setting and monitoring clear service standards, provide the context. The role of local clinical governance arrangements within the system is to ensure 'dependable local delivery' of these standards, and provide information to support assurance internally and externally. Self-regulation within this system needs to be 'rigorous' i.e. tied firmly to the local delivery of national targets, rather than an ethical code and cornerstone of professional autonomy. From this perspective, clinical governance represents a new balance between oversight ('checking') and mutuality ('trusting') modes of governance in service accountability.

Yet the twin objectives of assurance and improvement, related to oversight and mutuality modes of governance respectively, result in significant tensions. Clinical governance requires the delivery of a central agenda on one hand, while nurturing devolved continuous quality improvement on the other. These two aims require different sorts of information, for use in different ways, by different groups of people, and consequently they are not easy to run in parallel. Within devolved provider organisations the temptation to gain performance indicators is very high, given the potential rewards of reduced scrutiny and funds for improvements given to those scoring well. Furthermore, there is empirical evidence that providers may emphasise performance management at the expense of the quality improvement agenda (Freeman *et al.* 2001), which is understandable in an environment in which the CEO's job and development monies are dependent upon attainment of performance targets set by central government.

The tension between the needs of assurance and improvement is reflected in the difference between the short- and medium-term targets for clinical governance outlined in the discussion document, *A first class service: quality in the new NHS* (DoH 1998). While the medium-term agenda emphasises the need for cultural transformation including greater openness and avoidance of unnecessary blame, the short-term targets relate to committee structures. There is a danger that as the structural work is completed, organisations will feel that they are now 'doing' clinical governance, leaving the long-term quality improvement agenda underdeveloped.

Such a critical understanding of the policy of clinical governance highlights its political, contested nature. It sets out a terrain containing a mixture of motivations (e.g. clinical improvement, political control) with a diverse set of mechanisms (e.g. quality assurance, continuous quality improvement). Within this context, we should not expect research to find a direct relationship with service development across the national and local levels of the NHS automatically.

References

6, Perri. New Labour's project for modernising public services presentation to the annual congress of the Centre for Mental Health Services Development, Shrigley Hall, Cheshire, July 6th 2000.

Ball, A., Broadbent, J. and Moore, C. (2002). Best value and the control of local government: challenges and contradictions. *Public Money and Management*, 22, 9–15.

Bourne, M. and Ezzamel, M. (1986). Organisational culture in the National Health Service. *Financial Accountability and Management*, 2, 203–23.

Broadbent, J. (2003). Comprehensive performance assessment: the crock of gold at the end of the performance rainbow? *Public Money and Management*, 23, 5–7.

Buetow, S.A. and Roland, M. (1999). Clinical governance: bridging the gap between managerial and clinical approaches to quality of care. *Quality and Safety in Health Care*, 8, 184–90.

Campbell, S.M., Sheaff, R., Sibbald, B., Marshall, M.N., Pickard, S., Gask, L., Halliwell, S., Rogers, A. and Roland, M.O. (2002). Implementing clinical governance in English Primary Care Groups/Trusts: reconciling quality improvement and quality assurance. *Quality and Safety in Health Care*, 11, 9–14.

Clarke, J. and Newman, J. (1997). *The managerial state.* Sage, London.

Clarke, J., Gewirtz, S. and McLaughlin, E. (eds). (2000). *New managerialism, new welfare?* Sage, London.

Cullen, R., Nicholls, S. and Halligan, A. (2000). Reviewing a service – discovering the unwritten rules. *British Journal of Clinical Governance*, 5, 4, 233–9.

Davies, H.T.O. and Mannion, R. (1999a). *Clinical governance: striking a balance between checking and trusting.* Centre for Health Economics, University of York, York.

Davies, H.T.O. and Mannion, R. (1999b). The rise of oversight and the decline of mutuality? *Public Money and Management*, 19, 55–9.

Davies, H.T.O. and Mannion, R. (2000). Clinical governance: striking a balance between checking and trusting. In *Reforming markets in health care: an economic perspective* (ed. Smith, P.C.). Open University Press, Buckingham.

Davies, H.T.O. and Mannion, R. (2001). Treading a third way for quality in health care. *Public Money and Management*, 21, 6–7.

Davies, J.S. (2002). The governance of urban regeneration: a critique of the 'governing without government' thesis. *Public Administration*, 80, 2, 301–22.

Department of Health. (1997). *The new NHS: modern, dependable.* HMSO, London.

Department of Health. (1998). *A first class service: quality in the new NHS.* HMSO, London.

Department of Health. (1999). *Health Act 1999.* HMSO, London.

Department of Health. (2000). *Clinical governance in London trusts: taking stock: the 1999 London Region stocktake of clinical governance: an overview of activities across all London trusts.* NHS London Regional Office, London.

Department of Health. (2000). *The NHS plan.* HMSO, London.

Department of Health. (2001). *Shifting the balance of power.* HMSO, London.

Department of Health. (2002a). *NHS Foundation trusts.* HMSO, London.

Department of Health. (2002b). *National service framework for diabetes: delivery strategy.* HMSO, London.

Emsley, S. (2002). Governance and internal control. *Health Care Risk Report*, **6**, 20–1.

Ferguson, B. and Lim, J.N.W. (2001). Incentives and clinical governance: money following quality? *Journal of Management in Medicine*, **15**, 6, 463–87.

Freeman, T., Latham, L., Walshe, K., Wallace, L. and Spurgeon, P. (2001). How do trusts intend to measure progress in clinical governance? *The Journal of Clinical Governance*, **9**, 1, 37–43.

Freeman, T. (2002). Using performance indicators to improve health care quality in the public sector: a review of the literature. *Health Services Management Research*, **15**, 126–37.

Geddes, M. and Martin, S. (2000). The policy and politics of Best Value: currents, crosscurrents and undercurrents in the new regime. *Policy and Politics*, **28**, 3, 379–95.

Goddard, M., Mannion, R. and Smith, P. (2000). Enhancing performance in health care: a theoretical perspective on agency and the role of information. *Health Economics*, **9**, 2, 95–107.

Goodman, N. (1998). Clinical governance. *British Medical Journal*, **317**, 1725–7.

Hackett, M., Lilford, R., Jordan, J. (1999). Clinical governance: culture, leadership and power – the key to changing attitudes and behaviours in trusts. *International Journal of Health Care Quality*, **12**, 98–104.

Halligan, A. and Donaldson, L. (2001). Implementing clinical governance: turning vision into reality. *British Medical Journal*, **322**, 1413–7.

Ham, C. (1999a). Improving NHS performance: human behaviour and health policy. *British Medical Journal*, **319**, 1490–2.

Ham, C. (1999b). The third way in health reform: does the emperor have any clothes? *Journal of Health Services Research and Policy*, **4**, 3, 168–73.

Harrison, S. and Dowswell, G. (2000). The selective use by NHS management of NICE-promulgated guidelines: a new and effective tool for systematic rationing of new therapies? In *NICE, CHI and the NHS reforms: enabling excellence or imposing control?* (eds. Miles, A., Hampton, J.R. and Hurwitz, B.), Aesculapius Press, London.

Harrison, S. and Lim, J.N.W. (2000). Clinical governance and primary care in the English National Health Service: some issues of organization and rules. *Critical Public Health*, **10**, 3, 321–9.

Hoggett, P. (1996). New modes of control in the public service. *Public Administration*, **74**, 9–32.

Hood, C., Scott, C., James, O., Jones, G. and Travers, T. (eds) (1999). *Regulation inside government: waste watchers, quality police and sleaze busters.* Oxford University Press, Oxford.

Jobanputra, R. and Buchan, J. (2003). Power sharing. *Heath Service Journal*, **13**, 5853, 26–7.

Klijn, E.H. and Koppenjan, J.F.M. (2000). Public management and policy networks: foundations of a network mode of governance. *Public Management*, **2**, 2, 135–58.

Kooiman, J. (1993). Findings, speculations and recommendations. In *Modern governance* (ed. Kooiman, J.) Sage, London.

Latham, L., Freeman, T., Walshe, K., Spurgeon, P. and Wallace, L. (2000). Clinical governance in the West Midlands and South West regions: early progress in NHS trusts. *Clinician in Management*, **9**, 83–91.

Lee, R. (1999). Clinical governance and risk management. *Journal of the Medical Defence Union*, **15**, 2, 9–12.

Lowndes, V. and Skelcher, C. (1998). The dynamics of multi-organizational partnerships: an analysis of changing modes of governance. *Public Administration*, **76**, 313–33.

McLaughlin, V., Leatherman, S., Fletcher, M. and Wyn-Owen, J. (2001). Improving performance using indicators. Recent experiences in the United States, the United Kingdom, and Australia. *International Journal for Quality in Health Care*, **13**, 6, 455–62.

Martin, V. (2001). Service planning and governance. *Nursing Management*, **8**, 2, 32–6.

Mayntz, R. (1993). Governing failures and the problems of governability: some comments on a theoretical paradigm. In *Modern governance* (ed. Kooiman, J.). Sage, London.

Miles, A., Hampton, J.R. and Hurwitz, B. (2000). *NICE, CHI and the NHS reforms: enabling excellence or imposing control?* Aesculapius Press, London.

Newman, J. (2000). Beyond the new public management? Modernising public services. In *New managerialism, new welfare?* (eds. Clarke, J., Gewirtz, S. and McLaughlin, E.), pp. 45–61. Sage, London.

NHS Executive. (1999). *Clinical governance: quality in the new NHS.* HMSO, London.

Nicholls, S., Cullen, R., O'Neil, S. and Halligan, A. (2000). Clinical governance: its origins and foundations. *British Journal of Clinical Governance*, **5**, 3, 172–8.

Osborne, D. and Gaebler, T. (1992). *Reinventing government: how the entrepreneurial spirit is transforming the public sector.* Addison-Wesley, Reading, MA.

Ouchi, W.G. (1979). A conceptual framework for the design of organizational control mechanisms. *Management Science*, **25**, 9, 833–48.

Ouchi, W. (1991). Markets, bureaucracies and clans. In *Markets, hierarchies and networks: the co-ordination of social life* (eds. Thompson, G., Frances, J., Levacic, R. and Mitchell, J.). Sage, London.

Peck, E. (2001). Modernising the NHS: a game of two halves. *British Journal of Health Care Management*, **7**, 5, 198–201.

Power, M. (1997). *The audit society: rituals of verification.* Oxford University Press, Oxford.

Rhodes, R.A.W. (1996). The new governance: governing without government. *Political Studies*, **44**, 4, 652–67.

Rhodes, R.A.W. (1997). *Understanding governance: policy networks, governance, reflexivity and accountability.* Open University Press, Buckingham.

Rhodes, R.A.W. (1999). Foreword: governance and networks. In *The new management of British local governance* (ed. Stoke, G.), pp. xii–xxvi. Macmillan, Basingstoke.

Robinson, R. (2003). Change it or leave it. *Health Service Journal*, 113, 5852, 16.

Robinson, R. (2002). Who's got the master card? *Health Service Journal*, 112, 5824, 22–4.

Roland, M., Campbell, S. and Wilkin, D. (2001). Clinical governance: a convincing strategy for quality improvement? *Journal of Management in Medicine*, 15, 3, 188–201.

Salter, B. (2001). Who rules? The new politics of medical regulation. *Social Science and Medicine*, 52, 871–83.

Scally, G. and Donaldson, L. (1998). Clinical governance and the drive for quality improvement in the new NHS in England. *British Medical Journal*, 317, 61–5.

Schama, S. (2000). *A history of Britain: at the edge of the world? 3000 BC–AD 1603*. BBC Worldwide, London.

Sharma, S. (1997). Professional as agent: knowledge asymmetry in agency exchange. *Academy of Management Review*, 22, 3, 758–98.

Shortell, S.M., Waters, T.M., Clarke, K.W.B. and Budetti, P.P. (1998). Physicians as double agents: maintaining trust in an era of multiple accountabilities. *Journal of the American Medical Association*, 280, 12, 1102–8.

Smith, P. (1995). The unintended consequences of publishing performance data in the public sector. *International Journal of Public Administration*, 18, 2, 277–310.

Smith, P.C. (2002). Performance management in British health care: will it deliver? *Health Affairs*, 21, 3, 103–15.

Smith, P.C., Stepan, A., Valdmanis, V. and Verheyen, P. (1997). Principal–agent problems in health care systems: an international perspective. *Health Policy*, 41, 37–60.

Springings, N. (2002). Delivering public services under the new public management: the case of public housing. *Public Money and Management*, 22, 4, 11–17.

Streek, W. and Schmitter, P. (eds) (1985). *Private interest government*. Sage, London.

Sweeney, G., Sweeny, K., Greco, M. and Stead, J. (2002a). *Developing clinical governance in primary care: Briefing paper 1: The experience of primary care clinical governance leads*. University of Exeter and Exeter and North Devon NHS Research and Development Support Unit.

Sweeney, G., Sweeny, K., Greco, M. and Stead, J. (2002b). *Developing clinical governance in primary care: Briefing paper 2: Exploring the implementation and development of clinical governance within primary care in the Southwest*. University of Exeter and Exeter and North Devon NHS Research and Development Support Unit.

The NHS plan. (2000). The Stationery Office, Cm 4818 Norwich.

Thompson, G., Frances, J., Levacic, R. and Mitchell, J. (eds) (1991). *Markets, hierarchies and networks: the co-ordination of social life.* Sage, London.

Trinder, L. and Reynolds, S. (eds) (2000). *Evidence-based practice: a critical reader.* Blackwell, Oxford.

Wallace, L.M., Freeman, T., Latham, L., Walshe, K. and Sprurgeon, P. (2001). Organisational strategies for changing clinical practice: how trusts are meeting the challenges of clinical governance. *Quality and Safety in Health Care*, **10**, 76–82.

Walsh, M.J. and Small, N. (2001). Clinical governance in primary care: early impressions based on Bradford South and West Primary Care Group's experience. *British Journal of Clinical Governance*, **6**, 2, 109–18.

Walshe, K. (2000). Developing clinical governance: leadership, culture and change. *Journal of Clinical Governance*, **8**, 166–73.

Walshe, K., Freeman, T., Latham, L., Wallace, L. and Spurgeon, P. (2000). *Clinical governance: from policy to practice.* Health Services Management Centre, Birmingham.

Walshe, K. (2002). The rise of regulation in the NHS. *British Medical Journal*, **324**, 967–70.

Williamson, O. (1985). *The economic institutions of capitalism.* Free Press, New York.

Part III

Methods and frameworks

12

Dementia plus

David Jolley and Kate Read

UK NETWORK OF DEMENTIA SERVICES DEVELOPMENT CENTRES

The Dementia Service Development Centre, which Mary Marshall developed at the University of Stirling, was a truly visionary initiative. It was set up predominantly to support Scots people striving to develop high-quality dementia services. However, the centre soon found itself overwhelmed by enquiries from the rest of the UK and the world beyond, and called on to support endeavours in many localities. There came a point at which Mary and her colleagues felt strongly that others could add to the body of expertise available in a complementary manner.

Thus, with Mary's encouragement and guidance, the Department of Health has supported the development of a network of Dementia Services Development Centres (DSDCs) to cover the whole of the UK (Fig. 12.1). Likewise, centres providing some or similar services are also beginning to identify themselves throughout Europe and other parts of the world.

The funding of the UK DSDCs has come from a variety of sources, including the NHS, academic bodies, charitable funding research grants and direct commissions. For some, the funding streams have been difficult to identify and precarious to sustain but the intention remains to have centres in Scotland, Ireland and Wales and in each of the old NHS 'regions'. It is felt that this will extend and enrich the range and depth of expertise available and will also facilitate the collection and

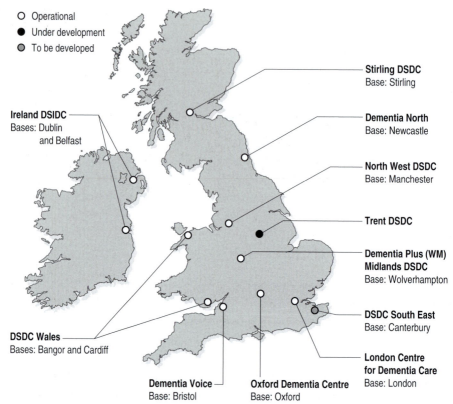

Figure 12.1   Dementia Services Development Centres in the UK

collation of materials which will be of particular interest to neighbouring trusts and other agencies.

THE DEVELOPMENT OF DEMENTIA PLUS

Enthusiasm for a West Midlands Dementia Services Development Centre was generated within health and social care agencies, voluntary sector and academic circles. The West Midland NHS Executive had decided to use monies identified for a modernisation programme in mental health to develop three Learning, Education, Development Centres (LEDS): one focused on Child and Adolescent Mental Health (CAMHS), a second focused on mental health for adults of working age, and another on the mental health of older people. It seemed logical to bring together the concepts of Dementia Services Development Centre and Learning

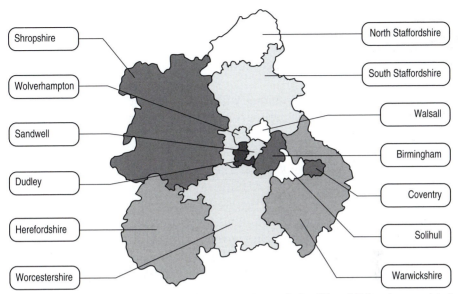

Figure 12.2 Health and social care communities of the West Midlands supported by Dementia Plus

Education Development Centre to produce something for the West Midlands, which combined the benefits of both for Older People with Mental Health problems. Thus it was that a collaborative partnership of Wolverhampton Health Care NHS Trust, the Social Services department of Wolverhampton Metropolitan Borough Council and the University of Wolverhampton tendered successfully to develop the centre for older people.

Dementia Plus was established in Wolverhampton, with a remit to provide the activities of a DSDC within the West Midlands in liaison with other members of the UK Dementia Services Development Centre network, but with a broader vision and responsibility to encompass all mental health issues of late life, thereby contributing to the all age vision of the Learning Education Development Centres.

The overall objective of Dementia Plus is:

> *'To measurably improve the quality of the care and treatment of older people with mental ill health by working with the staff throughout the West Midlands.'*

In common with all of the Dementia Services Development Centres this is approached through activity in four core areas:

- Information
- Education and training
- Research and evaluation
- Service development and consultancy.

Dementia Plus is currently unique within the dementia network in accepting a remit to cover aspects of mental health/mental illness in late life.

Regional office funding enabled Dementia Plus to become operational from October 2000 to March 2003. The disappearance of the regional tier of administration from the NHS, in April 2002, produced uncertainties for the future but the West Midlands Primary Care Trusts Levy Board has provided core funding for the year 2003/4. Alternative long-term sponsorship within the current framework of services and agencies is being explored. Additional revenue has been attracted from the start through commissions, conferences, grants and from other sources.

The three partnership organisations, Wolverhampton City Primary Care Trust, Wolverhampton Social Services and Wolverhampton University provide accommodation and supportive infrastructure. A core team includes the Executive Director (a social scientist), Director (consultant old age psychiatrist) and secretary. Other staff are employed on shorter contracts in response to specific commissions and funding opportunities and have included nurses, a management consultant and several research assistants from various backgrounds. The National Institute for Mental Health has attached its 'Old Age' Fellow to Dementia Plus. This is a very significant appointment and has been strengthened by additional sponsorship by the University of Wolverhampton where the Fellow has been awarded a personal Chair. A number of academics, clinicians and other practitioners contribute their time and skills, part-time, to enhance the activity and expertise of the core team.

In addition to its links into the formal NHS structure and the Dementia Centre network, Dementia Plus has a steering group originally set up and chaired by the West Midlands NHS Executive with people of all relevant professions and organisations drawn from all localities across the West Midlands. This steering group is vital both to ensure that activities are relevant and responsive to the issues, which are of interest and concern to staff in commissioning and provider organisations, and to disseminate information about activities and findings.

Core activities

Information

The success or failure of Dementia Plus will be determined by its being recognised and used by professionals across the region to improve their competence, raise their confidence and improve services.

The approach to communication has been to be multi-faceted. A newsletter, reaching approximately 3,000 people (mainly mental health care professionals) across the West Midlands, has appeared approximately every six months. It offers hard copy and can be kept for reference, photocopied and/or passed between colleagues. Latterly, a joint circulation with the West Midlands-based Institute of Health and Ageing has begun. This has the potential to bring mental health interest to those involved with physically ill older people and information about treatments for physical illness to those caring for the mentally ill. A further variation should see a linkage with the newsletter of the recently established West Midlands Centre of the National Institute for Mental Health in England (NIMHE). This will bring together news of mental health initiatives and opportunities across the age spectrum.

A website has been created in partnership with the LED for adults of working age and enabled the first version of the site to include linked pages for the other West Midlands Mental Health Partnership as well as networking with other DSDCs. The website continues to evolve and has proved to be an effective channel by which the centre has become known and can give and receive information flexibly and responsively.

Regular emailing to key individuals can be a useful means of reminding them of interesting projects, meetings and things to look out for. Email messaging and sharing of ideas is developing as being at least as important as the more traditional exchange of correspondence.

Personal contact, however, remains the most potent of mechanisms. Consultant psychiatrists of the region have an established network with regular meetings. Dementia Plus has been welcomed at these and uses the network for easy exchange of ideas and promotion of initiatives. Clinical psychologists in the region have a special interest group but there were no similar pre-existing forums for nurses, occupational therapists or other disciplines. First meetings of a nurse interest group have been stimulated and this and similar ventures will, hopefully, thrive.

A good deal of time was committed in the early weeks to visits to key individuals in agencies throughout the region. These led to opportunities to speak to larger, representative groups or to contribute to local projects and programmes. People have been encouraged to visit the centre, and staff have issued invitations to interested parties when invited to speak at meetings and conferences. These have been accepted with particular enthusiasm by people in training or with special responsibilities to develop new services or variations in services in response to national guidance.

The telephone is busy and allows immediate and personalised discussion of interests and particular problems or quandaries.

The centre is eager to receive enquiries and requests for information and help from professionals across the West Midlands (colleagues from elsewhere are usually redirected to their own DSDC). The number of enquiries fluctuates from 7 to 15 per month and they have come from all localities across the West Midlands. Most enquiries come from health professionals with lesser numbers from social services and independent sector staff (ratio 2:1:1). Some come from students registered on training courses and an interesting minority from other indirectly related organisations such as the police. In two-and-a-half years, there have been over 250 enquiries relating to nearly a hundred different topics. These range from questions about latest insights in the biological substrate of disorders to mental health implications of recent government initiatives. Most arise from uncertainties about how to offer the best, most up-to-date service for particular groups and in defined circumstances and with restricted budgets. Early onset dementia, design for dementia, care practice in hospital or care settings, day care and community mental health teams are amongst the most frequent areas of interest. Table 12.1 lists the topics for information sought most frequently during the first two-and-a-half years of Dementia Plus' operation.

Some enquirers seek advice on a literature search or ask that Dementia Plus undertake such a search for them. One facility that can be offered is access to the shared electronic database of literature held by the DSDCs, particularly the long-established library at Stirling. This relates mainly to Dementia, though Dementia Plus has begun to collect materials on other mental disorders in late life to complement the dementia literature. It includes unpublished work and local publications (the 'grey literature') with brief summaries and interpretations of its significance and applicability. There is also capacity to obtain copies or loans of much of the literature held which makes it a rich source of material.

Other callers want to talk through issues and dilemmas with someone who has experience of the situation they find themselves in, or

Table 12.1 Information requests	
Topic	No. of information requests
Early onset dementia	28
Training for nursing/residential homes	18
Ethnicity and dementia	16
Models of good practice (intermediate care)	12
Design for dementia	11
Assessment	9
Memory clinics	8
Carer support	8
Care standards in nursing/residential homes	7
Inpatient resources	7
Sexuality	6
Environmental technology	6

something similar. Dementia Plus staff may be able to fulfil this role themselves or make contact with others who can.

It became clear early in the development of Dementia Plus that a compendium of the style, volume and nature of services in all localities across the West Midlands would be helpful. This goes some way to providing an overview of the complexity of needs encountered and the variety of responses demonstrated. It is a resource to help people network with colleagues who are striving to tackle similar problems and who could learn from each other. Putting together the first edition of this compilation proved to be a taxing undertaking, particularly at a time of radical change within the NHS and additional changes in other agencies. It provides, however, an information base upon which Dementia Plus can draw now and from which potentially change in the future and its varied impact can be monitored. It has the capacity therefore, to inform the research agenda.

EDUCATION AND TRAINING

The range of training and education opportunities available across the West Midlands was scoped in 2001/2 (available on the website). This enables staff and enquirers to identify courses, which might satisfy particular demands. It has also revealed a number of gaps in provision when set against the needs for training and education arising from developments in knowledge, practice and guidance.

Dementia Plus has begun to attempt to fill these gaps by organising some training directly and encouraging other agencies to address others. The review identified no courses providing post-qualification training in ageing and mental health. This has encouraged Dementia Plus to work with its partners in the University of Wolverhampton to develop a Masters programme in Ageing and Mental Health which will be provided on a modular basis, allowing students to study part time to gain a certificate, two years for a diploma and three years for the MSc. This is being taught predominantly by practising clinicians in association with academics. It aims to be attractive to professionals of all disciplines, including doctors and nurses working in primary care and general hospitals as well as specialist mental health services, social services and the independent sector. The validated programme will run from September 2003.

Two themes have emerged from scoping and networking in the West Midlands and from national studies as requiring the most urgent attention:

- The identification and management of mental health problems in older people in primary care
- The care of older people with mental health problems who are in nursing or residential care.

These themes find echoes in the standards which were identified by the Department of Health's 'National Service Framework for Older People' and the Audit Commission's 'Forget-me-Not'. It is clear from colleagues in other DSDCs that these are needs that are shared throughout the country.

Whilst the Masters programme and other developmental initiatives within the West Midlands may begin to address the needs of qualified professionals working in primary care and specialist services in secondary care, the challenge of education and training for unqualified staff and volunteers who give day-to-day care to old people in their own homes or in residential and nursing homes is even more complex and massive in scale. A number of agencies are exploring approaches. Amongst these, the DSDC network is attempting to develop an accredited programme of training for care staff which focuses on the specialist needs of older people with mental health problems and which can be mapped against NVQ requirements.

Training for both qualified and unqualified staff will be informed by the research findings in the understanding of older people and the conditions encountered, good practice in care and service delivery and in educational method. This will mean that students' time will be used optimally and they will become agents of change toward better services and iteratively improved training.

In addition to these major programme developments, bespoke courses are prepared at the request of organisations or groups. Thus, courses have been provided with success to residential and nursing facilities, very sheltered and sheltered housing schemes, community mental health teams and others.

There is an evolving pattern of conferences. Some have used the expertise of Dementia Plus in partnership with another organisation. In other instances Dementia Plus has organised all aspects of the conference as a West Midlands initiative. Events have usually been open to all disciplines though there may be advantage in also offering smaller events for individual professions to explore topics in greater depth or in facilitating multi-professional events focused on a single topic. Seminars and publicly accessible open lectures are organised in conjunction with the University of Wolverhampton.

RESEARCH AND EVALUATION

Despite progress made in services for older people with mental health problems over the past forty years there remains opportunity to research a wide range of questions about the natural history of the disorders and the impact of specific treatment and therapeutic approaches, services or components of services on the lives of older people with mental illness, families and the wider community.

One of Dementia Plus' roles is to glean the most relevant findings from the work of other researchers, distil them and make them available in a useable form within the care communities of the West Midlands; however, it can and does contribute to research in the field as a research unit and in liaison with others.

As indicated by the enquiries for information early onset dementia was quickly identified as a topic of concern in the West Midlands. One of the first commissioned pieces of work was a review of the needs of younger people with dementia and their families in Worcestershire from which a series of recommendations for service development were made

(Dementia Plus 2000). This work has linked to another West Midlands initiative involving the Alzheimer's Society and the creation of a regional early onset forum. This meets regularly and is encouraging the systematic commissioning and development of specialist services for Early Onset Dementia tailored to the characteristics of the differing communities and including better liaison with neurology services and wider appreciation of the potential contributions to be made by the clinical genetics service.

Another early venture investigated the understanding of people with dementia from black and minority ethnic communities and their views of the services, which should support them. Many of the towns and cities of the West Midlands have substantial minority populations, which are beginning to generate larger cohorts of old people. This work enabled Wolverhampton's health and social care community to develop a five-year strategic approach to make services better informed, more sensitive to cultural issues and to engage in an on-going programme of mutual education (Dementia Plus 2001). The information achieved in this study is of interest and application for other communities in the Midlands and elsewhere. A follow-on study reviewed progress one year on and compares and contrasts the Wolverhampton initiative and its outcomes with those in Bradford. Bradford Social Services have adopted a predominantly 'in-reach' approach in equipping its mainstream domiciliary care service to meet the needs of South Asian elders, whilst the Wolverhampton model is essentially based on 'out-reach' into the community networks from established specialist services.

There are strengths and weaknesses to both the 'in-reach' and 'out-reach' approaches, which are clarified in the research. This learning will be applied to improve developments in Bradford and Wolverhampton and will be of interest to other communities with similar minority population issues.

Intermediate care is another area where Dementia Plus is contributing research findings. With publication of the *National service framework for older people* (2001) came the aspiration that funding for new developments would follow. In reality, the only additional funding was ring-fenced to be spent on 'intermediate care'. Intermediate care built on established concepts of rehabilitation, bringing together approaches which help older people avoid unnecessary institutionalisation and recover their independence so that they can return to the community after a period of acute ill health which has left them disabled/unable to live independently (6).

The *National service framework for older people* laid down very specific criteria to which services seeking to access funding had to adhere. Whilst the criteria did not specify that older people with mental health problems should be excluded from intermediate care, the first generation of such services often did exclude people with dementia and other psychiatric disorders. They justified this by citing evidence that people with cognitive difficulties were less likely to benefit from therapies of such short duration. (The *National service framework for older people* criteria specify that interventions should be for less than six weeks and usually be for only one to two weeks). It was not until the Department of Health issued further guidance (DoH 2002), which emphasised the importance of including people with dementia, that services began to equip themselves to respond to the mental health components of people's needs.

It was therefore of great interest that Dementia Plus had the opportunity to evaluate the implementation of the intermediate care service developed in Telford and Wrekin, which had included mental health professionals in the core team from inception (Dementia Plus 2003). The design of this study included an interim evaluation within the first year, which allowed feedback to both the steering group and the intermediate care team so that modifications of practice could be agreed and incorporated at this stage. The evaluation team were then commissioned to revisit the service a year later to identify outcomes and outputs demonstrated and from the perspectives of the whole health and social care system and service users points of view. (9). Again the evaluative process was able to contribute to the ongoing development of the service.

Other projects have continued investigation of the work patterns and stress profiles of staff working with older people with mental illness, facilitated description and evaluation of memory clinic activity and measured the effectiveness of a brief training experience for probationer police recruits to raise their awareness of mental health problems and to allow them to discuss their role in relationship to other agencies caring.

Research assistants from Wolverhampton University, supervised by Dementia Plus and university staff are involved with studies of: nursing home care, continuing care of people with severe dementia, and the implementation of guidance in best practice in the care of people who enter old age with a long-standing or relapsing psychosis.

Other projects are in preparation in association with the University of Wolverhampton, University of Birmingham, University of Kentucky and other DSDCs. An element of the research work undertaken has to combine expertise with opportunity presented by funding bodies. It is, never the less, important to Dementia Plus that the research and evaluative work it undertakes is relevant to practice development within the West Midlands and can inform consultancy and education activity.

SERVICE DEVELOPMENT CONSULTANCY

The model upon which Dementia Plus activity is based is a continuous four-themed cycle, with each area or activity being informed by, and generating information for, the other elements of the cycle. (See Fig. 12.3.)

Service development consultancy is the fourth aspect of the cycle, which, to promote high quality service, needs to be firmly based on experience, the evidence base of research activity and the corresponding literature. Whilst much of the developmental work undertaken has been in response to requests from localities or agencies gearing up to implement the standards of the *National service framework for older people*, there are opportunities to undertake more thematic and strategic initiatives.

Examples include:

I. Working with Primary Care Trusts and Mental Health Trusts to develop expertise and resource to improve the effectiveness of their primary/secondary care interface.

II. Partnership work with the charity For Dementia to establish Admiral Nursing Teams in specific localities throughout the West Midlands. For Dementia have recognised that there is a limited evidence base underpinning the development of this approach and the

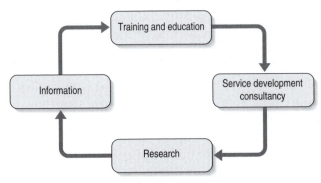

Figure 12.3 Dementia Plus cycle of activity

organisation has identified that a robust research approach is required, to which Dementia Plus has become an adviser.

III. Review of plans to remodel services which carry an implication that some existing facilities will close and some very disabled residents will be required to move from their home of some years to another environment.

CONCLUSION

It is early days for Dementia Plus. The aspiration is to build on the innovation of Mary Marshall's Dementia Service Development Centre at Stirling in encouraging improvements of services for dementia by supporting professionals involved in care work and to expand that vision to encompass all the mental health needs of older people.

The range and breadth of the *National service framework for older people* has confirmed this aspiration to be entirely appropriate and relevant for the population of the West Midlands, and might be applied in other parts of England and Wales.

References

Audit Commission. (2000). *Forget me not. Mental health services for older people.* Audit Commission, London.

Dementia Plus. (2000). Early onset dementia in Worcestershire (1999/2000). Dementia Plus, Wolverhampton.

Dementia Plus. (2001). *Twice a child: dementia care for African-Caribbean and Asian older people in Wolverhampton.* Dementia Plus, Wolverhampton.

Dementia Plus. (2002). *Intermediate Care Team Telford and Wrekin: Interim Evaluation.* Dementia Plus, Wolverhampton.

Dementia Plus. (2003). *Intermediate Care Team Telford and Wrekin: Second Evaluation.* Dementia Plus, Wolverhampton.

Department of Health. (2001). *National service framework for older people.* HMSO, London.

Department of Health. (2002). *Intermediate care: the way forward.* HMSO, London.

13

Early intervention in psychosis: research, clinical practice and service reform

Elizabeth Newton and Max Birchwood

INTRODUCTION

The aim of this chapter is to explain the rationale for early intervention through a review of past and current literature and to explain how this relates to clinical practice. We will go on to give an example of how this research informs current clinical practice by describing Birmingham Early Intervention Service. Finally, we will discuss the impetus for government reforms, which recommend that for every one million of the population there should be an early intervention service comprising three to four early intervention teams. This will ensure that young people with psychosis receive fast and easily accessible treatment within the early, critical phase, of psychosis which should lead to an improved, long-term prognosis.

EARLY INTERVENTION IN PSYCHOSIS: THE RESEARCH

Intervening early in the course of psychotic illness is 'intuitively appealing and ethically justified' (Malla and Norman 2002). The current research evidence for early intervention is extremely promising and is continuing to grow with a wide range of new, international studies now in progress. This body of research will be considered here under the following subheadings: the early detection of psychosis; reducing treatment delay; the early phase of psychosis as a 'critical period'; and evidence-based interventions in psychosis.

The early detection of psychosis

The possibility of identifying psychosis before the emergence of positive symptoms has been an ambition of psychiatry for generations, but is only now being afforded serious consideration. It is now understood that most individuals with broadly defined schizophrenia experience a lengthy 'prodrome' involving non-specific symptoms, behaviour change and increasing functional impairment prior to the emergence of more diagnostically specific psychotic symptoms (Yung and McGorry 1996a; 1996b). This has recently been translated into a workable research paradigm. From a series of naturalistic prospective studies, the PACE clinic in Melbourne, Australia, have defined operational criteria for an 'ultra high risk' group of individuals based on attenuated psychotic symptoms, transient psychotic symptoms or genetic risk, in the context of functional decline (Yung *et al.* 1998). These have been used as the inclusion criteria for research which targets a group at possible 'high risk' of developing psychosis. Studies using these criteria have found that 40% of those defined using these criteria will proceed to develop a 'full blown' psychosis (Yung *et al.* 1998). This rate has remained consistent at follow-up (McGorry 2000), and has been independently replicated (Phillips *et al.* 1999; McGlashan *et al.* 2001).

Using the PACE ultra-high-risk paradigm, McGorry *et al.* (2002) identified 59 individuals at incipient risk of progression to first-episode psychosis. The sample were randomly assigned to one of two conditions: 'needs-based intervention' (supportive psychotherapy, vocational and family interventions, plus needs-led assistance in areas such as accommodation and education) or 'specific preventative intervention' (needs-based intervention, plus six months of low-dose Risperidone and cognitive behavioural therapy, focusing on understanding, coping with symptoms and reduction of associated distress). The main outcomes indicated that there were significantly more benefits to the specific prevention treatment than the needs-based treatment immediately following the intervention ($P = .01$). This significant difference was lost, however, at six months post-intervention, as three more people from the specific preventive-intervention group made transition to first-episode psychosis. It is important to note that in cases where individuals remained Risperidone-adherent the treatment benefits continued. In addition, all individuals in the study improved symptomatically and functionally after treatment (irrespective of treatment group) – this was also true for the 'false-positives' who received anti-psychotics and did not become psychotic. Furthermore, no other harm as a result of treatment was detected in terms of stigmatisation, side-effects of anti-psychotic medication or anxiety caused due to being informed of a risk of progression to psychosis (the investigators noted that individuals were aware that something potentially serious was happening to them even before entering the study).

This study is of importance as it was the first to suggest that it is possible to delay, and potentially avert, progression across the full diagnostic threshold for psychotic disorder. McGorry *et al.* (2002) point out that although these findings are not necessarily generalisable, they should be investigated more rigorously, with larger sample size, and over longer follow-up periods before medication is used as standard treatment in ultra-high-risk individuals. EPOS is a collaborative study which aims to do just this. It is the first European multi-centre study on early recognition and intervention for persons at risk of developing psychosis. This prospective, longitudinal field-study involves a multi-level assessment which aims to validate the predictive factor of the PACE 'ultra high risk' criteria. It covers a total population area of five million people (estimated cases = 3,600) and is expected to provide extensive data to determine a 'risk profile' with regard to the transition to psychosis. Systematic monitoring of received interventions (e.g. psychological or pharmacological treatments) and their outcomes will form an empirical evidence-base for controlled clinical trials in the future (www.epos5.org).

There is ongoing debate over the risks and benefits of such early detection (McGlashan, Miller and Woods 2001; Verdoux and Cougnard 2003), particularly as the usefulness of early detection from a public health perspective has not yet been demonstrated (Verdoux and Cougnard 2003). Ethical issues are raised in such prevention strategies, particularly because interventions might target 'false–positive' cases, and depending on the type of treatment might increase the risk of side-effects from medication or may cause unnecessary exposure to distress, stigmatisation and other potential psychosocial consequences of 'being at risk of psychosis' (Warner 2001; Verdoux and Cougnard 2003). However, the ultra-high-risk paradigm focuses on distressed, help-seeking individuals who already have low-level psychotic symptoms and for whom a protocol of treatment does not yet exist. Thus, the concept of false-positive is something of a misnomer; what is needed is a protocol of treatment that can both prevent exacerbation of these low-level symptoms, and also reduce the distressing symptoms themselves. Drug treatments have low engagement at this stage (McGorry *et al.*

2002) and there is the problem of knowing how long to continue drug treatment in those who do not experience a transition to psychosis. Studies using psychological approaches to lowering distress such as CBT (e.g. French *et al.* 2004) show promise in reducing both transition rates and distress caused by low-level psychotic symptoms. They may also be more acceptable to service users than drug treatments.

The general consensus appears to be that evidence for benefits of early detection and intervention is not yet strong enough to justify pre-onset treatment as 'standard practice', but that the benefits found to date '... outweigh risks to a degree that justifies continued, well-controlled investigation' (McGlashan, Miller and Woods 2001, p. 569). Therefore, the high-risk paradigm remains primarily a research area, and service implications are yet to be established.

Reducing treatment delay

The relationship between long duration of untreated psychosis (DUP) and poorer clinical outcome is a 'cornerstone' argument in favour of early intervention (Verdoux and Cougnard 2003). Beginning with the *UK Northwick Park study of first episodes of schizophrenia in 1986* (Johnstone *et al.* 1986), a number of studies have demonstrated the delay between onset of psychosis and first treatment, averaging approximately a year (Birchwood *et al.* 1992; Norman and Malla 2001).

Longer DUP has been found in some research to have a positive correlation with both a poorer outcome and a longer time prior to symptomatic remission (Wyatt 1991; Loebel *et al.* 1992; Norman and Malla 2001). Long delays have also been found to increase the use of the Mental Health Act (1983) in the UK (compulsory detention), which in turn increases likelihood of disengagement – approximately 50% of people in routine mental health services are 'lost' within 12 months (McGovern *et al.* 1994). In addition, long DUP is frequently associated with severe behavioural disturbance, sometimes including harm to self or others, and family difficulty (Johnstone *et al.* 1986).

There are some inconsistencies in research findings, and although most retrospective studies of DUP do confirm a relationship between longer DUP and poor outcome, findings are generally correlational, and do not confer causality (Norman and Malla 2001). There is also evidence that other factors are at play which partly account for this link, for example, that negative symptoms in the prodrome (a known prognostic factor) lead to a delay in help-seeking and to first treatment. However, studies which have attempted to allow for this (Loebel *et al.* 1992;

Drake *et al.* 2000) still find that DUP emerges in a robust fashion. Randomised control designs to establish causality would require a deliberate (and ethically unacceptable) delay in treatment, and therefore can not be conducted. An early placebo-control study of drug treatment in first-episode psychosis (May *et al.* 1981) has shown that those with longer DUP due to allocation to a placebo condition, have a poorer long-term outcome than those treated immediately with neuroleptics, despite prescription of neuroleptics following completion of the trial.

Two major studies are currently investigating the possibility of reducing DUP, and the effect of this on outcome. The TIPS project in Norway aims to reduce DUP using an epidemiological 'case-control' design comparing Rogaland County in the west of Norway with control areas in Oslo (Norway) and Roskilde County (Denmark) (see Johannessen *et al.* 2001 for a description). TIPS consists of a low-threshold detection team established to assess individuals who may be experiencing a first-episode of psychosis, and a large-scale educational/awareness campaign to encourage early identification of psychotic individuals. Following detection, individuals are included in the project for two years, this involves assessment and treatment based on medication, psychotherapy and family work. The project aims to establish optimal treatment programmes by conducting follow-up studies assessing outcome. Early results have shown that increasing awareness of psychosis amongst the general public, schools and primary mental health services can dramatically reduce DUP. The early detection group had a median DUP 21.5 weeks less than that of the 'usual' detection group (Larsen *et al.* 2001). This has led to significant improvement in service engagement and decreased use of compulsory detention (www.tips-info.com). The anti-stigmatising and informative campaign has also changed help-seeking behaviours (Johanessen *et al.* 2001).

The REDIRECT project in Birmingham, UK, aims to reduce DUP by increasing the detection of those experiencing a first-episode psychosis in primary care. Recognition and treatment of individuals in the early stages of psychosis has been found to be poor (Lincoln and McGorry 1999) and the REDIRECT project aims to improve this by providing an intensive training programme for GPs to increase awareness of early warning signs and high-risk 'individuals' by using video vignettes and interview practice. The cluster-randomised study covers all GP practices in inner-city Birmingham (population 350,000). The project aims to reduce the referral and treatment delay arising from within primary care (by increasing detection rates) and by improving the interface with secondary care (by direct access to the Birmingham early intervention service intake team). Data on the impact of reducing DUP and consequent impact on early outcome are pending.

In summary, although early, optimistic claims of the impact of DUP on the natural course of psychosis are presented more cautiously in recent literature (Verdoux and Cougnard 2003). It is evident that there are at least short-term deleterious effects of delays in treatment (Norman and Malla 2001). Harrison *et al.* (2001) have found that short-term outcomes and illness course are the best predictors of long-term outcome and illness course. Treatment delay also causes major distress and difficulty for service users and for their families and is, in itself, sufficient to justify a focus on this group of young people with serious mental illness. Shorter DUP should minimise distress experienced by service users and their families, and reduce the burden imposed on health care systems. Reducing DUP must therefore be viewed as a high service priority. Early intervention services are now being set up across the world, with this as a primary aim. Services and research studies have tackled this difficulty successfully in different ways. For example, some studies have aimed to make access to services easier for individuals potentially suffering from psychosis (Jorgensen *et al.* 2000), others have taken a more active, outreach approach to community case detection (Johannessen *et al.* 2001).

The early phase of psychosis as a 'critical period'

It is now widely acknowledged that the early stage of psychosis 'sets the scene' for long-term illness trajectories, social disabilities and psychological co-morbidities. The first five years following the onset of psychosis have been posited as a 'critical period' (Birchwood and MacMillan 1993; Birchwood, Todd and Jackson 1998) during which most deterioration occurs and when long-term trajectories are established. The 'critical period' hypothesis is supported by evidence which links early outcomes to long-term outcomes and also by evidence which shows that psychotic symptoms plateau within the first few years following onset.

In a comprehensive study of 15- and 25-year outcomes from a first-episode psychosis, Harrison *et al.* (2001) found early (two-year) course patterns to be the strongest predictors of 15-year outcomes. The strongest predictor of all long-term outcome variables was the duration of positive psychotic symptoms within the first two years of illness (the shorter the percentage of time with psychotic symptoms, the better both symptom scores, disability scores and overall course of illness were at long-term follow-up). This research has strengthened the case for early clinical intervention, aimed at reducing the amount of time experiencing psychotic symptoms within the first two years after their onset, which may improve long-term prognosis and outcome. OPUS is a randomised control trial designed to investigate this relationship. Integrated treatment (assertive community treatment; low-dose, second-generation, anti-psychotic medication; family treatment and social skills training) is being compared with standard treatment (anti-psychotic medication plus some psychoeducation) for first-episode psychosis (Jorgensen *et al.* 2000). The study has begun to yield some interesting results regarding treatment in the early phase of psychosis. The integrated treatment has been found to show significant benefits in reducing positive and negative symptoms in individuals experiencing first-episode psychosis, as well as increasing client satisfaction, an essential prerequisite for engagement (Nordentoft *et al.* 2002a). However, with most early intervention services still in their infancy, the case for early intervention is not yet proven. Early indications are promising and outcome data are now being collected across the world, which will allow us to evaluate the effectiveness of early intervention and its effects on long-term trajectories.

Another argument in favour of early intervention comes from Bleuler's classic follow-up study in which he observed that patients reach a plateau of psychopathology and disability early in the course of illness, contrary to the Kraepelinian notion of relentless, progressive deterioration. It has become apparent from consequent research that early deterioration in many individuals stabilises, and that favourable outcomes are achieved at long-term follow-up (Carpenter and Strauss 1991; Harrison *et al.* 2001). Generally, the prospective first-episode studies have not addressed this 'plateau' hypothesis, the one exception being a multiple follow-up investigation in Madras (Thara *et al.* 1994; Eaton *et al.* 1995). This unique investigation discovered a steep decline in the prevalence of both positive and negative syndromes during the first year of follow-up, and a stabilisation of such prevalence to about 20–25% after two years. Another study, which bears on the plateau hypothesis, is Harrison *et al.*'s (1996) analysis of the Nottingham (UK) sample of first-episode cohort. The addition of information about the two-year course type, 'complete or near complete remission' versus 'continually psychotic' (defined as more than one relapse and/or residual personality change), substantially increased prediction of outcome at 13 years in terms of social activity and psychopathology, with the latter of the course types predicting unfavourable outcome.

These two studies provide the strongest evidence yet for the concept of a 'plateauing out' of schizophrenia and supports McGlashan's view that deterioration, though variable, does occur in the pre-psychotic period and early in the course of psychosis (whether treated or untreated), but this will stabilise between two and five years (McGlashan 1988). Such a notion gives much needed therapeutic optimism and an alternative to the chronicity paradigm that dominated thinking throughout much of the twentieth century. Again, these data suggest that within the first two to five years, interventions, particularly for variables, which may be predictors of long-term outcome such as medication adherence, substance misuse, relapse, family support and so forth, may have a beneficial effect on the long-term outcomes of the illness. Some of these interventions are discussed further below.

Evidence-based interventions in early psychosis

Above, we have summarised the evidence, which supports and continues to investigate the notion of early intervention in psychosis. It seems that the key research question has now shifted from: Is early intervention effective? to: What kind of early intervention is most appropriate and effective? In order to put early intervention into clinical practice, services need to incorporate therapeutic interventions, which have been demonstrated to be effective in research studies. There is now a reliable body of evidence, which supports medical, psychological and family interventions in psychosis, and based on a thorough review of the evidence these interventions are recommended by the NICE guidelines (2002).

Pharmacological interventions

The aim of pharmacotherapy in the treatment of young people with first-episode psychosis is to maximise the therapeutic benefit whilst minimising adverse effects. Spencer *et al.* (2001) reviewed the literature on drug treatments in first-episode psychosis and have made six recommendations for medical intervention:

1. An initial anti-psychotic-free observation period should be used to confirm that psychosis is present and to discount organic causes by carrying out routine medical examinations.
2. Use of atypical antipsychotics is recommended as fewer side-effects make them more tolerable for clients, resulting in greater compliance with treatment.

3. Low doses of atypical anti-psychotics are recommended and benzodiazepines for the treatment of hostility. The positive symptoms experienced by people with first-episode psychosis have been demonstrated to respond well to 2–3 mg haloperidol equivalents per day or 2–4 mg risperidone. There is therefore no response advantage in prescribing higher doses, which increase the likelihood of side-effects.
4. Anti-psychotic medication should be changed when no significant response is made. Research has demonstrated that symptoms will improve significantly in the vast majority of cases (Lieberman *et al.* 1993). However, several different medications may need to be tried to achieve success.
5. Remission of positive psychotic is believed to stabilise between three and six months after their first onset (Edwards *et al.* 1998). Failure to respond to treatment by this time should trigger prompt action, such as a review of organic factors, chlozipine treatment for persistent symptoms and the introduction of cognitive behavioural therapy for distressing residual symptoms.
6. It is currently unclear how long patients should be prescribed anti-psychotic medication for following a first-episode. Spencer *et al.* (2001) suggest at least one to two years following remission of symptoms.

Psychological interventions

Since the early 1990s, cognitive behavioural therapy (CBT) for psychosis has been used in clinical practice in the UK. This approach draws on Beck's approach to depression (1979) and on a multifactorial formulation of psychotic symptoms that takes into account neuropsychiatric theories of psychosis, stress-vulnerability models and cognitive theories of psychotic symptomotology (Fowler, Garety and Kuipers 1995). CBT for psychosis concentrates on positive psychotic symptoms and their meaning to the individual. Its main aims are to reduce the distress and disability associated with these symptoms, to reduce emotional disturbance such as anxiety and depression associated with the symptoms and to help the individual arrive at their own formulation of their difficulties, which should reduce risk of relapse (Garety, Fowler and Kuipers 2000).

CBT for psychosis is a long-term individual therapy; it is suggested that at least six assessment sessions are required followed by a median of twenty therapy sessions (Garety *et al.* 2000). A number of recent meta-analyses (Rector and Beck 2001; Pilling *et al.* 2002) have concluded that cognitive approaches produce large clinical effects and are effective in reducing or eliminating both positive and negative psychotic symptoms.

As yet, evidence for the effectiveness of CBT in reducing positive symptoms in early psychosis is sparse because trials have mainly included only those participants who have experienced treatment-resistant positive symptoms for a number of years. In a randomised controlled trial of CBT for acute psychosis, which included a number of young people with recent-onset psychosis, Drury *et al.* (1996) demonstrated that, as an adjunct to treatment as usual, cognitive therapy led to faster recovery and significantly fewer residual positive symptoms at nine months. Although this significant difference between groups had disappeared by the time of a five-year follow-up (Drury *et al.* 2000), the CBT group in this study continued to report greater perceived control over their illness than the non-cognitive therapy group. For those participants who had suffered one (or less) relapse, self-and-observer reported delusional beliefs were significantly reduced in the CBT group. More recently, preliminary reports from the SOCRATES trial in Manchester have suggested that early intervention using CBT in the acute phase of psychosis, following a first or second episode, can accelerate the resolution of positive symptoms. However, at the six-week follow-up, both the CBT and the routine-care groups had recovered to the same degree (Lewis *et al.* 2002). Longer-term outcomes, yet to be published, will examine the possibility that the CBT group will benefit more significantly later on, in terms of residual symptoms and relapse rates. These data alone are not enough to argue for the efficacy of CBT in early intervention, although a review of the evidence so far suggests that CBT clearly has some benefits. For example, studies show increased perception of control over symptoms, faster recovery from acute episodes and success in the treatment of residual, more persistent symptoms. However, until more evidence is available, treatment in early intervention services is guided by the promising results of CBT studies conducted on adult populations, and young people are, as suggested by NICE (2000), offered CBT as a part of routine clinical practice.

Family interventions
Between 60% and 70% of people with schizophrenia return from hospital after a first episode to live with their families (Stirling *et al.* 1991). Reports have associated living with families with greater risk of relapse. The mediating factor that has been demonstrated to increase the

likelihood of relapse is 'expressed emotion' (EE), the amount and intensity of positive or negative emotion, hostility and critical comments directed towards the person with schizophrenia. There has been much research in this area and a review of studies reported that a higher rate of relapse is consistently found in high EE groups (Bebbington and Kuipers 1994). Clearly, this is of particular concern for young people with psychosis, who are more likely to live with their families and may never progress to the stage of independent living. There is now a large and consistent body of evidence demonstrating the effectiveness of psycho-educational family interventions (for reviews see Fadden 1998; Dixon *et al.* 2000; Pilling *et al.* 2002). Family interventions have been shown to reduce relapse rates (e.g. Falloon *et al.* 1985; Tarrier *et al.* 1989), decrease frequency of hospitalisation (e.g. Mari *et al.* 1996), reduce costs of care (Fadden 1998), improve effective communication (Tarrier *et al.* 1994), increase understanding of difficulties (Szmuckler *et al.* 1996) and decrease the burden felt by carers (e.g. Posner *et al.* 1992).

Summary

A great deal is now known about the short- and long-term trajectories of psychosis and their biological and psychosocial influences. Delay in first treatment is robustly linked to poor early outcome (Norman and Malla 2001) and long-term follow-up studies show clearly that the outcome at two to three years strongly predicts outcome twenty years later (Harrison *et al.* 2001). The implication of these findings is that psychosis, even in its prodromal stages, needs to be recognised, monitored and treated. The possibility of predicting individuals at high risk for psychosis and averting or delaying transition to 'full-blown' psychosis is now becoming a real possibility. Once a person has been diagnosed with first-episode psychosis interventions need to be intensive during the 'critical' early stage in order to influence long-term outcomes and these interventions should be evidence-based. It is now widely recognised that psychological, family and social interventions in addition to pharmacological treatments are both efficacious and necessary in the treatment of psychosis if the best possible outcome is to be achieved.

Not only is the potential human benefit from early intervention enormous, it has been calculated that the annual cost of schizophrenia in England is £2.6 bn (Knapp *et al.* 1997). Therefore there is also an economic case for pursuing policies, such as early intervention, which may reduce the lifetime costs of care. The rationale for a greater concentration of therapeutic and service resources to the onset and early phase of psychosis seems overwhelming.

CLINICAL PRACTICE: THE BIRMINGHAM EARLY INTERVENTION SERVICE

Aims and guiding principles

The Birmingham Early Intervention Service (EIS) was the first early intervention service in the UK, established in 1989. It has played an integral role in influencing health policy and in developing guidelines for early intervention across the UK and was awarded 'beacon' status by the DoH providing the blueprint for the reform of services.

Referrals to the Birmingham EIS come from two functionalised teams working within Birmingham (home treatment, primary care liaison) and from local GPs. Referrals are accepted if the young person falls within the catchment area, is between the ages of 16 and 30 years and in their first year of treatment by mental health services for a psychotic illness (regardless of any diagnosis that has been given). The EIS uses a bio-psycho-social, multi-disciplinary approach to treatment. The intensive nature and wide range of interventions provided, aim to promote recovery in many different aspects of service users' lives to optimise recovery within the 'three-year critical period' (Birchwood *et al.* 1997). For example, to improve mental and physical health, psychological well-being and social and vocational performance. The primary aims of the Birmingham EIS are summarised in Table 13.1 below.

The service structure

Figure 13.1 gives an overview of the service structure, which is made up of four integrated component parts: ED:IT (the Early Detection and Intervention Team); the early intervention community assertive outreach teams; the vocational program; respite services.

ED : IT

In 2002, the Early Detection and Intervention Team (ED:IT) opened. This team works alongside the EIS providing support for young people felt to be at high risk of psychosis; for example those who have had attenuated psychotic symptoms or those with familial risk of psychosis

Table 13.1 Aims in the management of first-episode psychosis	
Aim	Implementation
1. To reduce the duration of untreated psychosis	● Close liaison with functionalised teams ● The REDIRECT project ● Early Detection and Intervention Team (see below) ● A 'no waiting list' policy
2. To accelerate recovery through effective biological and psychosocial interventions	● Multi-disciplinary formulation of clients needs and regular team reviews to ensure holistic care-plan and appropriate interventions ● Commitment to providing evidence-based interventions ● Adherence to NICE guidelines ● Regular and assertive-outreach style contact with service users (average one visit per week) so that treatments can be changed/implemented as soon as required ● Regular medication reviews ensuring change when something is not working
3. To reduce the individual's adverse reactions to the experience of psychosis and of treatment	● Youth-focused service in a non-stigmatising community setting ● Flexibility to meet at clients homes or in community settings by providing an outreach-style service ● Emphasis on engagement with one primary worker (case manager) for the whole period that a person is with the service ● Community respite facilities and home treatment as an alternative to admission ● Cognitive behavioural therapy for trauma symptoms ● Psycho-education aimed at normalising and destigmatising psychosis ● Recovery focused service
4. To work with families to give information, reduce likelihood of relapse and to ease the burden of care	● Regular family contact ● Psycho-education with every family ● Provision of literature on psychosis ● Family assessment and family therapy offered to all families ● Monthly carers group

Table 13.1 Continued	
Aim	Implementation
5. To maximise social and work functioning	● Case manager conducts individual work with clients ● Regular social and activity groups provided ● Individual and group psychological therapy for loss of social confidence, low self-esteem, social phobia, etc. ● Vocational worker in every team ● Regular vocational assessment for each client and individual vocational plan ● Early intervention community activity centre
6. To prevent relapse and treatment resistance	● Reduction of duration of untreated psychosis ● Relapse work and plan undertaken with each client and family ● Prompt intervention as soon as symptoms increase ● CBT for residual psychotic and co-morbid symptoms ● Regular medication reviews ensuring change when something is not working e.g. if two atypicals have not improved symptoms client is offered chlozipine

who themselves have had a recent deterioration in functioning. The aim of ED : IT's clinical service is threefold:

1. To educate other health services and statutory youth services about psychosis and therefore to pick up vulnerable people early
2. To work with young people believed to be 'at risk' from psychosis by using psychological techniques, supportive counselling and by providing practical support and by doing so to prevent or delay the transition to psychosis
3. To reduce duration of untreated psychosis by immediately referring those people who meet the criteria for a first psychotic episode onto the Early Intervention Service.

The research arm of the ED : IT service forms part of the European EPOS study investigating risk factors for transition to psychosis and the utility of psychological therapy and case management in reducing transition rates.

The early intervention community assertive outreach teams

The early intervention service currently comprises two community based, assertive outreach teams: one covering the north of the inner city

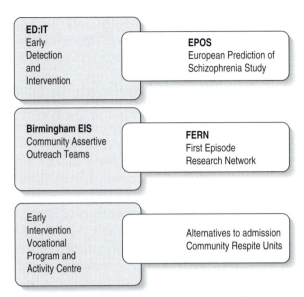

Figure 13.1 The structure of the Early Intervention Service and associated research projects

and one covering the eastern locality (population, 310,000). By 2005, there will be five community teams, covering the whole of Birmingham and Solihull (1.2 m population). The bulk of each clinical team consists of case managers who come from either a nursing or a social work background. The role of the case manager is multi-faceted. For example, case managers are involved in engagement, psycho-education, relapse prevention work, care planning, helping to enhance new and lost skills, family therapy, medication monitoring and helping with practical difficulties such as financial benefits or housing. A number of support workers are employed to assist case managers in the day-to-day management of clients, with some of these support-workers having specialist skills (for example an Asian family support worker to help with the engagement of Asian clients and to advise the teams on cultural issues).

One of the difficulties with traditional models of mental health care has been the disengagement of clients with psychosis (McGovern *et al.* 1994). Problems with engagement have been particularly highlighted in young people, who tend to doubt the usefulness of professional help and hold negative stereotypes of mental illness and mental health services (Lincoln and McGorry 1995). This has led to treatment non-compliance and 'revolving door' situations (when clients are treated in in patient units when in crisis, are discharged once their symptoms have reduced, disengage from community service, stop treatment, relapse and are again admitted to hospital in crisis), poor recovery and high levels of risk.

High levels of engagement and treatment retention are predictors of good symptomatic and functional outcomes in psychosis (Frank and Gunderson 1990). It is therefore essential that clients' and families' first impressions of the EIS and its staff are positive, in order to maximise future engagement with the service. We achieve this by allocating a case manager, who will remain with the client for the full three years that they are treated by the EIS. Each case manager has a small caseload of between 10 and 15 clients, which allows workers to spend a great deal of time getting to know new service users and their carers and to build trusting relationships with them. During their three years with the service, clients will be seen by many other members of the team, the case manager will remain the first point of contact for both the service user and other professionals involved in the service user's care (e.g. psychologist, vocational worker). This ensures a well-co-ordinated and structured care package. Sometimes a service user is non-adherent to treatment and reluctant to engage with their case manager. In these situations we do not reduce contact or discharge the client, as in more traditional models of mental health care. Instead, the case manager and the wider team increase their attempts to engage the service user and where possible will continue to work with their carers. By doing this signs of relapse can be caught early and treatment can be started promptly should relapse occur. Such intensive case management has demonstrated good outcomes. The service currently engages with 90% of clients successfully, has a lower than average use of the Mental Health Act and there has been only one suicide since the service opened in 1989.

In addition to case managers, each community team has two medical staff, one consultant and one staff grade. Medical practitioners in the EIS employ a symptom approach to treatment and follow closely the guidelines set out by Spencer *et al.* (2001). Very early diagnosis has been demonstrated to be both unreliable (Werry *et al.* 1991) and harmful (McGorry 1995). The symptom-based approach used in the EIS, and the use of the umbrella term 'psychosis', means that diagnoses are unlikely to be changed over time. This is less confusing for service users, families and medical professionals. Rather than specific diagnoses (e.g. schizophrenia or bipolar affective disorder) the term 'psychosis' is used to explain symptoms to service users and relatives who usually find this more tolerable and hopeful. Booklets are given to explain psychosis symptoms, treatment and expected outcome (Reading and Jackson 2003). A diagnosis that is more specific is only given once a stable pattern of symptoms has emerged.

Each early intervention team has one full-time clinical psychologist and two assistant psychologists who carry out psychological assessments and implement evidence-based psychological interventions. These begin with a full psychological assessment and formulation. The team psychologist provides psychological interventions in a number of different ways. Appropriate psychological interventions may be individual (for example, providing CBT for delusions and hallucinations or for co-morbid difficulties such as anxiety, depression, and social phobia and, neuropsychological assessment and therapy to improve cognitive difficulties); systemic (e.g. work with families, staff groups, colleges, etc.); group work (for example, cognitive behavioural groups to reduce the distress caused by auditory hallucinations) or indirect interventions (advising a care co-ordinator or staff about psychological issues affecting a client and supervising psychological interventions). In addition, the clinical psychologist plays a full part in multi-disciplinary team life by acting in a consultancy role at all team meetings and client reviews to provide a psychosocial perspective and to highlight areas where psychological interventions may have utility. The clinical psychologist and assistants also have a research and clinical governance role within the team; for example, in carrying out specific, clinically related research projects.

Research forms an integral part of the EIS, both guiding and stemming from clinical practice. The Birmingham Early Intervention Service have a commitment to evidence-based practice. It bases its clinical service on the latest research evidence and each team is involved in a number of research projects which both evaluate the effectiveness of interventions and aim to further the evidence base for early intervention in psychosis. Current research includes REDIRECT and EPOS as described earlier. Two (of many) further research projects are summarised below:

First episode research network
Assistant psychologists are employed to evaluate and audit the clinical service provided by the EIS continuously as a part of the national first episode research network initiative. Clinical data (e.g. measures of psychopathology and co-morbid symptoms) are collected from each client treated within participating early intervention services, at entry

to the service and later at yearly intervals. Data collected may be used to examine the clinical outcomes for young people treated within dedicated specialist early intervention.

Asian service users' and families' experiences of early intervention
Ethnicity and cultural beliefs need to be carefully considered when providing an early intervention service in Birmingham because the services cover areas of wide-ranging ethnic diversity. Research has demonstrated that Afro-Caribbean patients, in particular, may be poorly engaged with traditional mental heath services and that clients from ethnic minorities tend to report more adverse experiences with mental health services (McGovern *et al.* 1991; Goater *et al.* 1999). The team aspires to provide equal access for all people with psychosis and to provide a culturally appropriate service. This qualitative research is examining the experiences of Asian service users and their families, which will enable us better to understand their perceptions of psychosis and early intervention and their service requirements, so that we can target future interventions appropriately for this group of clients.

Vocational program and activity centre
Vocational workers conduct assessments of the employment and training needs of every service user twice a year. Regular assessments mean that service users are encouraged to re-engage in activities or to seek employment as soon as they are well enough to do so, and ensures that their vocational goals are given high priority as demanded in the NICE guidelines. Vocational workers work closely with service users to help them find suitable employment or courses and they also run a job-club for those who are thinking about beginning work. Talks are given on topics such as how to write a CV, how to prepare for an interview and service users are supported in writing job applications. To begin with, voluntary work or work with an employer with an understanding of mental health problems may be used to enable service users to build confidence at work prior to full-time, main-stream, employment. When a service user starts a new job, or course, vocational workers can provide outreach work, both liasing with the employer and meeting the client to give support and help where necessary.

For those not yet ready for work or education, a pre-vocational program is provided in a day service, based in a community building in Birmingham city centre, which can be accessed by all EIS clients. The service is run along the lines of a structured 'youth club', providing an informal social meeting place and structured activities such as cookery, basic living skills, art and craft, and information technology. It is supported by national employment schemes, including Learn-Direct and Connexions.

Respite services

The EIS has two community 'respite' units, each with four to six beds. The units are houses within the community, where service users have their own bedrooms and cater for themselves. Nurses and support-workers staff the respite facilities. They are available 24-hours a day and fulfil a number of important roles. These include: assessment of mental state and medication monitoring, introduction or re-introduction to social activities and assessment and help with daily skills. Service users are employed as support-workers within the respite units. Their presence contributes to a strong sense of optimism for recovery. Narrative studies of recovery from psychosis suggest that meeting other recovering individuals is a source of hope, and provides much needed social contact and support. In addition, service users often feel more comfortable socialising with people who have had similar experiences and interests to themselves, and who may also be able to provide valuable support and practical advice (Leete 1989; Ridgeway 2001).

The respite units are able to provide care in a number of different situations:

- When clients' show the early signs of relapse but do not require in-patient hospital care
- When the consultant would like a client to have a medication-free observation period or to change medication which may require being carefully monitored
- When housing breaks down the respite unit can be used as a temporary place to stay until new, satisfactory accommodation can be found
- In situations when carers or service users themselves need a short break
- Following hospital admission, once high risk and symptoms have remitted, to shorten length of stay in an acute in-patient unit.

Summary

Birmingham Early Intervention Service was developed with the aim of providing high-quality care to young people who are within the early, crucial phase of psychosis. Clinicians, with an understanding of the evidence-base summarised at the beginning of this chapter, felt that a dedicated early intervention service would lead to improved prognosis. They realised that there was no team able to provide such a service and that young people with psychosis were not satisfied with the treatment that they were receiving from general adult mental health services. Therefore, the Birmingham service was set up to provide a dedicated, specialist, early intervention service for young people in Birmingham. It opened in 1989 and has since moved to a comprehensive community service under the 'assertive outreach' model. It includes community teams, respite units, a vocational service and a specialist early detection and intervention team. The service has successfully engaged and treated young people with psychosis who have been traditionally difficult to engage in mainstream mental health services. By doing so, Birmingham Early Intervention Service has played an integral role in influencing health policy and in developing guidelines for early intervention across the UK and was awarded 'beacon' status, providing the blueprint for the reform of services, discussed below.

THE REFORM OF SERVICES FOR YOUNG PEOPLE WITH PSYCHOSIS

National policy has recently incorporated recommendations in its agenda for services for young people with first-episode psychosis. These national changes were brought about by a combination of three vital ingredients: firstly, government advisors reviewed the research evidence documented in this chapter. Secondly, this evidence was brought to the Health Secretary's attention by the formation of the 'Initiative to Reduce the Impact of Schizophrenia' (IRIS) group who lobbied parliament for changes in the structure and provision of services for young people with psychosis. Thirdly, the most powerful case for UK service reform has come from consumers of mental health care themselves.

Awareness of the evidence for intervening early in the course of psychosis and the poor state of services for the young severely mentally ill was first promoted in England by the efforts of the 'Initiative to Reduce the Impact of Schizophrenia' (IRIS) group formed in the West Midlands, UK in 1994. Members of the IRIS group included Professor Max Birchwood, who developed Birmingham Early Intervention Service; Dr. Fiona MacMillan, one of the researchers involved in the Northwick Park study; Dr. David Shiers, a GP and carer whose daughter developed schizophrenia; the National Schizophrenia Fellowship (a campaigning

UK mental health charity now called 'RETHINK'); and other clinicians and service users, who shared a vision of how services should be improved for young people with schizophrenia. The IRIS group made presentations all over England, and organised two major conferences (in 1997 and 2000) at which international experts in early psychosis presented their work. Among others, Professor Pat McGorry described the successful work of the Melbourne EPPIC early intervention service. The impact of this international work on opinion in the UK was very significant in securing the inclusion of early psychosis services in the National Service Framework for significant government and health service investment.

In 2002, RETHINK launched their campaign, Reaching People Early (www.rethink.org/reachingpeopleearly) to bring to wider attention the poor state of services for the young severely mentally ill. They described a catalogue of concerns. For example, they highlighted the delay of twelve months between the onset of the positive symptoms and first treatment (Norman and Malla 2001) and their members described how some of this delay occured due to problems at the interface of primary and secondary care, including the lack of an 'assertive' response when the diagnosis was first raised. RETHINK pointed out that the incidence of schizophrenia begins to rise during the 15–18 age range and does not respect the often impermeable service boundaries between child and adolescent and adult services. Young people surveyed by RETHINK found adult services stigmatising, therapeutically pessimistic and youth-insensitive (e.g. access to employment and training are high on young peoples' agendas, but are not one of the priorities of the services). They invited us to consider: would we be happy with our children receiving care from our services? Our impression is that many mental health professionals are still dissatisfied with the current quality of care but provide a caring and professional service within the constraints that service pressure and resources allow. These are reasons enough to 'rethink' our services to young people suffering from severe mental illnesses.

This combination of consumer dissatisfaction and professional pressure has raised awareness of the evidence for early intervention and of our failure to provide evidence-based care during the 'critical period'. By doing so it brought about the zeitgeist in the UK that paved the way for radical service reform. Early intervention is now placed firmly and highly on the Government's and Mental Health Services' list of priorities. The need for specialist early intervention services is now beginning to be addressed through the NHS' commitment to deliver such services throughout the UK. The early intervention services are to be funded by a major Government initiative; guidelines for these services are set out in the *National service framework for mental health (NSF)*, *NHS plan* and NICE guidelines for schizophrenia.

The *NHS plan*

In July 2000, the government published the *NHS plan* (DoH 2000), setting out its intentions for the following three years. Much of the *NHS plan* concerned structural and cultural changes for services as a whole, but it identified three clinical priorities: coronary heart disease, cancer, and mental health. The government announced in the *NHS plan* an extra annual investment of over £300 m by the year 2003/4 to 'fast-forward' the National Service Framework for Mental Health. Commitments on early intervention became more specific:

● Fifty early intervention teams will be established over the next three years to provide treatment and active support in the community to these young people and their families
● By 2004 all young people with a first episode of psychosis such as schizophrenia will receive the early and intensive support they need. This will benefit 7500 young people each year.

There are a number of models for delivering early intervention, ranging from the 'specialised services' model adopted in the NHS Plan to the 'mainstream services' model in which appropriate interventions are delivered by staff entirely integrated within mainstream psychiatric services. The specialised team approach (as adopted by Birmingham Early Intervention Service) has a number of advantages, which are described by IRIS as follows:

> . . . *staff expertise and team coherence are encouraged by the consistent experience of managing similar clients and the informal supervision and sharing of ideas that occur when a team is housed on one site; the creation of a concrete 'service' allows easy identification of the service by the referrers (who might include other clients and families): it is possible to create a separate point of entry for direct referrals, thus increasing ease of referral; the existence of a concrete team with a physical location allows the creation of an actual youth-friendly space which may promote client engagement.*
>
> (IRIS 2001)

An additional advantage, from the government's perspective, is that by creating separate and identifiable early intervention teams, the delivery of early intervention across the UK can be easily monitored to see whether targets have been reached by the dates specified.

The National Institute for Clinical Excellence guidelines

In 2002, the National Institute for Clinical Excellence (NICE) published the first comprehensive, evidence-based guidelines addressing the treatments and services for people with schizophrenia. These build upon the NSF and service development plans for England and Wales. The aim of these guidelines is to help to improve the experience of people with schizophrenia and to improve outcomes in terms of the degree of symptomatic recovery a person makes and their quality of life. NICE recommend that in order to reach acceptable standards a thorough multi-professional assessment of medical, social, psychological, occupational, economic, physical and cultural needs is necessary for every person with psychosis.

The guidelines have been divided into three phases, the first of these being 'initiation of treatment in the first episode'. They suggest that specialist early intervention services should be used assertively to engage young people with a first episode of psychosis who may otherwise find difficulty getting help or treatment. Such teams should provide the correct mix of specialist treatments including: pharmacological, psychological, social occupational and educational interventions. In crisis stages, NICE recommend that early intervention works in conjunction with home treatment teams, day care facilities, and crisis resolution or in-patient units until the crisis is resolved. First-line treatments should be with oral atypical anti-psychotic medications which have been proven to cause fewer side-effects than older typical anti-psychotic medications, therefore they are often more tolerable to service users which in turn may increase compliance and engagement with services and reduce the risk of relapse. NICE also provide many general guidelines that also have implications for early intervention (see NICE 2002).

Summary

Presentation of the evidence for early intervention to the Government by the IRIS group and increasing consumer pressure to review services for young people with psychosis has focused Government attention on the need for early intervention services similar to Birmingham EIS, but every part of the UK Government guidelines now specify that by 2004 every young person with psychosis should receive early intervention from a specialist team and the NICE guidelines set out clearly the type of service and interventions that service users should expect to receive. The preferred model for delivery of specialist early intervention services is a multi-disciplinary team approach which enables each team to provide a range of specialist treatments including: pharmacological, psychological, social, occupational and educational interventions.

CONCLUSION

As we have seen at the beginning of this chapter the evidence for early intervention is overwhelming. For example, longer durations of untreated psychosis are frequently associated with poorer outcomes, and evidence suggests that time spent experiencing psychotic symptoms within the first two years of psychotic illness is the best predictor of outcome fifteen years later (Harrison *et al.* 2001). This has led to the 'critical period' hypothesis (Birchwood *et al.* 1997) which suggests that providing comprehensive, evidence-based treatment early on in the course of the illness may lead to better long-term prognosis. This is now widely accepted, and dedicated early intervention services have begun to be set up both nationally and internationally. Outcome data from such services are still in the early stages. In addition, the detection of psychosis in prodromal stages through the study of high-risk groups is now being afforded serious consideration. Studies offering both medical and psychological interventions during the 'pre-psychotic' stage have demonstrated promising preliminary results (McGorry *et al.* 2000; French *et al.* 2004). It seems that the key research question has now shifted from: Is early intervention effective? to: What kind of early intervention is appropriate and effective? As noted previously, the evidence base in this area is scant, but developing. In this chapter we have outlined some of the key interventional studies now addressing this issue.

A review of the evidence for early intervention by clinicians led to the opening of the first early intervention service in the UK, in Birmingham in 1989. This chapter described the structure of this service and the interventions which it provides, with reference to the evidence base. Finally, the chapter reviewed the current early intervention reforms, backed by the *NHS plan* and *National service framework for mental health.* These reforms were driven largely by the IRIS group who brought the evidence for early intervention to the Government's attention. This evidence has led to a major shift in the way we conceptualise schizophrenia by demonstrating that long-term difficulties develop quickly and aggressively in the early phase but that this deterioration may be averted by effective treatment during and following the first episode. Change has also arisen out of consumer involvement in service reform and a recognition that we fail to engage service users in a sustained way in our current service structures, at what is a critical phase in the development of the illness. Service engagement, consumer satisfaction and the provision of evidence-based interventions are now key outcomes of the UK service reforms in early psychosis.

The national reforms of services for the young people with severe mental illnesses are radical and create major challenges for implementation. When completed, they will transform the consumer experience of services. By 2004, it is hoped that every young person who develops psychosis will be treated within a specialist early intervention team similar to the Birmingham Early Intervention Service. These services will set the stage for future research to determine *what kind* of early intervention is appropriate for achieving the best outcomes possible given our current and developing range of treatments (Birchwood 2003).

ACKNOWLEDGEMENTS

We would like to thank Bethan Reading, Beth Spencer, Michael Larkin and Chris Jackson for their work and suggestions, which have informed this chapter.

References

Bebbington, P. and Kuipers, E. (1994). The predictive utility of expressed emotion in schizophrenia. *Psychological Medicine*, 24, 707–18.

Beck, A., Rush, A., Shaw, B. and Emery, G. (1979). *Cognitive therapy for depression.* Guilford. New York.

Birchwood, M. (1992). Family factors in psychiatry. *Current Opinion in Psychiatry*, 5, 295–9.

Birchwood, M. and McMillan, F. (1993). Early intervention in schizophrenia. *Australia and New Zealand Journal of Psychiatry*, 17, 374–8.

Birchwood, M., McGorry, P. and Jackson, H. (1997). Early intervention in schizophrenia. *British Journal of Psychiatry*, **170**, 2–5.

Birchwood, M., Todd, P. and Jackson, C. (1998). Early intervention in psychosis: the critical period hypothesis. *British Journal of Psychiatry*, **172**, supp. 33, 5–9.

Carpenter, W. and Strauss, J. (1991). The prediction of outcome in schizophrenia. V: eleven-year follow-up of the IPSS cohort. *Journal of Nervous and Mental Disease*, **179**, 517–25.

Department of Health. (1999). *A national service framework for mental health.* London, England.

Department of Health. (2000). *The NHS plan.* London, England.

Department of Health. (2001). *Mental health policy implementation guide.* London, England.

Dixon, L., Adams, C. and Lucksted, A. (2000). Update on family psychoeducation for schizophrenia. *Schizophrenia Bulletin*, **26**, 5–20.

Drake, R.J., Haley, C.J., Akhtar, S. and Lewis, S.W. (2000). Causes and consequences of duration of untreated psychosis in schizophrenia. *British Journal of Psychiatry*, **177**, 511–15.

Drury, V., Birchwood, M.J., Cochrane, R., Macmillan, F. (1996a). Cognitive therapy and recovery from acute psychosis: a controlled trial. 1. Impact on psychotic symptoms. *British Journal of Psychiatry*, **169**, 602–7.

Drury, V., Birchwood, M.J. and Cochrane, R., Macmillan, F. (1996b). Cognitive therapy and recovery from acute psychosis: a controlled trial. 11. Impact on recovery time. *British Journal of Psychiatry*, **169**, 602–7.

Drury, V., Birchwood, M. and Cochrane, R. (2000). Cognitive therapy and recovery from acute psychosis: a controlled trial: 3. Five-year follow-up. *British Journal of Psychiatry*, **177**, 8–14.

Eaton, W., Thara, R., Federman, B., Melton, B. and Liang, K.-Y. (1995). Structure and course of positive and negative symptoms in schizophrenia. *Archives of General Psychiatry*, **52**, 127–34.

Fadden, G. (1998). Family intervention in psychosis. *Journal of Mental Health*, **7**, 115–22.

Falloon, I. and Pederson, J. (1985). Family management in the prevention of morbidity of schizophrenia: the adjustment family unit. *British Journal of Psychiatry*, **147**, 156–63.

Frank, A. and Gunderson, J. (1990). The role of therapeutic alliance in the treatment of schizophrenia: relationship to course and outcome high engagement. *Archives of General Psychiatry*, **52**, 127–34.

French, P. and Morrison, A.P. (2004). *Early detection and cognitive therapy for people at high risk of developing psychosis – a treatment approach.* John Wiley and Sons Limited, Chichester.

Garety, P., Fowler, D. and Kuipers, E. (2000). Cognitive-behavioural therapy for medication-resistant symptoms. *Schizophrenia Bulletin*, **16**, 73–86.

Goater, N., King, M., Cole, E., Leavey, G., Johson-Sabine, E., Blizard, R. and Hoar, A. (1999). Ethnicity and outcome of psychosis. *British Journal of Psychiatry*, **175**, 34–42.

Harrison, G., Croudace, T., Mason, P., Glazebrook, C. and Medley, I. (1996). Predicting the long-term outcome of schizophrenia. *Psychological Medicine*, 26, 697–705.

Harrison, G., Hopper, K., Craig, T., *et al.* (2001). Recovery from psychotic illness: a 15- and 25-year international follow-up study. *British Journal of Psychiatry*, **178**, 506–17.

Initiative to Reduce the Impact of Schizophrenia. (2000). Early Intervention in Psychosis: Clinical Guidelines and Service Frameworks. Available at: www.iris-initiative.org.uk

Jablensky, A., Sartorious, N., Emberg, G., Anker, M., Korten, A., Cooper, J. and Bertelson, A. (1992). *Schizophrenia: manifestations, incidence and course in different cultures.* A World Health Organisation ten country study. Psychological Medicine. Monograph Supplement 20.

Johnstone, E., Crow, T., Johnson, A. and Macmillan, F. (1986). The Northwick Park study of first episodes of schizophrenia. 1. Presentation of the illness and problems relating to admission. *British Journal of Psychiatry*, **148**, 115–20.

Johannessen, J.O., McGlashan, T.H., Larsen, T.K., Homeland, M., Joa, I., Sigurd, M., Kvebraek, R., Friis, S., Melle, I., Opjordsmoen, S., Simonsen, E., Ulrick, H. and Vaglum, P. (2001). Early detection strategies for untreated first-episode psychosis. *Schizophrenia Research*, **51**, 39–46.

Jorgenson, P., Nordentoft, M., Abel M., Gouliaev, G., Jeppesen, P. and Kassaw, P. (2000). Early detection and assertive community treatment of young psychotics: the OPUS Study. Rationale and design of the trial. *Social Psychiatry and Psychiatric Epidemiology*, **35**, 283–7.

Knapp, M. (1997). Costs of schizophrenia. *British Journal of Psychiatry*, **171**, 509–18.

Larsen, T.K., Moe, L.C., Vibe-Hansen, L. and Johannessen, J.O. (2000). Premorbid functioning versus duration of untreated psychosis in 1-year outcome in first-episode psychosis. *Schizophrenia Research*, **45**, 1–9.

Larsen, T., McGlashan, T., Johannessen, J., Friis, S., Guldberg, C., Haahr, U., Horneland, M., Melle, I., Moe, L., Opjordsmoen, S., Simonsen, E. and Vaglum, P. (2001). Shortened duration of untreated first episode of psychosis: changes in patient characteristics at treatment. *American Journal of Psychiatry*, **158**, 11, 1917–19.

Leete, E. (1989). How I perceive and manage my illness. *Schizophrenia Bulletin*, **15**, 197–200.

Lewis, S., Tarrier, N., Haddock, G., Bentall, R., Kindeman, P., Kingdon, D., Siddle, R., Drake, R., Everitt, J., Leadley, K., Benn, A., Grazebrook, K., Haley, C., Akhtar, S., Davies, L., Palmer, S., Faragher, B. and Dunn, G. (2002). Randomised controlled trial of cognitive-behavioural therapy in early schizophrenia: acute-phase outcomes. *British Journal of Psychiatry*, **181**, suppl 43, 91–7.

Lincoln, C.V. and McGorry, P.D. (1999). Pathways to care in early psychosis: clinical and consumer perspectives. In *Recognition and management of early psychosis. A preventative approach* (eds. McGorry, P. and Jackson, H.J.). Cambridge University Press, Cambridge.

Loebel, A.D., Lieberman, J.A., Alvir, J.M.J., Myerhoff, D.I., Geisler, S.H. and Szymanshi, S.R. (1992). Duration of untreated psychosis and outcome in first episode schizophrenia. *American Journal of Psychiatry*, **149**, 1183–8.

Malla, A.K. and Norman, R.M.G. (2002). Early intervention in schizophrenia and related disorders: advantages and pitfalls. *Current Opinion in Psychiatry*, **15**, 17–23.

Mari, J., Adams, C. and Streiner, D. (1996). Family intervention for those with schizophrenia. In *Schizophrenia module of the Cochrane database of systematic reviews* (eds. Adams, C., De Jesus, M. and White, P.), The Cochrane Library. The Cochrane Collaboration, Oxford.

May, P.R.A., Tum, H., Dixon, W.J., Yale, C., Thiele, D.A. and Kraude, W.H. (1981). Schizophrenia: a follow-up study of the results of five forms of treatment. *Archives of General Psychiatry*, **38**, 776–84.

McGorry, P. (1995). Psycho-education in first episode psychosis: a therapeutic process. *Psychiatry*, **58**, 313–28.

McGorry, P., Krstev, H. and Harrigan, S. (2000). Early detection and treatment delay: implications for outcome in early psychosis. *Current Opinion in Psychiatry*, **13**, 1, 37–43.

McGorry, P., Yung, A., Phillips, L., Yuen, H., Francey, S., Cosgrave, E., Germano, D., Bravin, J., McDonald, T., Blair, A., Adlard, S. and Jackson, H. (2002). Randomized controlled trial of interventions designed to reduce the risk of progression to first-episode psychosis in a clinical sample with subthreshold symptoms. *Archives of General Psychiatry*, **59**, 10, 921–8.

McGorry, P.D., Edwards, J., Mihalopoulos, C., Harrigan, S.M. and Jackson, H.J. (1996). EPPIC: an evolving system of early detection and optimal management. *Schizophrenia Bulletin*, **22**, 305–26.

McGovern, D. and Cope, R. (1991). Second generation Afro-Caribbeans and young whites with a first admission diagnosis of schizophrenia. *Social Psychiatry and Psychiatric Epidemiology*, **26**, 95–9.

McGovern, D., Hemmings, P. and Cope, R. (1994). Long-term follow-up of young Afro-Caribbeans and white Britons with a first admission diagnosis of schizophrenia. *Social Psychiatry and Psychiatric Epidemiology*, **29**, 8–19.

McGlashan, T.H. (1988). A selective review of recent North American follow-up studies on schizophrenia. *Schizophrenia Bulletin*, **14**, 515–42.

McGlashan, T.H., Miller, T.J. and Woods, S.W. (2001). Pre-onset detection and intervention research in schizophrenia psychoses: current estimates of benefit and risk. *Schizophrenia Bulletin*, **27**, 4, 563–70.

National Institute for Clinical Excellence. (2002). *Schizophrenia: core interventions in the treatment and management of schizophrenia in primary and secondary care.* www.nice.org.uk NICE, London.

Norman, R.M. and Malla, A.K. (2001). Duration of untreated psychosis: a critical examination of the concept and its importance. *Psychological Medicine*, **31**, 381–400.

Nordentoft, M., Jeppesen, P., Abel, M., Petersen, L., Thorup, A., Christensen, T., Ohlenschlaeger, J. and Jorgensen, P. (2002). Opus-project: a randomized controlled trial of integrated psychiatric treatment in first-episode psychosis – clinical outcome improved. *Acta Psychiatrica Scandinavica, Supplementum*, **106**, Supplement 413.

Phillips, L., Yung, A.R., Hearn, N., McFarlane, C., Hallgren, M. and McGorry, P.D. (1999). Preventative mental health care: accessing the target population. *Australian and New Zealand Journal of Psychiatry*, **33**, 912–17.

Pilling, S., Bebbington, P., Kuipers, E., Garety, P., Geddes, J., Orbach, G. and Morgan, C. (2002). Psychological treatments in schizophrenia. I. Meta-analysis of family intervention and cognitive behavioural therapy. *Psychological Medicine*, **32**, 763–82.

Posner, C., Wilson, Kral, M., Lander, S. and McIlwraith, R.D. (1992). Family psycho-educational support groups in schizophrenia. *American Journal of Orthopsychiatry*, **62**, 206–18.

Reading, B. and Jackson, C. (2003). *Getting back on your feet*. Birmingham and Solihull Mental Health Trust.

Rector, N. and Beck, A. (2001). CBT for Schizophrenia: an empirical review. *Journal of Nervous and Mental Disorders*, **189**, 278–87.

Ridgeway, P. (2001). Restoring psychiatric disability: learning from first person recovery narratives. *Psychiatric Rehabilitation Journal*, **24**, 335–43.

Spencer, E., Birchwood, M. and McGovern, D. (2001). Management of first-episode psychosis. *Advances in Psychiatric Treatment*, **7**, 133–42.

Stirling, J., Tantum, D., Thonks, P., Newby, D. and Montague, L. (1991). Expressed emotion and early onset schizophrenia. *Psychological Medicine*, **21**, 675–85.

Szmuckler, G., Herrman, H., Colusa, S., Benson, A. and Bloch, S. (1996). A controlled trial of counselling intervention for caregivers of relatives with schizophrenia. *Social Psychiatry and Psychiatric Epidemiology*, **31**, 149–55.

Tarrier, N., Barrowclough, C., Porceddu, K. and Fitzpatrick, E. (1994). The Salford family intervention project. Relapse rates of schizophrenia at 5 and 8 years. *British Journal of Psychiatry*, **165**, 829–32.

Tarrier, N., Barrowclough, C., Vaughy, C., Bamrah, J., Porceddu, K., Watts, S. and Freeman, H. (1989). Community management of schizophrenia: a 2-year follow-up of behavioural interventions with families. *British Journal of Psychiatry*, **154**, 625–8.

Thara, R., Henrietta, M., Joseph, A., Rajkumar, S. and Eaton, W. (1994). Ten-year course of schizophrenia – the Madras longitudinal study. *Acta Psychiatrica Scandinavica*, **90**, 329–36.

Verdoux, H. and Cougnard, A. (2003). The early detection and treatment controversy in schizophrenia research. *Current Opinion in Psychiatry*, **16**, 175–9.

Warner, R. (1994). *Recovery from schizophrenia: psychiatric and political economy.* Routledge, London.

Wyatt, R.J. (1991). Neuroleptics and the natural course of schizophrenia. *Schizophrenia Bulletin*, **17**, 325–51.

Werry, J., McClellan, J. and Chard, L. (1991). Childhood and adolescent schizophrenic, bipolar and schizoaffective disorders: a clinical and outcome study. *Journal of the American Academy of Child and Adolescent Psychiatry*, **30**, 457–65.

Yung, A. (1998). The prodomal phase of first-episode psychosis: past and current conceptualisations. *Schizophrenia Bulletin*, **22**, 353–70.

Yung, A.R. and McGorry. P.D. (1996b). *The initial prodrome in psychosis: descriptive and qualitative aspects. Australian and New Zealand Journal of Psychiatry*, **30**, 5587–99.

14

Evidence and argument in crisis care

Kevin M. Hogan and Sarah Orme

Following the adage 'those who cannot remember the past are condemned to repeat it' (Santayana 1905) we offer a discussion of the recent history of the development of crisis services in the UK. This chapter is also based upon a small programme of empirical work carried out at the University of Wolverhampton over the last five years. The subject of the work has been the organisation and delivery of crisis and home treatment services; our studies have included a case study evaluation of a single crisis service, a national survey of such services in the UK, a project examining the development of services in a single region – the West Midlands – and consultancy work in service development, again in the West Midlands. Parts of this work have been reported elsewhere; in this chapter, however, we will be focusing upon the impact of the ways in which crisis services have been developed for the future. Our purpose is to explore the nature of organisational change under government direction and guidance; research and development support flowing into the area of crisis care in the UK.

It would be otiose to suggest that crisis services reflect many of the problems and opportunities that confront the wider NHS today. It remains to be seen whether or not lessons have been learned from the past, or as sometimes seems to be the case, we are in some danger of simply putting the past behind us.

In order to proceed, we must first of all offer up some definition of what crisis services are, what it is they do, for whom and under what circumstances. This is, in part at least, an exercise in providing some rigid definition for our many areas of doubt and uncertainty. Which is to say that offering definitions in such an area presents considerable difficulties and may very well turn out to be a foolish enterprise. There are two problems that we must address at the outset in order not to add to the current confusion. Firstly, and perhaps most importantly, we do not wish to convey the impression that because we offer definitions of terms we are arguing that such definitions widely inform(ed) practice; indeed, there is rather more evidence for the converse position. Secondly, we also need to keep in mind the difference between a definition of a clinically salient element or elements of a service and a service configuration *per se.* The debate over crisis services, however named, has frequently revolved around the observation that crisis intervention need not be delivered by a crisis service; indeed some authors have argued that it should not be and others have pointed out that, logically, all of the interventions required cannot be delivered by a crisis service standing alone.

Typically, discussions concerning the origins of crisis intervention refer to the theory of psychiatric crises elaborated by Caplan (1964). In his text on preventative psychiatry, Caplan proposed a model of psychiatric crises which had much in common with the biological homeostatic principles that framed early attempts at theory building in the field of stress research (Selye 1956). It has been suggested that the theory proposed by Caplan is very much 'dated', influenced as it was by Freudian and biological thought (Sainsbury Centre 2001). It is interesting to note that the discussion of crisis services development does not include any recognised test of the validity of the model, hence it is difficult to argue for its rejection on scientific grounds.

It would appear that what has changed is the focus of those writing about services, who are no longer so much concerned with the theoretical model(s) that underpin innovations in community based psychiatric services such as those that flowed from the crisis concept (Caplan 1974), but rather upon describing and evaluating the services themselves.

Unfortunately, as we shall see, the services are severely heterogeneous, betraying both a lack of consistent theoretical underpinning and a willingness to adopt and adapt in the light of local circumstances. As was recently observed, 'Crisis intervention can no longer be seen as a unified strategy for care, as many divergent practices in different settings have developed since its origin' (Rosen 1998, p. 46). It is in the light of just these developments that it has become increasingly difficult to argue that there is a strong body of evidence concerning these services or 'strategies' that can safely be generalised to the development of new services. Indeed it has been argued (Sandor 2001) that no well-defined model of home treatment or crisis intervention exists, and consequently that there is no definitive list of the key elements of such services precluding much-needed testing of the implications of varying model fidelity.

CRISIS AND EMERGENCY

It is important to define what is meant by a crisis because the terms 'crisis' and 'emergency' can be confused, and a crisis needs to be identified clearly in order to be treated appropriately within the model.

> *. . . an emergency is an urgent situation that can occur repeatedly, requiring immediate action without necessarily bringing about a change in the person's life; whereas a crisis is a turning point that precludes the possibility of life going on as usual.*
>
> (Jacobs 1983, p. 172)

> *. . . a time-limited break in a person's capacity to cope with stimuli that have temporarily exhausted all of a person's problem-solving strategies.*
>
> (Dixon 1982, p. 26)

> *'Emergency refers to external situations requiring immediate action to prevent dire consequences'.*
>
> (Dixon 1982, p. 27)

A psychological crisis has been defined as an individual's response to a certain event that results in a qualitative change in their functioning (Renshaw 1989). Finally, Brimblecombe (1993) defines a crisis as:

> *. . . an internal disturbance resulting from a stressful event or a perceived threat to self, [that] arises when an individual's usual coping mechanisms are ineffective in dealing with a threat.*
>
> (Brimblocome 1993 p. 40)

From these descriptions, the question must be raised as to whether many crisis services are actually dealing with crises or emergencies, a point we will return to below.

WHAT IS CRISIS INTERVENTION?

Simply put, crisis intervention is providing appropriate help quickly to clients with identifiable psychological crises (Renshaw 1989) with the aim of returning clients to their pre-crisis level of functioning (Waldron 1989). Renshaw describes crisis intervention as mental health personnel identifying who is in crisis (for example a carer may be in crisis because of their charge's behaviour), what stage the crisis has reached and then providing an appropriate intervention.

Waldron (1989) describes the three phases of crisis identified by Caplan (1964). Phase one is the rise in tension when a person realises something is wrong; phase two is the point of crisis when a person's internal resources are exhausted and overcome; and phase three represents the resolution of crisis through either growth or stagnation. It is during the second phase, when people are most open to suggestion, that Caplan suggests is the appropriate time to intervene with therapy. Waldron continues that therapy at this point is active, focusing on solving problems and current difficulties, using, in the majority of cases, behavioural and cognitive techniques. She adds that crisis intervention should be short-term, as successful resolution should not involve clients becoming dependent on crisis personnel.

Newton (1989) describes three basic ways for crisis intervention services to operate. They can run in parallel to current services with referrals coming from the same sources. They may be integrated into local mental health provision with one point of entry for clients and referral on to the crisis service. Or a crisis service can target one particular population and select its referrals in terms of their suitability to the treatment offered. Newton adds that there is no blue print for a crisis intervention service and those local resources, demands and needs influence the development of a service and how it works. He states that:

> *It is essential to begin with a clear view of the principles of crisis intervention and to plan the service in conjunction with all the relevant agencies and professions in the area. Failure to obtain such working agreements at the outset will lead to conflict, division and confusion for customers.*
>
> (Newton 1989, p. 3)

It is important to note that there are some problems with the use of the term crisis intervention. Renshaw (1989) states that crisis intervention is a well-used term that is sometimes misused. Firstly, crisis intervention means different things to different people. For example, some advocates of crisis intervention believe its role is to avoid hospital admissions while others (e.g., Bengelsdorf, Church, Kaye, Orlowski and Alden 1993) are of the opinion that, as well as supporting clients in their own homes, crisis intervention should regard hospitalisation as a necessary and acceptable part of therapy in some cases. Both views are crisis intervention. As Hobbs (1984, cited by Warburton 1996) states:

there is very little consensus, even among practitioners, as to what constitutes crisis intervention. A variety of techniques are applied in a variety of settings to a wide variety of problems, by practitioners with a variety of skills and qualifications, and with a variety of aims.

(p. 32 in the original)

Secondly, Renshaw notes that just because a service calls itself a crisis intervention service does not mean it practices crisis intervention; providing a rapid response, for example, does not mean itself involve the application of crisis theory.

The work of Schnyder (Schnyder 1997) set out a seven point plan for the organisation of crisis intervention; one which moved away from the focus applied by Caplan (1964) and drew in an eclectic fashion upon a number of concepts such as social support, and coping theory. The model proposed by Schnyder is a process model describing how the client is moved from initial contact through the analysis on definition of the problem into the definition of goal(s), actively working upon the problem with termination and follow-up. Rosen (1998) who elaborates a detailed picture of a variety of types of crisis summed up the position: 'A psychological crisis is a brief, non-illness response to severe stress. When maladaptive responses to crisis are detected, crisis intervention is employed to achieve a more adaptive resolution and a more effective learning experience.' (Rosen 1998, p. 44).

CRISIS OF DEFINITION

It is hard to escape the conclusion that the best definition of crisis services is an operational definition: namely, a crisis service is defined by what it does. In this we follow the Sainsbury Centre (2001) where they have listed the core characteristics of a crisis service as being: intensive short-term interventions, rapid response, frequent daily visits, availability of medical staff and medication, social issues addressed and support and education provided. Crisis services have the role of gatekeeper for acute care resources with involvement after crisis resolution when patients have been referred on. It is important to remember that this definition was designed to reflect the provision of home-based care. As others have noted, however, many of these characteristics can be provided by an integrated acute and community mental health care system that does not include a separate crisis team

(Pelosi and Jackson 2000), nor can we be certain which of them are essential for success (Burns and Catty 2002).

It is legitimate to draw the conclusion that services have not been driven by the accumulation of evidence upon which to base their practice, notwithstanding the existence of a number of studies (e.g., Scott and Starr 1981; Davis *et al.* 1985; Parkes 1992; Minghella *et al.* 1998) that purport to show the benefits of early intervention and crisis resolution strategies by a reduction in admissions and improved bed use, better retention and similar or improved clinical outcomes. The fact is, given the lack of definition and validation of the individual components of services, the diversity of services themselves, not to mention uncertainty concerning how, if it all, theory is applied in terms of the activities undertaken by services, precludes any argument based upon the accumulation of robust evidence. These points have been made in great detail elsewhere (Burns 2000; Burns and Catty 2002). Our suggestion is that we concentrate on understanding what has driven the development of services in the 'crisis' field; this is perhaps best achieved by examining what is delivered by whom and to which clients.

WHAT DO CRISIS SERVICES ACTUALLY DO?

As noted above, Caplan (1964) proposed crisis intervention as a form of preventative psychiatry designed to reduce the incidence of mental ill health in the community (primary prevention), reduce the duration of disorders that occurred (secondary), and reduce the amount of impairment resulting from the disorder (tertiary). The provision of crisis and home-treatment-based services increased rapidly during the 1990s (McMillan 1997), a development encouraged by the NHS. Government guidelines (DoH 1994) emphasised multi-disciplinary working and crisis response services as core components in the delivery of comprehensive mental health services. Service providers were encouraged to develop joint strategies for services that offer speedy assessment, fast effective care and fast action when crises occur (DoH 1996).

Faulkner *et al.* (1994) carried out a survey of 49 district health authorities to establish the provision of hospital, residential and community support services. Community provision was considered in terms of the presence of crisis intervention teams, continuing care teams for people with long-term mental health problems and residential alternatives to hospital admission. The survey found that three (6.5%) of the Units or Trusts had established crisis intervention teams and three

(6.5%) had residential alternatives to admission in place. A further five (11%) areas were in the process of considering the development of crisis services. Continuing care teams were more established with 41% of the Units or Trusts having community or hospital-based teams offering services to those with long-term mental health problems.

Johnson and Thornicroft (1995) conducted a survey to determine how emergency services in England and Wales were organised and staffed. Their questionnaire survey of managers of mental health units and local MIND representatives revealed that outside of office hours, A&E departments and hospital wards were most frequently used for emergency assessments, and home assessments relied on district duty psychiatrists and social workers. The weaknesses of this situation were felt by staff to lie in the poor out-of-hours service, too few staff and a lack of crisis intervention teams. User representatives identified difficulties in gaining access to emergency services, poor service outside office hours and no crisis beds as the greatest weaknesses.

Subsequently, in *Modernising mental health services* (DoH 1998) it was suggested that service development should focus on 24-hour, seamless services and the National Service Framework would,

> . . . *consider the implications of inequities and service gaps for service planning and service configuration. This will ensure that those responsible for delivering services have the benefit of clear information about how to achieve greater consistency and higher standards.*
>
> (DoH 1998, p. 33)

Subsequent to the publication of *Modernising mental health services* (DoH 1998), it was decided by the present authors to investigate what services had already developed in light of government guidelines and also to see how far provision had to progress in order to meet the requirements of the then forthcoming *National service framework for mental health* (DoH 1999).

Starting in June 1998 every health authority and board in the UK was approached and asked what crisis, home treatment and other emergency mental health services they purchased. Detailed information was sought from each provider, Trust and social services department; all were asked to provide background information, an operational policy for services and, where available, a service evaluation report. The initial request for data was followed up with subsequent letters and telephone requests until a return rate of 89% was achieved. A database was designed in the light of the information obtained, to support an analysis of the aims and objectives of the services that provided data. A set of categories were developed and then applied to the data set as a whole and frequencies calculated.

The definition of a crisis service employed in the study was pragmatic, services were included in this analysis on the basis of the self-descriptions provided by Trusts or services. The researchers did not apply a theoretical model of crisis or crisis services as a basis for inclusion in the analysis. For the purposes of this study, a crisis service was considered to exist where one or more of the following criteria were met in the service description provided to the researchers:

1) The service used the term crisis in the title of the service
2) Accepted users in crisis
3) Offered crisis intervention and/or management
4) The service accepted crisis referrals
5) Included a service to clients in crisis in the aims of the service.

Services were excluded from our definition of crisis services if they were restricted to clients already on a specific service caseload e.g. home treatment services – data from these services were published separately (Orme 2001).

RESULTS

The survey received 144 sets of documentation from 77 different health authorities; of these, 87 services were classified as a crisis service. The first issue of interest in the context of the design and operation of crisis services was the date of the inception of services. Of those crisis services that provided the information ($n = 83$), the majority (72%) had been established since 1995. In fact, the years 1996 to 1997 account for the start of 37% of all the crisis services included in the database.

Funding

Of the 87 services classified as crisis services, 42 provided details of funding. Once again the importance of initiatives in the late 1990s is apparent. The tendency appears to be for services to have been established as pilot projects using special funding arrangements or grants before some go on to be consolidated into the regular purchasing of health authorities. It is also clear that a significant proportion of services were funded by, or included within their arrangements, a contribution from social services departments.

Table 14.1 Date of service inception: all records

Year	All services		Crisis	
	n	%	n	%
1989	1	1	1	1
1990	1	1	0	0
1991	3	2	1	1
1992	0	0	0	0
1993	8	6	5	6
1994	7	5	2	2
1995	12	9	9	11
1996	17	12	12	15
1997	32	23	19	23
1998	19	14	14	17
1999	7	5	6	7
unknown	30	22	14	17
Total	137*	100	83*	99[†]

*Four services were established prior to 1989 or only the date of the termination of the service was provided.
[†]May not add to 100 due to rounding.

Table 14.2 Sources of funding

Source of funding	n	%
Mental health challenge fund	9	21
Specific mental illness grant	4	10
Health authority	12	29
Joint health authority/social services	6	14
Joint health authority/mental health challenge fund	4*	10
Joint health authority/specific mental illness grant	2	5
Social services	3*	7
Winter pressures initiative	1	2
Grant (Sainsbury Centre, Mental Health Foundation)	2	5
Total	42	103[†]

[†]May not add to 100 due to rounding.

Table 14.3 Staff composition of crisis teams

Staff team	n	%
Nurses alone	42	53
Nurse and OT	3	4
Nurse and social worker	11	14
Nurse and psychiatrist	7	9
Nurse and social worker and psychiatrist	6	8
Nurse, social worker, psychiatrist, psychologist and OT	3	4
MIND and volunteers	2	3
Social services staff	3	4
Community mental health team	3	4
Total	80	103[†]

[†] May not add to 100 due to rounding.

Staffing

Eighty of the 87 services (92%) provided sufficient detail on the staffing of their crisis service provision for subsequent analysis. The most notable feature of the staffing arrangements for crisis services is the dominance of teams that consist of nursing staff alone (53%) or small teams where nurses work with staff from one other profession (26%). A small number of teams also made reference to the purchase of psychiatry staff on a sessional basis or the availability of psychiatric consultants where necessary.

A total of 63 (73%) services specified the grade of nursing staff involved in the provision of the service (see Table 14.4). From these data it is clear that the preponderance of nursing staff were G, E and F grades. In fact, Table 14.4 indicates that larger services employed multiples of E and F grade nurses whereas G grades were mentioned in the make-up of most services. Four services reported the presence of H grades in their teams at a senior management level. It is very clear that the majority of services rely upon nurses as the major source of interventions, especially bearing in mind that 53% of services are comprised of nursing staff alone.

Table 14.4 Nurse grades			
Nurse grade	Total no. (WTE)	Services involved	
		n	%
G	51	23	out of how many?
E	42.5	14	
F	33	14	
C	1	1	
B	19	9	
A	2	2	

Operation of the service

Of the 87 services that were identified as providing a crisis service only 22 could be identified as offering a 24-hour service. However, it is clear that even services that are set up to provide a 24-hour service tend to operate at a much reduced level overnight and at weekends (see Table 14.5: one did not provide any additional details regarding provision). The route to referrals at night and weekends must vary from day-time practice as the majority of these services are in fact offering only telephone access to the service and some explicitly stated that visits would not be made overnight.

Referrals

Of 87 services, 27 (31%) stated that they had an open referral system, and of these, several identified the service as being 'open' to known clients only. A total of 78 crisis services (90%) provided sufficient detail of their referral system such that researchers could identify exactly who was allowed to make referrals and under what circumstances. As can be seen from Table 14.6, the number of open referrals is somewhat lower than at first seemed to be the case.

Of those services that accepted client referrals, 54% specified that the client must have been previously known to the service. A proportion of these further specified that such contact could only occur as part of a previously arranged care plan. Services accepting referrals from the police sometimes specified the Police surgeon as the acceptable source of referrals. The largest group of referrals not included in the table came from services that accepted referrals from hospital staff: 9% of services. A small number of services also accepted referrals from managers of day centres and staff working at a similar level in hostels.

Table 14.5 Service hours of operation

Hours	Days	Out-of-hours cover	Weekends and BH
8.30am–10pm	7	10.00am–8.30pm	YES
9am–9pm	5+	OOH telephone	1pm–9pm Sat/Sun
8am–5pm	7	OOH telephone	–
On-call	7	1900–1900	YES
24 hours	–	–	–
24 hours	7		YES
9am–5pm	5	OOH 5.00pm–9.00am Duty psychiatrist	YES duty psychiatrist
On-call 24	7		YES (known clients)
9am–12pm		OOH telephone	
10am–10.30pm		OOH telephone	
24 hours (residents)	7	On call 5pm–9am 7 days	YES
9am–5pm	7	OOH telephone	1 worker
7am–10pm	7	Reduced roster	YES
8.30am–10.00pm	7	On call OOH	YES
9.00am–9.00pm	7	On call OOH	YES
24 hours	7	Reduced roster	YES
10.00am–3.00pm	7	OOH (known clients)	YES (known clients)
9.00am–5.00pm	7	OOH telephone OOH telephone	
9.00am–12.00pm	7	12.00pm–9.00am no visits	–
9.00am–5.00pm	7	5.00pm–9.00am on-call	–

Exclusions

Forty-five (52%) of the 87 crisis services reported that they operated some sort of client exclusion criteria and 86% reported that they targeted services at specific clients. Clients are targeted in terms of age (51%), resident locally (35%), CPA level (17%) and presence of severe (31%), enduring (17%) or acute (18%) mental illness. The significant role

Table 14.6 Referrals	
Source of referrals	Proportion of all services responding
GP	49%
CMHT	40%
Psychiatrist	41%
A&E	25%
Social services	26%
ASW	21%
CPN/Nurse	23%
Client	23%
Carer/Family	18%
Police	18%
Open	13%

of services in the context of primary mental health care is apparent from the referral data. When combined with the data on target clients and service exclusion policies a very clear picture is formed of the client for whom these services were designed.

Services were targeted at the existing population of severely mentally ill clients known to mental health services. In particular, these services were typically not addressing the needs of patients with multiple diagnoses, usually those with a history of substance misuse or deliberate self-harm. Nor were they designed to address the requirements of people presenting with severe mental illness for the first time or people entering a significant crisis as a result of life events.

Crisis intervention

Service protocols were examined for details of the intervention offered and the operation of discharge planning. Although these issues are dealt with in more detail in another paper they are relevant here. In total, 64 crisis services indicated whether or not crisis intervention was offered; of these, 46 (72%) reported that they did not offer a crisis intervention and a further 18 (28%) of the services reported that they did offer crisis intervention.

Table 14.7 Exclusions	
Exclusion criteria	Proportion of all services responding
Accommodation required	12.73
Not known to service	7.27%
Caseload limit	9.10%
Psychotic	3.64%
Personality disorder	3.64%
Learning disability	14.55%
Risk to self	16.36%
Minor disorder	7.27%
No MH crisis	5.45%
Organic disorder	29.09%
Not local	5.45%
Anti-social	1.82%
Over 65	12.73%
Under 18	3.64%
Under 16	20%
Alcohol	76.36%
Drugs	72.73%

Finally, 9 (10%) of the 87 crisis services considered here have ceased operating, or were being considered for closure, during the course of this work.

DISCUSSION

Given the timing of the development of these services, it would appear that many were established in response to policy developments outlined in the documents *Health of the nation mental illness handbook* (DoH 1994) and the *Spectrum of care* (DoH 1996). This would, in part at least, account for the widespread emphasis upon an out-of-hours provision as part of most services, even where the nature of provision precludes a traditional crisis response service. The significance of the staffing, hours of operation and referrals data would appear to be that although every one of these services is described as a crisis service, the majority do not include a significant element of theoretically driven crisis intervention. This can be argued despite the continuing reference to the importance of the work of Caplan and others and the theoretical underpinnings of crisis intervention in crisis service documentation. The organisation of the services described in this paper does not appear to be, in the main, able to deliver interventions that maximise the opportunities for significant therapeutic intervention. Such interventions are a key feature of crisis theory and, at least in the early stages of the development of crisis services within the UK (e.g., Scott and Starr 1981; Davis *et al.* 1985), were usually a central feature of their operation.

Neither do the majority of services appear to have been designed to help clients experiencing a psychiatric emergency. For example, few services offered psychosocial interventions to help with crises (training in coping strategies and problem solving is carried out by a minority of services). In a majority of services staff are not always, if indeed ever, available or equipped to offer this form of support. Also, in the main, interventions offered to clients are very time limited and cannot act to prevent or help with psychiatric emergencies, particularly as immediate action is not always readily available – for example, where referrals need to be forwarded in writing.

Service documents make it clear that in the majority of cases, rapid assessment, including out-of-hours provision, followed by referral to other elements of mental health services, predominates. This characteristic of the service provision as discussed here would appear to be driven by two different features of the then current mental health system. Firstly, the drive for an integrated approach dictated that provision is available when required by patients and that it should not be confined to the hours of operation conventional in a primary care setting. Hence, the services examined in this survey are frequently an extension of existing provision and not a crisis service as such. Secondly, is the perhaps more important aspect of the human resources required by such a rapid expansion in provision. It is clear that the majority of services relied upon Community Psychiatric Nurses and ward-based nurses. Although service teams include a variety of other professionals, not least psychiatrists, these are not usually providing first-line care for patients. Certainly this is the case with regard to the provision of services out-of-hours. There is general recognition of a shortfall in the number of suitably skilled staff available to undertake significant therapeutic work with regard to psychiatric and psychological disorders in a community setting. Indeed, a recent report (Duggan 1997) into the provision of trained mental health staff identified a number of significant deficiencies in current provision and identified both a skills shortage and a requirement for new approaches to training that emphasises new roles and the central importance of multi-disciplinary settings for mental health care practice (Gournay and Sandford 1998).

Regarding the addressing of client need, the majority of these crisis services could be considered as 'diversion from admission' services. It is fair to conclude that the majority of service protocols appear to be organised so as to identify which clients can benefit from the service. This is to be contrasted with an approach that emphasises what services can do for patients. The pattern of exclusions and referrals, combined with the absence of key aspects of crisis care identified by client groups e.g. respite and self-referral (Cobb 1995) serve to underline the organisation-centred pattern of provision revealed by the survey.

Next we turn to a project funded by the West Midlands NHS Executive concerning the provision of crisis services within the West Midlands region. The goal of the research was to identify how far localities had to develop in order to meet *National service framework for mental health* (DoH 1999) guidelines. Specific questions addressed by the project included how the need for crisis services was assessed and how services measured their impact, e.g., throughput of clients and effectiveness. The project sought to understand how crisis services were planned and developed and to explore the extent to which they were part of a system of local mental health service provision.

The framework for the research was based upon the methods reported by Wing *et al.* (1998) and Faulkner *et al.* (1994). Wing *et al.* (1998) developed a protocol for assessing mental health service development by allocating scores for the standards of commissioning and service provision. A questionnaire was developed to collect baseline information regarding the overall provision of mental health services by each West Midlands mental health service-providing NHS Trust and social service department. The questionnaire was based on that of Faulkner *et al.* (1994) but included indicators identified by Johnson *et al.* (1997) as important. Community provision was considered in terms of crisis intervention teams, continuing care teams for people with long-term mental health problems and residential alternatives to hospital admission. The provision of 24-hour access to specialist psychiatric care was measured in terms of the provision of eight types of service (crisis house, crisis team, 24-hour CMHT, intensive home-support team, telephone helpline, drop-in centre, on-call community mental health nurses and on-call doctors (Johnson and Lelliott (1997)). Morbidity indicators such as finished consultant episodes, admissions under the Mental Health Act (1983), length of acute admission stay, Mental Illness Needs Index and Jarman or York Psychiatric Index scores were also requested. The questionnaire also asked respondents to identify 24-hour services accessible by both new and established mental health service clients.

The questionnaire was sent to the Chief Executives of all the providing Trusts and mental health leads in all the social services departments in the region. Letters asked respondents to complete the questionnaire themselves or nominate someone to do so who would be prepared to be interviewed at a later date. The questionnaire requested respondents send operational service documentation for all crisis services identified on the questionnaire as well as joint policy documents, implementation plans, mental health strategy documents and other relevant documentation. Letters were also sent to the mental health leads of the 13 health authorities in the West Midlands region requesting service level agreements for crisis services. Two follow-up mailings were made to non-respondents.

The documentation obtained was read and entered into a database. Triangulation of returned questionnaires, documentary analysis and content analysis of operational documents was undertaken to identify key themes; issues identified from this analysis were followed up in interviews.

Questionnaire responses were received from 10 out of 14 social services departments (71%) and 12 out of 16 NHS Trusts (75%). Follow-up interviews were completed with 19 out of a possible 23 interviewees (83%).

Information concerning service configurations and operational arrangements were extracted from the data. For the purpose of illuminating our discussion, the following table contains a comparison between the overall service design drawn from the national survey referred to above and the West Midlands regional response.

Service documentation identified six (23%) services as being staffed by a single discipline, four (15%) were only staffed by nurses and two (8%) by nurses with support workers. Fourteen (54%) services were multidisciplinary, seven (27%) were staffed by nursing and social-work staff, two of these with support workers. Six (23%) services were staffed by nursing, social work and psychiatry staff with a mixture of other

Table 14.8 Comparison of national and regional service characteristics

Organisational characteristics present	National sample		Regional sample	
	n	%	*n*	%
Multidisciplinary	64	44	14	54
Operate 24 hours	34	24	2	8
Target clients	123	85	23	89
Open referrals	40	28	3	12
Client exclusions	72	50	16	62
Offer crisis intervention	21	15	6	23
Offer follow-up	37	26	6	23
Refer clients on	78	54	11	42
Liaison with other services	108	75	17	65
Feedback to involved professionals	83	58	10	39

disciplines including psychology, occupational therapy, physiotherapy and housing officers in different mixtures. Nursing and psychology personnel staffed one service jointly. Trained volunteers or support workers (no professional qualifications specified) staffed five (19%) services.

Only two services (8%) reported operating throughout the 24-hour period, 19 did not (73%), five did not provide details. Of the 19 that did not operate for 24-hours, 16 provided additional details of operating hours. No two services offered exactly the same pattern of opening hours.

A range of criteria was identified by services by which to both target and exclude clients. Target criteria included: clients at risk or facing in-patient admission (7 services), clients experiencing severe mental illness (7), clients in crisis (6), known clients (5), resident locally (4) and experiencing psychotic illness/severe depression (3). Six services were targeted in terms of lower or upper age limits, but these were the same for two services only. Exclusion criteria included: primary diagnosis of alcohol/drug problems (7), primary diagnosis of learning disability (5), organic (5) and relationship and domestic violence issues (4). Primary diagnosis of anxiety disorders (4), history of overdose (5) and homelessness/seeking accommodation (3) were also reasons for exclusion.

Open referrals were only operated in a small minority of cases. Of the 65% of services that did not operate an open referral policy, a variety of professionals could refer. This included mental health professionals for four services, mental health professionals and GPs (3), any statutory service and GPs (3), police or police surgeons (2) and Trust and social services personnel (2). In one service, clients had to have been assessed by a GP or other health professional within the previous 24 hours.

Interview data and service documentation were also examined to determine what had driven or informed the design of services.

In their earlier study, Wing *et al.* (1998) reported that there was a lack of the information required to develop plans and set targets, for example, estimate of local population need compared to other areas. Needs assessment exercises involving users and the independent and/or voluntary sector were few and few commissioners had developed a service specification based on solid information about costs, volumes and quality standards for the local service as this information was not available. To a very great extent these findings were replicated and extended in our study of services in the West Midlands region. In terms of defining a crisis, no consensus of opinion was generated from the interviewees. Indeed in some cases interviewees laughed at being asked this question and one requested the recording machine be turned off. The diversity of views concerning what constitutes a crisis translated into diverse views of who should be targeted by crisis services. However, when reporting the type of client existing services focused on, it became clear that these were current and known mental health service users, i.e. there was a focus on secondary rather than primary access to crisis services.

Regarding the factors that contributed to the development of crisis services other than the *National service framework for mental health* (1999), a recognition of the inadequacy of current provision out of hours, from whatever source, was apparent. Respondents were unable to identify specific research or guidelines used in crisis service development. In only one case was the research and support of the Sainsbury Centre for Mental Health acknowledged. Government guidelines in general and individual's own experiences, picked up through their own reading or knowledge of other services, were felt to be the main contributing factors.

The development of crisis services within localities was not planned in any strategic way in the majority of cases. In only one area was new provision part of a long-term strategic plan. In other areas local history was the main influence in terms of key individuals, gaps in current provision combining with the ability often derived from new sources of funding and opportunity to build on existing services.

The collection and consideration of a body of empirical data affording a clear picture of the level and range of mental health needs and requirements was a very rare feature in the planning of new service developments. Indeed, the quality and quantity of the data available to our respondents would seem to have precluded such a strategy in the majority of cases; significant though was the fact that several services were able to demonstrate a central role for local service users in their work of designing services, and most included user representation at some level. Rather, local need was interpreted in terms of the need of local providers to develop services in line with organisational structure and history. Ring-fenced monies for certain types of service requirement resulted in service developments that were service and history focused rather than client focused. It seemed that Mental Health Grant, Single Regeneration Budget and Health Action Zone monies acted in some ways to increase differences between areas in that service developments were not so much based on local need but on the need for a local 'response.'

It is clear that the recent policy developments presage massive change in the organisation and delivery of crisis and outreach services in particular. There is also a broad understanding that high-quality research and development work is required to underpin these changes (Ford, Minghella and Ryrie 2001). Those same authors, in drawing together the published work and views of other workers in the field, also highlighted the problems that face any such programme. Amongst these problems are, of course, the questions of definition, staff training, heterogeneous service configurations and the paucity of research on the question of service models and questions of fidelity. We would suggest, however, that this analysis only partially addresses the issues raised by the history of the last ten years or so. Setting aside the significant contribution of those authors arguing for more sophisticated and imaginative designs for evaluation studies, we agree that these initiatives will contribute to an enhanced understanding of crisis services (Catty *et al.* 2002). It is nevertheless an unspoken, but highly questionable implicit assumption, that published research will influence services; their actual configuration, clinical practices and relationships with the mental health community and those who use services.

It would appear that there is an implicit 'trickle-down' model of sorts in which research, it is hoped, will either influence strategic thinking at the highest levels and this will translate into local action and/or local initiatives will be built upon the evidence of quality research. It is readily apparent that this process has not governed practice in the arena of assertive outreach and crisis resolution in the UK in the recent past. It cannot be argued, for example, that recent policy initiatives such as the *National service framework for mental health* (DoH 1999) which have driven service developments were based on sound evidence, if only because researchers and practitioners did not then agree upon whether or not such evidence existed or indeed what research methods may yield such evidence. Furthermore, there is an abundance of evidence that considerations other than research or the diffusion of good practice have helped frame developments on the ground. We would offer from our own national and regional surveys the following points:

- Only very infrequently were working definitions for a 'psychiatric crisis' or 'crisis service' apparent in service specifications and operational guidelines
- Most commonly, no commissioning guidelines were referred to for the design, goals or operation of crisis services
- Crisis services were most frequently developed from recognition of the inadequacy of service provision rather than assessment of need
- There was a lack of data regarding certain issues (e.g. disaggregated spend, client contacts, service loads) which may have precluded strategic planning, a form of planning that was anyway not commonly associated with service development
- Crisis services have developed in an *ad hoc* manner dependent on local circumstances; driven by issues such as budgets, staff availability and existing service configurations.

Now it could be argued that this, what we would call the contingent design of services, is driven by the absence of good quality research. However, a more robust interpretation, making far fewer assumptions, would be that these data reflect how things are done. Moreover, given the pressures upon services to deliver rapid change, there is every likelihood that this will continue to be so.

We would argue therefore that the 'gold standard' of RCT research designs are, in the context of complex systems such as components of community based services, at best a malapropism and at worst a chimera. It is not enough to recognise that treatments are embedded within services and services are themselves components of dynamic and complex systems. What is required, are systems for planning and managing change within the health sector, which both reflect this 'reality' and seek to improve outcomes from the process.

We would argue, therefore, that the UK model of services designed, owned and organised at the local level implies a need for local evaluation. This does not mean that we are arguing solely for more effective clinical audit, although it is clear that well-organised and executed systems of audit can deliver service gains (Gillies 1997). In short, we need to move towards a standard of practice in which the model of research becomes something like that espoused by evaluation practitioners such as Pawson and Tilley (1997). We need to move towards locally organised, action-oriented research based on the collection and analysis of quantitative and qualitative data; a research process less oriented towards a medical or hypothesis-testing mode, where the RCT is seen not as the standard, but one option.

In order to produce effective change, clinical staff, managers, clients and carers must be capable of detecting variation from agreed and accepted standards of delivery and, of course, outcomes. These standards need to be articulated when services are designed and the tools and skills for acquiring and analysing those data chosen as measures, identified at the outset. Above all, strategies for acting upon the output from the evaluation process, itself a continuous activity, must be seen as a key feature of effective services.

Our own research (Hogan *et al.* 1997; Hogan and Orme 1999; Orme 2001) has led us to recognise that the design of services is best understood as a form of dialectic. A dynamic process whereby evidence and arguments are marshalled to the cause in a manner that is usually partial, even biased for want of a better word, by local sentiments, history and views. The detailed work by researchers such as Cohen (2001) has begun to unpack this process and revealed the complex system of balance and counterbalance in the form of professional boundaries, funding issues and politics that underpin the development and survival of services. What we would suggest, is that what is required is a raising of the standard(s) of evidence and argument that are applied to the commissioning and design of services. By acknowledging the dialectical nature of the process, we can open up a legitimate avenue for applying knowledge derived from the study of organisations to the task of developing and evaluating systems of mental health care.

References

Baldwin, B.A. (1978). A paradigm for the classification of emotional crises: implications for crisis intervention. *American Journal of Orthopsychiatry*, **48**, 3, 538–51.

Brimblecombe, N. (1993). Family crisis. *Nursing Times*, **89**, 44, 40–1.

Brimblecombe, N. (ed) (2001). *Acute mental health care in the community: intensive home treatment*. Whur Publishers, London.

Burns, T., Fiander, M., Kent, A., Ukoummene, O.C., Byford, S., Fahy, T. and Kumar, K.R. (2000). Effects of case-load size on the process of care of patients with severe psychotic illness. Report from the UK700 trial. *British Journal of Psychiatry*, **37**, 392–7.

Burns, T., Catty, J., Watt, H., Wright, C., Knapp, M. and Henderson, J. (2002). International differences in home treatment for mental health problems: results of a systematic review. *British Journal of Psychiatry*, **181**, 375–82.

Callahan, J. (1994). Defining crisis and emergency. *Crisis*, **15**, 4, 164–71.

Caplan, G. (1964). *Principles of preventive psychiatry*. Basic Books, New York.

Caplan, G. (1974). *Support systems and community mental health*. Behavioural Publications, New York.

Cobb, A. (1995). Crisis? What Crisis? *Health Service Journal*. **105**(5435), 22–3.

Cohen, B.M.Z. (2001). Providing intensive home treatment: inter-agency and inter-professional issues. In Brimblecombe, N. (ed). *Acute mental health care in the community: intensive home treatment*. pp. 163–86. Whur Publishers, London.

Davis, A., Newton, S. and Smith, D. (1985). Coventry Crisis Intervention Team: the consumer's view. *Social Services Research*, **14**, 1, 7–32.

Department of Health. (1994). *Health of the nation. Key area handbook. Mental illness*, (2nd edn). HMSO, London.

Department of Health. (1996). *The spectrum of care*. HMSO, London.

Department of Health. (1998). *Modernising mental health services. Safe, sound, supportive*. HMSO, London.

Department of Health. (1998a). *Partnership in action*. HMSO, London.

Department of Health. (1999). *National service framework for mental health*. The Stationery Office, London.

Department of Health. (2000). *The NHS plan*. The Stationery Office, London.

Dixon, K. (1982). Personal crisis and psychiatric emergency: commentary on case mismanagement in crisis clinics. *Crisis Intervention*, **12**, 1, 24–35.

Duggan, M. (1997). *Pulling together*. Sainsbury Centre for Mental Health, London.

Gournay, K. and Sandford, T. (1998). Training for the workforce. In C. Brooker and J. Repper (eds), *Serious mental health problems in the community. Policy, practice and research*, pp. 291–310. Ballière Tindall, London.

Gillies, A. (ed.) (1997). *Improving the quality of patient care*. Wiley, Chichester.

Faulkner, A., Field, V. and Muijen, M. (1994). *A survey of adult mental health services.* The Sainsbury Centre for Mental Health, London.

Ford, R., Minghella, E. and Ryrie, I. (2002). *Assertive outreach and crisis resolution: moving forward the research and development agenda.* The Sainsbury Centre for Mental Health, London.

Hogan, K., Crawford-Wright, A., Orme, S., Easthope, Y. and Barker, D. (1997a). Walsall Crisis Support Service. Final Report. Volume 1. Service Evaluation. Psychology Division, University of Wolverhampton. Unpublished Report.

Hogan, K., Crawford-Wright, A., Orme, S., Easthope, Y. and Barker, D. (1997b). Walsall Crisis Support Service. Final Report. Volume 2. Literature Review. Psychology Division, University of Wolverhampton. Unpublished Report.

Hogan, K. and Orme, S. (1999). The effectiveness of crisis services. In Tomlinson, D. and Allen, K. (eds), *Crisis services and hospital crises: mental health at a turning point.* Ashgate, Aldershot.

Hogan, K. and Orme, S. (Unpublished report.) An overview of crisis service provision in the UK: service design and organisation.

Jacobs, D. (1983). The treatment capabilities of psychiatric emergency services. *General Hospital Psychiatry,* 5, 3, 171–7.

Johnson, S., Brooks, L., Ramsay, R. and Thornicroft, G. (1997). The structure and functioning of London's mental health services. In Johnson, S., Ramsay, R., Thornicroft, G., Brooks, L, Lelliott, P., Peck, E., Smith, H., Chisolm, D., Audini, B., Knapp, M. and Goldberg, D. (1997). *London's mental health,* pp. 220–49. King's Fund, London.

Johnson, S. and Lelliott, P. (1997). Mental health services in London: evidence from research and routine data. In Johnson, S., Ramsay, R., Thornicroft, G., Brooks, L, Lelliott, P., Peck, E., Smith, H., Chisolm, D., Audini, B., Knapp, M. and Goldberg, D. (1997). *London's mental health,* pp. 167–92. King's Fund, London.

Johnson, S., Ramsay, R., Thornicroft, G., Brooks, L., Lelliott, P., Peck, E., Smith, H., Chisolm, D., Audini, B., Knapp, M. and Goldberg, D. (1997). *London's mental health.* King's Fund, London.

McMillan, I. (1997). Confidence in a crisis. *Mental Health Practice,* 1, 3, 4–5.

Minghella, E., Ford, R., Freeman, T., Hoult, J., McGlynn, P. and O'Halloran, P. (1998). *Open all hours, 24-hour response for people with mental health emergencies.* Sainsbury Centre for Mental for Mental Health, London.

Newton, S. (1989). Organisational models for crisis intervention. In Renshaw, J. (ed.) *Crisis intervention service information pack.* Good Practices in Mental Health, London.

Orme, S. (2001). Intensive home treatment services: the current position in the UK. In Brimblecombe, N. (ed.) *Acute mental health care in the community: intensive home treatment,* pp. 29–53. Whur Publishers, London.

Parks, C.M. (1992). Services for families in crisis in Tower Hamlets: evaluations by general practitioners and social workers. *Psychiatric Bulletin,* 16, 12, 748–50.

Pawson, R. and Tilley, N. (1997). *Realistic evaluation*. Sage, London.

Pelosi, A.J. and Jackson, G.A. (2000). Home treatment enigmas and fantasies. *British Medical Journal*, **320**, 308–9.

Renshaw, J. (1989). Crisis intervention: introduction. In Renshaw, J. (ed.) *Crisis intervention service information pack*. Good Practices in Mental Health, London.

Rosen, A. (1998). Crisis management in the community. *Medical Journal Australia: Practice Essentials*, **8**, 44–8.

Sainsbury Centre for Mental Health. (2001). *Crisis resolution*. The Sainsbury Centre for Mental Health, London.

Santayana, G. (1924). *The life of reason or the phases of human progress: reason in common sense* (2nd edn). Charles Scribner's Sons, New York, New York (originally published 1905 Charles Scribner's Sons).

Schnyder, U. (1997). Crisis intervention in psychiatric outpatients. *International Medical Journal*, **4**, 1, 11–17.

Scott, D. and Starr, I. (1981). A 24-hour family oriented psychiatric and crisis service. *Journal of Family Therapy*, **3**, 177–86.

Selye, H. (1956). *The stress of life*. McGraw Hill, New York.

Stroul, B. (1988). Residential crisis services: a review. *Hospital and Community Psychiatry*, **39**, 10, 1095–9.

University of Birmingham. (1999). Key Health Data for the West Midlands, 1999. From the West Midlands Public Health Office. Department of Public Health and Epidemiology, University of Birmingham.

Waldron, C. (1989). Crisis intervention: a persistent theme. In Renshaw, J. (ed.) *Crisis intervention service information pack*. Good Practices in Mental Health, London.

Warburton, J. (1996). A study into the effectiveness of a residential unit in managing mental health crises: the views of service users, residential staff and social workers. University of Central England, Birmingham. Unpublished MSc Thesis.

Wing, J. K., Rix, S., Curtis, R. H., Beadsmoore, A. and Lelliott, P. (1998). Protocol for assessing services for people with severe mental illness. *British Journal of Psychiatry*, **172**, 121–9.

15

Recovery
Piers Allott

BACKGROUND

It is remarkable that in the twenty-first century and with the 1990s 'decade of the brain' behind us that our understanding of 'mental illness', and hence recovery from 'mental illness', is still delineated and influenced by the work of Emil Kraepelin from 1887 when he formulated his understanding of 'schizophrenia' or dementia praecox as he termed it then. In *Recovery from schizophrenia* (1994) Professor Richard Warner recognised Kraepelin's work as 'continuing to serve us well, with some exceptions, as a picture of modern-day schizophrenia' (p. 8). However, central to Kraepelin's concept of schizophrenia was a belief that the condition would have a deteriorating course and with the adoption of his formulation around the world, the impression that this condition was inevitably progressive and incurable became accepted, despite evidence to the contrary.

Even today, many people when given a diagnosis of a serious mental disorder, and particularly a diagnosis of 'schizophrenia', are often given dire predictions of a future within which there is little hope for recovery. Many professionals believe that recovery from 'mental illness' is not possible. This is true across the 'developed' world. Mary O'Hagan, a Mental Health Commissioner in New Zealand, states:

> *One of the commonest complaints I have heard from service users about mental health workers is that they stole their hopes and dreams. Yet, people with mental illness often say the hope others had for them when they had lost it, was a key to their recovery.*

> (O'Hagan 1999, p. 5)

She presents a view from one of the pacific people in New Zealand:

None of the doctors, nobody said to me . . . 'You can do better, you can get well, you can beat this, you can still lead a normal life in spite of it.' If someone had said that to me, it would've made all the difference!

(O'Hagan 1999, p. 4)

The knowledge that recovery occurs is not new and Kraepelin's research identified complete recovery, defined by Warner (1994) as 'loss of psychotic symptoms and return to the pre-illness level of functioning' (p. 8) in some 10% of the people he followed up. Warner (1994) provides a very comprehensive table of eighty-five long-term follow-up studies and these are summarised by period in Fig. 15.1. From this it is clear that 'recovery rates from schizophrenia are not significantly better now than they were during the first two decades of the century' (p. 72) with complete recovery rates remaining around 20–25% and about 40–45% of people being socially recovered. Warner (1994) defines social recovery as 'economic and residential independence and low social disruption. This means working adequately to provide for oneself and not being dependent on others for basic needs or housing' (p. 59).

Years	Complete recovery				Social recovery
	No. of studies	Numbers followed up	% Recovered	Numbers followed up	% Recovered
1881–1900	2	207	12	182	15
1901–1920	12	1373	20	1850	41
1921–1940	27	4264	12	3761	29
1941–1955	17	3285	23	2818	44
1956–1994	37	3715	22	3388	44

Figure 15.1 Recovery rates from Schizophrenia. Adapted from Warner 1994, pp. 60–71

Eugen Bleuler, in 1911, provided case examples of recovery in his monograph, *Dementia praecox or the group of schizophrnias*, that make interesting reading even today:

> *Physician: Neurasthenia at twenty-nine. Then at thirty-one after typhoid fever, catatonic. At forty-seven, apparently 'cured'. He then resumes his practice, marries. Has been well for the past two years.*
>
> (Cited in Warner 1994, p. 10)

So why is it that in modern-day psychiatry with a significant knowledge about recovery from serious 'mental illness' that the concept of recovery has been so hard to promote? Perhaps a developing belief in the power of 'science', along with other medical technological advances, to find a biological aetiology for mental illness that could be resolved by new pharmaceutical discoveries has led psychiatry down a singular route of exploration when the issues are much more complex. Fulford (2003) points to the history of twentieth-century psychiatry as 'a history of fashions – psychoanalysis, community care, a narrowly conceived "biological" psychiatry, all started as good ideas that, lacking the perspective of history, deteriorated into ideologies.' (p. 327) Psychiatry should, therefore, recognise the lessons from history that many of these 'fashions' have excluded, such as 'recovery', and recognise the point made by Warner (1994) that 'recovery rates from schizophrenia are not significantly better now than they were during the first two decades of the century' (p. 72).

WHAT IS RECOVERY FROM 'MENTAL ILLNESS'?

The concept of recovery from 'mental illness' has only begun to emerge in the last decade in the UK – or re-emerge according to Roberts and Wolfson (2003) – so how might it be defined? The recent concept of recovery has been emerging since the 1980s in the US. It is, in large part, due to the courage of some people who had been diagnosed with 'mental illness' to recover, in spite of the system, and to tell their stories. Judi Chamberlin (1978) was one of the first although there have been a number of others as far back as the nineteenth century.

In the US, many States have been seeking more effective services and have begun to establish 'dialogues' with, listen to and hear people who use their services. As a result, those States now have recovery as a central guiding vision and philosophy included in State policy for mental health services. A similar process has been occurring in

New Zealand where in 1998 recovery became a central part of the *Blueprint for mental health services* (Mental Health Commission 1998). The *Blueprint* definition of recovery is:

> . . . the ability to live well in the presence or absence of ones mental illness (or whatever people choose to name their experience). Each person with mental illness needs to define for themselves what 'living well' means to them.

The *Blueprint* also identifies that,

> Recovery is a journey as much as destination. It is different for everyone. For some people with mental illness, recovery is a road they travel on only once or twice, to a destination that is relatively easy to find. For others, recovery is a maze with an elusive destination, a maze that takes a lifetime to navigate.
>
> Recovery is happening when people can live well in the presence or absence of their mental illness and the many losses that may come in its wake, such as isolation, poverty, unemployment and discrimination. Recovery does not always mean that people will return to full health or retrieve all their losses, but it does mean that people can live well in spite of them.

The *Blueprint* also recognises that,

> Some people have experienced recovery without using mental health services. Others have experienced recovery in spite of them.

And that,

> . . . most will do much better if services are designed and delivered to facilitate recovery. Virtually everything the mental health sector does can either assist or impede recovery.
>
> (pp. 1–2)

What is of central importance is that there is respect for, and valuing of, the differences between people that recognises each person's uniqueness as identified in the National Institute for Mental Health in England (NIMHE 2003) operational draft framework of values for mental health. For recovery to be facilitated, it is essential for people to have 'space' within which they are enabled to discover and own their experiences with no expectation that recovery will be achieved within a particular timeframe. The perception that people have similar mental health experiences does not mean that those experiences should be treated in the same way but in ways unique to each person, and this is perhaps one of the essential differences between traditional psychiatric practice and working in a way that supports recovery.

For example, the experience of 'hearing voices' had been assumed for many years to be one that should not be colluded with. However, as people listened to the experiences of voice hearers and became aware of the work of Romme and Escher (1993) that provided the research evidence on which a better understanding of these experiences emerged, practice has begun to change. Many people with voice-hearing experiences never attend psychiatric services and many people value their voice-hearing. However, we must recognise that for many 'voice-hearing' is very distressing because of the nature of the voices and it is usually this group of people who attend mental health services for assistance. However, we now know that whilst medication and professional support may be helpful, at the end of the day it is the individual who is the best expert in his/her own experiences and the task of service providers is to provide support and be able to walk the journey towards recovery with the person.

RECOVERY FROM WHAT?

It is interesting that both psychiatrists and survivors of psychiatry ask this same question. From the point of view of system survivors there is a fear that accepting the concept of recovery implies acceptance of the 'medical model' (Turner-Crowson and Walcraft 2002), or what will be referred to in this chapter as the 'biological model'. Many people who have been treated in the mental health system do not see themselves as experiencing a 'mental illness', and often the distress that brought them to the notice of mental health services in the first place may well have been the trauma of abuse, racism or many other situations in which people felt out of control of their lives. In these circumstances, what is often perceived by people as the coercive and punitive nature of in-patient admission – and in the case of African-Caribbean men, often the experience of entry to the system – does little to provide a safe environment for the person but provides a further experience of trauma. Hence, many people wish to see themselves as 'recovering' from psychiatry and mental health services rather than from 'mental illness' and many would agree with Thomas Szasz (1960) that 'mental illness' is a myth.

From the point of view of many psychiatrists, recovery from the 'illness' is not considered a possibility, contrary to the follow-up studies identified above, as exemplified in the following anonymous quote from *Roads to recovery* (Baker and Strong 2001, p. 23):

> *A professor of psychiatry I work with (who doesn't know my past history) told me he doesn't believe it's possible for patients diagnosed as suffering from chronic schizophrenia to ever fully recover. They would at the least he said always have some degree of 'oddness' about them (I wondered what he'd think if he found that I, his secretary for many years, was once given that diagnosis – he doesn't seem to perceive me as odd, but). These attitudes make it very difficult for an ex-patient like myself to find the courage to speak out about their experience, but the irony is that not speaking out does not help the attitudes to change.*

RECOVERY TO WHAT?

There can only be one person to identify 'to what' and that is the person 'in recovery' from 'mental illness', themselves.

However, psychiatry has for so long been the arbiter for defining people as having a 'mental disorder' or 'psychiatric illness' that it is understandable that people should be concerned that expectations of 'psychiatry defined normality' will soon follow in the footsteps of 'recovery' and, as a consequence, issues raised about people who do 'not recover'.

On the other hand, perhaps a movement should be formed that is genuinely about 'mental health' rather than 'mental illness' and recognise that there are many ways in which 'mental health' can be defined. Mental health and mental wellness are more than an absence of mental illness. All of us have experiences of 'mental illness/distress' at some point in our lives, and the experience of 'mental illness' or even clinically diagnosable psychosis is much more common in the continuum of mental experience in our societies than has previously been identified. Van Os' (2000) study of a population of 7,076 people in the Netherlands found a significantly different occurrence of psychosis in the general population of 17.5%: some fifty times more than expected. This indicates that within that community a significant proportion of the population have experiences of 'the psychosis phenotype' indicating the continuum of 'mental illness' in our communities, and therefore, that even those forms of mental disorder considered the most serious are significantly more prevalent than previously identified. Therefore, if some 17% of people with clinically diagnosable 'psychosis' are not in contact with mental health services, we must assume that a person who can be clinically diagnosed as having a 'mental illness' can also be 'mentally healthy'. This will be particularly so if in addition to their symptoms of 'mental illness' they experience 'a state of psychological wellness characterised by the satisfactory fulfilment of basic human needs' that Prilletensky (2001) defines as mental health. They may have high self-esteem and feel good about who they are, they may have loving relationships and family lives and be successful in their chosen occupation, in spite of diagnosable symptoms. So the presence of symptoms in itself is not sufficient to determine 'mental illness' or to exclude 'mental health'. This view is supported by Repper and Perkins (2003) who contend that approaches that focus on deficits limit our view of people who experience mental health problems. They point out that 'People whose symptoms continue or recur can, and do live satisfying lives and contribute to their communities in many different ways and the alleviation of such symptoms does not necessarily result in the reinstatement of former, valued, roles and relationships' (Repper and Perkins 2003, p. viii).

RESEARCH

As has previously been identified, the concept of recovery is relatively new within the field of psychiatry and mental health services with much of the current research emanating from the field of psychosocial rehabilitation and focusing on evidence-based treatments such as family psychoeducation (Faloon and Fadden 1995; McFarlane 1997), employment (Stein *et al.* 1999) and assertive community treatment (Stein and Santos 1998). All of these tend to focus on finding ways of coping with, and managing, perceived pathological experience rather than to focus on issues of resilience and recovery. It was only in the latter part of the twenty-first century that some research has begun to examine issues of recovery, although there are very few such studies that are easily accessible or that have been well publicised.

Topor (2001) completed an in-depth study of the factors that contributed to the recovery experiences of 16 people in Sweden and identified the complexity of these and the difficulty of establishing a connection between the frequency and course of recovery and specific psychiatric interventions. He identified factors that are known to have an impact on the recovery process as being 'medication, the person's own volition and determination, and support from the persons surroundings'.

Topor highlights complexity as being the overarching category that has as its most distinguishing feature 'the idea of "both, simultaneously", not "either, or"' and states that 'This characterises both the individuals concerned, the people around them and the places and means that facilitate recovery. It encompasses the possibility to be both mad and rational at the same time' (p. 318). This raises significant methodological issues for research into recovery and highlights the uniqueness of each person's experience. On the one hand, there will be people who may feel that their needs are met by a biological approach to their experiences, supported by a psychiatric classification system such as ICD10 or DSMIV. On the other hand, this approach is meaningless to people who find alternative non-biological ways of recovering from their experiences and get on with their lives.

The core issue is one of contradictions. What helps at one point in time may not help, and may even hinder, at another. What may be perceived as negative and unsupportive experiences that trigger frustration and anger can also be the catalysts for purposeful action and recovery.

Topor (2001) states that

> *Managing contradictions is neither a method nor a treatment programme. The recovery process seems to depend on and consist of opportune coincidences that occur at times when the person is in a position to take advantage of the opening that is created to break with his/her one-dimensional identity as a mental patient and accommodate a more complex identity.*

(p. 319)

In an unpublished English pilot study (Allott and Loganathan 2002), many of the characteristics identified above are corroborated. This study involved six people in semi-structured interviews with participants identifying recovery as a 'step up in consciousness', 'a perception change' and 'having to change me'. One participant stated that 'doctors can't change ya, prison systems can't change ya' and the drugs can't change ya, you can change yourself' (Allott and Loganathan 2002, p. 9).

The issues raised above have been covered before but one of the aims of this study was to include a number of people from black and ethnic minority communities, and we have included two women from

Asian communities and one man who came from an African-Caribbean community. It was noticeable from the narratives of the people from black and ethnic minority communities that issues of poverty, cultural identity and experience were more significant with the issue of 'psychiatry' being seen to be as much about socio-economic and political factors and a form of behaviour control as about mental illness. Lack of education, lack of opportunity and deprivation were seen as elements that contribute to the potential for people to experience mental illness.

A further piece of research, completed in England, was that by Hermione Thornhill (2002) as part of her training as a clinical psychologist. Thornhill has her own experience of psychosis as a teenager and therefore states that she has something of an 'insiders perspective'. Fifteen people talked with her about their experiences of recovery, some of whom had written about their experiences and been public about them already. The aim of the study was to focus on the emotional and psychological themes in individuals accounts of their recovery that excluded some of the more concrete themes such as financial resources, employment and housing.

Themes fell into three clusters. The first was identified as, 'Making sense: how mad was I really?' and included understanding experiences in ways that made sense to the subjects and recognition of different realities and the different aspects of being human. The second theme was identified as '"Beating-up" versus "tea and sympathy": responses to psychosis' and included three sub-themes identifying how individuals respond to themselves, helpful relationships and the helpful and unhelpful mental health system. The third theme is identified as 'Telling stories' and included deception and silences on both the side of the individual and of the mental health service highlighting lack of trust and coercion rather than collaboration. Also meaningful to people in this research was working out where they stand, particularly with regard to human rights and responsibilities.

Compared to the non-UK research projects, both pieces of UK-based research seem to indicate greater differences between the mental health system and the identified needs of people who use services. This may be indicative of a less user-centred mental health system than in Sweden or the United States. It may also reflect the lack of a recognised, enabled and adequately funded service-user movement that can make a difference to the way in which services are delivered. The importance of 'putting the service user at the centre of everything we do', an essential stated ingredient of Government policy, is highlighted in the importance given to peer-operated services elsewhere. Peer-operated services in the UK are few and far between except for a significant number of local poorly supported and under-funded user groups (Walcraft, Read and Sweeney 2003).

One of the largest and most recent studies on recovery is that being undertaken for the National Association of State Mental Health Program Directors (NASMHPD) entitled *Mental health recovery: what helps and what hinders? A national research project for the development of recovery facilitating performance indicators*. The Phase I report was produced in October 2002 (Onken *et al.* 2002). The aims of this study are to:

- Increase knowledge about what facilitates or hinders recovery from psychiatric disabilities
- Devise a core set of systems-level indicators that measure critical elements and processes of a recovery-facilitating environment
- Integrate items that assess recovery-orientation into a multi-site 'report card' of mental health system performance measures, in order to generate comparable data across state and local mental health systems and encourage the evolution of recovery-oriented systems.

The following are the key implications from the findings of the Phase I report:

- Since persons are at the core of a dynamic interplay among themselves, other people, the resources available in the environment, and other forces, mental health services must recognise and allow for self-agency while bolstering, or at least not undermining, such efforts. Seeing people as whole persons, beyond their labeled identity, is integral to recovery.
- A shift to a recovery orientation will require attention to wellness and health promotion, not simply attention to symptom suppression or clinical concerns. Attention must be paid to basic needs in safe and affordable housing, health care, income, employment, education and social integration.
- A recovery orientation will require close attention to fundamental rights and needs.
- Re-orientation away from coercion requires alternative resources as well as training.
- There needs to be a continual evolution in our thinking, and for development of knowledge concerning recovery among diverse communities. For example, the balance of autonomy and self-reliance

versus group or family focus may differ in recovery based on such factors as ethnicity and culture. Special attention is needed for people who have experienced trauma or who have substance-use disorders.

- Resources for re-educating families, consumers, the professions and paraprofessional providers, young people, and the public at large, on the potential for recovery are called for, and will take significant investment. Stigma and misinformation must be countered through a variety of strategies (with attention to incorporating active roles for consumer/survivors) that target many audiences.
- Hope and empowerment are critical and their relationship to recovery warrants further research attention.
- True parity of decision-making power and respect through mutual and supportive partnership among consumer/survivors, professionals, administrators, and policy makers can become the basis of collaborative efforts to design and implement action strategies that will move America's mental health systems toward a recovery orientation.
- Adequate resources are needed to fund and support consumer voice and consumer leadership development.

RECOVERY THEMES

The search for themes that may help in understanding the process of recovery from 'mental illness' only began in the mid to late 1990s, although in the past ten to fifteen years there have been a growing number of recovery narratives written by people that recount individual recovery journeys. In addition, a small but growing number of research projects have attempted to explore the experiences of people in recovery. Knowledge from both these sources has begun to identify common themes. Ridgway (2001) analysed four early narratives. Ralph, Lambric and Steele (1996) and Ralph and Lambert (1996) reported themes from two groups of people who used mental health services in Ohio and Maine in the US.

In Australia, Tooth, Kalyansundaram and Glover (1997) broke down the one hundred and eleven themes identified in their research into the following broad themes:

1. *Process*: where people spoke about the process of coming to terms with the illness

2. *Activities*: where people spoke about a variety of activities that facilitated their recovery
3. *Environment*: where people spoke about various aspects of their environment that facilitated their recovery
4. *Medication*: where people spoke about the effects of medication in their recovery
5. *Self*: where people spoke about aspects of themselves that helped in their recovery and also about the coping strategies they used to aid in their recovery
6. *Network*: where people spoke of the role of their various networks of people and how they helped in their recovery
7. *Hospitalisation*: and its role in the person's recovery process
8. *Non-facilitatory*: where people spoke about things that hindered the recovery process.

These are reflected in the thesis of Topor (2001). The role of self was the most frequently reported theme in the Tooth *et al.* (1997) study with the person's determination to get better and manage their illness being of significant importance. Topor (2001) provides a very helpful analysis that recognises the complexity of self in the process that he describes as 'the successive gaining of control over one's life, of feeling secure in interpersonal relationships' (pp. 244–75). This is important because it confirms the significance of an 'expert patient' approach (DoH 2001b) to self management.

The following is an attempt to summarise and bring together the range of themes that appear to emerge from recovery narrative writings and research.

1. Recovery is a process that is unique for each person
2. Discovering hope for recovery is essential
3. Finding a persistent and resilient self enables recovery
4. Recovery means taking personal responsibility for instituting purposeful action and active coping
5. Finding meaning in 'mental illness' experiences promotes recovery
6. Recovery involves finding personal supports, activities and an environment that will support growth and development
7. Recovery is a non-linear process with spirals and difficult passages
8. Recovery is not simply about symptom elimination but is an active on-going process of self-directed healing and transformation
9. Thriving can be the result of recovering from experiences due to 'mental illness' and other adverse experiences.

DEVELOPING RECOVERY-ORIENTED SERVICES

As a result of their work in the early 1990s, the Ohio Department of Mental Health (ODMH 1999) 'recognised the right of people with severe and persistent mental illness to live in the community and participate in a lifestyle of their choice'. In order to deliver this they developed a recovery process model and emerging best practices in mental health recovery. The model and emerging best practices were developed by people with lived experience of recovery from 'mental illness'. They identified a core set of nine service domains they considered essential for a community to provide effective services and supports to people with 'mental illness'. The domains are:

1. Clinical care
2. Family support
3. Peer support and relationships
4. Work/meaningful activity
5. Power and control
6. (Combating) stigma
7. Community involvement
8. Access to resources
9. Education.

The role of each stakeholder was identified. Stakeholders include the person with lived experience, the clinician and the community in each of these service domains and at each of the four stages of recovery below:

1. Dependent/unaware
2. Dependent/aware
3. Independent/aware
4. Interdependent/aware.

For people identified as 'dependent/unaware', the framework recognises that multiple factors influence dependency and identifies the following possible influences:

a) Degree of illness experienced
b) The positive/negative impact and/or intervention of others, including the mental health system
c) An individuals interaction and/or reactions to experiences with traumatic events, such as hospital admissions, medication reactions, prisons, interpersonal relations
d) The impact of the illness on their daily lives.

They established a set of guiding principles (see Fig. 15.2) that formed the basis for the development of the recovery process model and emerging best practices that underpin the development of recovery-oriented services:

All of these principles are supported by current government policy including *Modernising mental health services: safe, sound and supportive* (1998), *The national service framework for mental health: modern standards and service models* (1999) and the *NHS plan: a plan for investment, a plan for reform* (2001a).

RESILIENCE AND THRIVING

Ridgway (1999) described resilience as:

- An innate human capacity
- The ability to contend successfully with and overcome personal vulnerabilities and external adversities
- A complex set of self-righting capacities that exist within stressful life circumstances
- The capacity for positive growth and transformation across the life span despite difficult challenges.

Many of the narratives of people who have been identified as experiencing 'mental illness' attest to resilience and thriving. O'Leary and Ickovics (1995) argued that theorists, researchers, and practitioners need to recognise that adversity can eventually bring benefits as the experience of facing adversity in itself can promote the emergence of a quality that makes the person better off afterward than beforehand (Carver 1998). Mary O'Hagan (1999) puts it like this:

> *Yet, I would not have missed that experience for anything, because hidden somewhere inside all the pain I felt, were the seeds of the person I went on to become. A person with a fuller understanding of life, a greater ability to overcome adversity, an enduring appreciation of the privilege of wellness, and a much more interesting career than I might otherwise have had. In the end my mental illness gave me as much, if not more, than it took away.*
>
> (p. 2)

Principle I	Principle VI
The service user directs the recovery process; therefore, service-user input is essential throughout the process.	In order to reflect current 'best practices' there is a need to merge all intervention models, including medical, psychological, social and recovery.
Principle II	**Principle VII**
The mental health system must be aware of its tendency to enable and encourage service-user dependency.	Clinicians' initial emphasison 'hope' and the ability to develop trusting relationships influences the service user's recovery.
Principle III	**Principle VIII**
Service users are able to recover more quickly when their • Hope is encouraged, enhanced and/or maintained • Life roles with respect to work and meaningful activities are defined • Spirituality is considered • Culture is understood • Educational needs as well as those of their family/significant others are identified • Socialisation needs are identified.	Clinicians operate from a strengths/assets model. **Principle IX** Clinicians and service users collaboratively develop a recovery management plan. This plan focuses on the interventions that will facilitate recovery and the resources that will support the recovery process.
Principle IV	**Principle X**
Individual differences are considered and valued across life span.	Family involvement may enhance the recovery process. The service user defines his/her family.
Principle V	**Principle XI**
Recovery from mental illness is most effective when a holistic approach is considered.	Mental health services are most effective when delivery is within the context of the service-user's community. **Principle XII** Community involvement as defined by the service user is important to the recovery process.

Figure 15.2   Guiding principles for recovery based mental health services. ©1999 Ohio Department of Mental Health

CONCLUSION

We know from research and personal narratives that recovery from serious mental disorders is a reality. We know that resilience and thriving are possible in spite of significant experiences of trauma and illness.

We must work to change practices that will increase the opportunities for recovery for the majority, not the minority, and we must carry out research that will inform and change practice. Research needs to focus on resilience and recovery; what helps, what hinders and how to change it, and it needs to recognise the wealth of experience and knowledge that 'experts by experience' hold, and develop and build on this in recognition that peer support and self-management are essential components of a recovery oriented mental health system.

References

Allott, P. and Loganathan, L. (2002). *Experiences of recovery.* Report of West Midlands personal narratives from a pilot study for the West Midlands Mental Health Development Team. University of Central England, Birmingham.

Allott, P., Loganathan, L. and Fulford, K.W.M. (2002, in press). Discovering hope for recovery from a British perspective: a review of a selection of recovery literature, implications for practice and systems change. In *International innovations in community mental health [special issue].* (eds. Lurie, S., McCubbin, M. and Dallaire, B.), *Canadian Journal of Community Mental Health,* **21**, 3.

Baker, S. and Strong, S. (2001). *Roads to recovery – how people with mental health problems recover and find ways of coping.* MIND, London.

Beale, V. and Lambric, T. (1995). The recovery concept: implementation in the mental health system- a report commissioned by the Community Support Program Advisory Committee. Dept. of Mental Health, Columbus, Ohio.

Carver, C.S. (1998). Resilience and thriving: issues, models, and linkages. *Journal of Social Issues,* **54**(2), 245–66.

Chamberlin, J. (1978). *On our own: patient-controlled alternatives to the mental health system.* McGraw-Hill, New York.

Department of Health. (1998). *Modernising mental health services: safe, sound and supportive.* HMSO, London, UK.

Department of Health. (1999). *National service framework for mental health. Modern standards and service models.* HMSO, London, UK.

Department of Health. (2001a). *NHS plan: a plan for investment. A plan for reform.* HMSO, London, UK.

Department of Health. (2001b). *The expert patient: a new approach to chronic disease management.* HMSO, London, UK.

Faloon, I.R.H. and Fadden, G. (1995) *Integrated Mental Health Care, A comprehensive community-based approach.* Cambridge. Cambridge University Press.

Fulford, K.W.M. (2003). Report to the Chair of the DSM-VI Task Force from the Editors of Philosophy, Psychiatry, and Psychology, 'Contentious and Noncontentious Evaluative Language in Psychiatic Diagnosis' (Dateline 2010). In *Descriptions and prescriptions – values, mental disorders, and the DSMs* (ed. Sadler, J.Z.), The Johns Hopkins University Press, Baltimore and London.

McCubbin, M. and Cohen, D. (2003). *Empowering practice in mental health social work: barriers and challenges. GRASP Working Papers Series, 31.* University of Montreal (GRASP). Available: http://www.grasp.umontreal.ca/documents/WP-An-31.pdf

McFarlane, W.R. (1997). Family psychoeducation: basic concepts and innovative applications. In *Innovative approaches for difficult-to-treat populations* (eds. Henggler, S.W. and Scott, W.), American Psychiatric Press, Washington, DC.

Mental Health Commission. (1998). *Blueprint for mental health services in New Zealand – how things need to be.* Wellington, New Zealand.

NIMHE. (2003). A Draft National Framework of Values for Mental Health. Available at www.connects.org.uk/conferences Values in Mental Health.

O'Hagan, M. (1999). Realising recovery. Six challenges to the mental health sector. Keynote address to Realising Recovery Conference. Mental Health Commission, Auckland, New Zealand.

Townsend, W., Boyd, Griffin, G. and Hicks, P.L. (1999). *Emerging best practices in mental health recovery.* Ohio Department of Mental Health, Columbus, Ohio.

O'leary, V.E. and Ickovics, J.R. (1995). Resilience and thriving in response to challenge: an opportunity for a paradigm shift in women's health. *Women's health: Research on Gender, Behavior, and Policy,* 1, 121–42.

Onken, S.J., Dumont, J.M., Ridgway, P., Dornan, D.H. and Ralph, R.O. (2002). Mental health recovery: what helps and what hinders? A national research project for the development of recovery facilitating system performance indicators. NTAC (National Technical Assistance Center), Alexandria, VA.

Polak, P. and Kirby, M. (1976). A model to replace psychiatric hospitals. *Journal of Nervous and Mental Disease* 162(1), 13–22.

Prilleltensky, I. (2001). Cultural assumptions, social justice, and mental health. In *Cultural cognition and psychopathology* (eds. Shumaker, J. and Ward, T.), pp. 251–65. Praeger, Westport, CO.

Prilleltensky, I. and Nelson, G. (2002). *Doing psychology critically: making a difference in diverse settings.* Macmillan, Toronto.

Ralph, R.O. and Lambert, D. (1996). *Needs assessment survey of a sample of AMHI consent decree class members.* Edmund S. Muskie School of Public Service, University of Southern Maine, Portland, ME.

Ralph, R.O., Lambric, T.M. and Steele, R.B. (1996). Recovery issues in a consumer developed evaluation of the mental health system. Paper presented at the 6th Annual Mental Health Services Research and Evaluation Conference, Arlington, VA.

Repper, J. and Perkins, R. (2003). *Social inclusion and recovery: a model for mental health practice.* Bailliere Tindall, London.

Ridgway, P.A. (2001). Re-storying psychiatric disability: learning from first person narrative accounts of recovery. *Psychiatric Rehabilitation Journal,* **24,** 335–43.

Roberts, G. and Wolfson, P. (2004). The rediscovery of recovery: open to all. *Advances in Psychiatric Treatment,* **10,** 37–49.

Romme, M. and Escher, S. (1993). *Accepting voices.* MIND Publications, London.

Stein, L.I., Barry, K.L., Van Dien, G., Hollingsworth, E.J. and Sweeney, J.K. (1999). Work and social support: a comparison of consumers who have achieved stability in ACT and clubhouse programs. *Community Mental Health Journal,* **35**(2), 193–204.

Stein, L.I. and Santos, A.B. (1998). *Assertive community treatment of persons with severe mental illness.* Norton, New York.

Stewart, E. and Kopache, R. (2002). Use of the Ohio Consumer Outcomes Initiative to Facilitate Recovery: Empowerment and symptom distress. Available: http://www.mhrecovery.com/ Boston%20Poster%20full%20version%20PDF.pdf

Szasz, T.S. (1960). The myth of mental illness. *American Psychologist,* **15,** 113–18.

Thornhill, H., Clare, L. and May, R. (2002). Recovery from psychosis: stories of escape, enlightenment and endurance presented by Thornhill, H., Holloway, J. and Weaver, Y. to the MIND Annual Conference.

Topor, A. (2001). *Managing the contradictions: recovery from severe mental disorders. SSSW no 18.* Department of Social Work, Stockholm University, Stockholm.

Turner-Crowson, J. and Wallcraft, J. (2002). The recovery vision for mental health services and research: a British perspective. *Psychiatric Rehabilitation Journal,* **25**(3), 245–54.

Van Os, J., Hanssen, M., Bijl, R.V. and Ravelli, A. (2000). Strauss (1969) revisited: a psychosis continuum in the general population? *Schizophrenia Research,* **45,** 11–20.

Walcraft, J., Read, J. and Sweeney, A. (2003). *On our own terms – users and survivors of mental health services working together for support and change.* The Sainsbury Centre for Mental Health, London.

Warner, R. (1994). *Recovery from schizophrenia: psychiatry and political economy* (2nd ed.). Routledge, New York.

16

Developing a local research network for mental health

David Rogers

INTRODUCTION

The Department of Health and the National Health Service as a whole spends close to half a billion pounds per year on research (DoH Website 2004). This represents a small proportion of the total UK health R&D expenditure, which recent estimates set at £4 billion for research alone (Harrison and New 2001) – although much of this is commercial research driven by the pharmaceutical industry and related sectors. In the late 1980s, the UK Government, reacting to general public concern about the state of publicly funded health-related research, set up a Parliamentary Review (House of Lords 1988). The Review argued that the NHS, like industry, 'should ensure that the fruits of research are systematically transferred into service'. The current NHS R&D funding programme is a product of that review. However, over the last ten years, a growing literature on implementing research and evidence-based practice in health care is being supplemented by a larger, critical literature on the notable fact that although much research and development is undertaken, little of this has had much impact on the work of practitioners and the care that consumers of the health service receive. A large and costly gap is still evident between research and practice. Nowhere is this more evident than in mental health service provision: there are still large gaps between what our researchers have found, and what practitioners do. Intriguingly, there are still aspects of mental health that are not as well investigated as they could be. In particular, the fields of mental health promotion, primary care management of mental ill health, access to services and the needs of carers are all under-researched (DoH 2002).

One aspect of this is that research can easily become uncoupled from clinical practice and clinical need (Haynes 1990; Haines and Jones 1994). Recently, however, a number of influential reviews and strategies have recommended closer partnership working between Higher Educational Institutions and NHS organisations. So, while in the context of research, it is often argued by practitioners that the competing demands of the Research Assessment Exercise (RAE) and the NHS R&D agenda uncouple institutional agendas – there is now real recognition of the need for closer dialogue and integrated working.

In the out-patient department, on the ward, and in the community team, there still, however, needs to be closer links between researchers and practitioners, so that research is relevant to practitioners' needs, so that practitioners are willing to participate in research and increasingly to ensure that clinical priorities are recognised as research priorities. While there is evidence that some researchers can promote their own work and do engage with practitioners, in general researchers have not been systematically involved in the implementation of their own findings and may not be well equipped to do this (Haines and Donald 1998).

By bringing researchers, clinical practitioners and other stake holders together, the potential for high-quality research that is relevant to the needs of the NHS is increased. Furthermore, while the NHS remains a national health service it continues to be a service that is provided locally – where variations in practice, service delivery and local contexts are notable. Nowhere is this more clear than in the Clinical Governance Review reports by the Commission for Health Improvement, and the widely reported NHS star rating system. With such wide variations, researchers need to be experts at dissemination and contextualising their work for practitioners. An overview of systematic reviews of interventions to promote the implementation of research findings found that the passive dissemination of research through publication and related strategies, while the most common approaches adopted by researchers, is generally ineffective. The authors argue for the use of specific strategies to implement research-based recommendations and highlight that more intensive efforts to alter practice are generally more successful (Bero *et al.* 1998). One of the more alluring models that has been proposed to enable research to influence practice is the conceptual framework for implementing evidence-based practice by Kitson *et al.* (1998). In their work, the authors identified that most successful implementation of evidence occurs when the evidence is high quality, but notably, where the context is receptive to change, with sympathetic cultures and appropriate monitoring and feedback mechanisms. The context is critical, and Kitson *et al.* delineate 'culture', 'leadership' and 'measures' as key indicators of context. Facilitation of evidence was also highlighted as a crucial feature of successful implementation (Kitson *et al.* 1998).

POLICY BACKGROUND

The UK Government is implementing the most comprehensive programme of modernisation the National Health Service has seen since its inception. The modernisation agenda was articulated in the publication of the *NHS plan* [DoH 2000), and for mental health services, in the *National service framework for mental health* (DoH 1999). *The NHS plan* articulated the need for new and smarter ways of working. Implicit within this was highlighted the need for more innovative responses to the demands placed on services by patients and the public, with a growing expectation for greater choice. With such great pressure for change, it is evident that existing models of service delivery need to change. Ferlie and Pettigrew (1996), in a key paper, argue that the shift towards a modernised service through policy and management initiatives is consistent with a shift towards a networked approach to service delivery. The needs of patients and the complexity of their problems, require service responses that cut across existing structural, geographical and professional boundaries. The development of managed clinical networks are such a response. The concept emerged from the Calman-Hine report on cancer services (Expert Advisory Group on Cancer 1995), the Scottish Office for the NHS, and Acute Services Review (Scottish Office 1998). It was further defined by the Scottish Executive in a response to the Acute Services Review, as linked groups of health professionals and organisations from primary, secondary and tertiary care, working in a co-ordinated manner, unconstrained by existing professional and health board boundaries, to ensure equitable provision of high-quality, clinically-effective services throughout Scotland (MEL 1999). In 2000, the South-East Regional Office produced a discussion paper on managed clinical networks noting that such networks can add value, but also noting that there is no one model for them and that there is a need to learn from experiences of establishing these networks.

Because managed networks can operate across organisational, geographical, and professional boundaries they are ideally suited to the development of research and the implementation of research findings. The Department of Health has funded the development of the National Cancer Research Network, the Mental Health Research Network, and the development of regional primary care research networks. These funded networks are beginning to provide impetus and influence both research and clinical practice. It is clear that they are bringing together both clinicians and academics in ways that are leading to new perspectives on services enabling innovation to happen, and for a high-quality and relevant research agenda to be developed. A wide range of informal and some formal local research networks exist. These are mostly in the form of research alliances within districts, or across strategic health authority regions. A good example of one such network is the Nottinghamshire, Derbyshire, and Lincolnshire Research Alliance, whose website is found at http://www.research-alliance.org.uk/. The Alliance aims to improve research collaboration between different health sectors, increase external research income and increase research output and quality. On a practical level, it aims to avoid unnecessary overlap and duplication, share R&D management resources and skills and initiate 'cross-boundary' events. In mental health, two events were organised under its auspices – a seminar to develop the research agenda around the issue of patients with unexplained physical symptoms, and the launch of a primary mental health care research network within the region. The critical mass that is created through the involvement of 16 NHS, academic and statutory organisations has enabled a greater shared understanding of research at the interface across all of these organisations, but, more importantly, has enabled the beginning of a whole systems approach to research at regional level.

Local, organisation-wide research networks also have a powerful role in enhancing research capacity and capability and are ideally placed to drive innovation and evidence-based practice within services.

Nottinghamshire Healthcare NHS Trust has been developing the concept of 'innovation networks'. These are networks of researchers, practitioners, service users, and managers. The inclusion of health care practitioners and academic researchers from different disciplines and contexts will bring different interpretations of problems to research and of evidence to implement. As a consequence, negotiation between disciplines and organisational groups will be required to find a way of researching or putting into practice, whatever new idea or innovation is embodied in the problem identified, or the 'evidence' being introduced to practice. Thus, an innovation process will be stimulated when the individuals in the network decide to adopt the new idea, practice or technology. The key for us is the 'newness' to the network (Rogers 1983), so that anything perceived as new by the people doing it is relevant. Moreover, this approach recognises that the process of innovation will be different for other networks or organisations introducing the new idea, practice or technology (Downs and Mohr 1976).

PHILOSOPHICAL BACKGROUND

The research process, including the diffusion of research knowledge into practice is essentially a socially orientated process. As discussed earlier, critics of research highlight the lack of integration between academic researchers and clinical practitioners and services. The difficulty, cited earlier, of getting research into practice, and of researchers undertaking clinically relevant research is a product of this lack of integration.

DIFFUSION OF INNOVATION

A growing range of research in the fields of innovation diffusion has highlighted the role of social networks in the diffusion of new ideas and products. One of the early studies of diffusion was a classic study of the spread of the use of a new antibiotic among doctors in Illinois in the early 1950s. It showed that the innovative early adopters of a new antibiotic were more integrated and less socially isolated than those who were later adopters. They had attended more medical meetings out of town and had more extensive social networks than did those who adopted the drug later (Menzel and Katz 1955).

Rogers describes the adoption of innovation in his seminal work, *Diffusion of innovations* (Rogers 1983), in which he shows how interpersonal networks are essentially homophilous in nature. Homophily is the degree to which individuals who communicate with each other, are similar in certain attributes such as beliefs, education, social status and so forth. This concept originates in the work of Lazarsfeld and Merton (1964), and earlier, in the work of Gabriel Tarde (1903) who noted that social relations are much closer between those individuals who resemble each other in occupation or education. Heterophily is the degree to which individuals differ. Homiphily and effective communication are bound together in a self-perpetuating cycle. Differences in language, beliefs, education, social status or technical awareness lead to disagreement and mistaken meaning. Heterophilous communication has qualities that can add advantage to networks. For example, heterophilous network links often connect quite different networks or groups and are important in spreading information about ideas and other innovations. The work of Mark Granovetter (1973) highlights that while homophilous networks consist of individuals with similar characteristics and results in strong ties that bind them to the network, they tend to circulate the same information, ideas and innovations. Weak ties, however, are more apt to have different characteristics and social links than the core members of a network and are more likely to spread the information, innovations and ideas. In his study of Boston job seekers, he found that individuals had often heard about their positions from hetereophilous individuals who were not close colleagues or acquaintances. Crucially, Granovetter argued that weak ties were much more important than strong network links because an individual's close friends and colleagues seldom know much that the individual does not also know. Close friends and colleagues also usually tend to form close-knit groups or cliques that form an interlocking personal network that, while sustaining the relationships, tend to perpetuate existing ideas and information, making newer ideas and information harder to be accepted and implemented. Granovetter argues that if weak ties were somehow removed from a system or network, the result would be a series of unconnected and separate cliques. Homophily, therefore, can be a barrier to the diffusion of innovation, the development of research and the implementation of best practice and research evidence as it can lead to a closed network that absorbs and is slow to adopt new ideas due to this more closed and inherently conservative social environment.

The concepts of homophily and hetereophily in social networks are helpful in understanding the diffusion of innovation and the growth of research cultures. This is particularly the case in mental health services where a wide range of professionals vie for ascendancy and ownership of the intellectual territory embodied in research evidence and research practice. A striking addition to the concept of homophily is what

Halliday (1985) describes as the power of 'knowledge mandates'. These are, effectively, how professions create and reinforce bastions of information that only they are privileged to own and apply. Typically, such information is embodied as know-how and 'evidence' and such 'knowledge mandates' are used to consolidate their positions in organisations and society as a whole. It is useful to note that such knowledge mandates are driven and strengthened through the informal networks that exist and in which issues such as clinical evidence and research are negotiated and appropriated. The continuing challenge of implementing evidence-based practice is made harder when such evidence is 'out in the open', for example, in NICE guidelines, research papers, and other forms of guidelines – and where all professions position themselves to challenge the mandate of each other to own whatever knowledge is being promoted.

A great deal of research suggests that formal reporting relationships, codified knowledge such as guidelines, protocols, and procedures – and the diffusion of such knowledge – are only a small part of actual management, and that informal networks influence organisations in many ways more powerfully through informal influence and lobbying. Information networks are in a position to influence through the relationships of people in four key roles. These roles are hubs, boundary spanners, information brokers and peripheral experts (Cross and Prusak 2000). 'Hubs' are individuals who seem to know everyone, and who put individuals in touch with each other in a network through their tacit knowledge of others' expertise and knowledge. 'Boundary spanners' connect informal networks with external groups, for example with other agencies, or health care services or types of organisation. Through their relationships with external agencies they are well positioned to access and disseminate useful information. 'Information brokers' connect groups and networks within the organisation rather than outside the organisation. They provide and share information across organisational structures and hierarchies. 'Peripheral experts' act as outsiders in any given network. They are typically brought into the network to provide advice or to complete tasks. Business consultants, advisers and specialists are a good example of peripheral specialists, as they are not typically members of staff but contribute expertise and skills at crucial times and places within a network. Within mental health services, an example of a 'boundary spanner' is a psychologist to three community mental health teams. Because the psychologist is not a core member of the team, he or she is in a powerful position to convey information to and from each of the teams, for example, about innovative approaches to practice, and what works or doesn't work within each of the other teams.

SOCIAL CAPITAL

Networks have the potential to generate a high degree of social capital. Social capital refers to the ability of organisations, networks, alliances or groups, to engage and empower the individuals within, in ways that are inclusive and meaningful. High levels of trust, reciprocity, participation and informal support are key indicators of successful networks and organisations with high levels of social capital. The more included and supported individuals feel: the greater is their sense of autonomy. A major advantage to organisations with high social capital is that individuals with a greater sense of autonomy are in a position to take responsibility, be proactive and innovate, generating creative responses to organisational and clinical challenges. Amabile (1988) argues that people are at their most creative when they are motivated primarily by the interest, enjoyment, satisfaction and challenge of the work itself, and not by external pressures. Also noteworthy is the idea that, where there is a high degree of role autonomy for individuals, networks are move effective in sustaining a high degree of social capital.

INTELLECTUAL CAPITAL

One of the leading proponents of the concept defines intellectual capital as the sum of everything and everybody in an organisation: it is the knowledge of a workforce (Stewart 1997). In the context of mental health services this refers to the stock of knowledge from the 'ward to the board'. Intellectual capital incorporates the knowledge that individuals have acquired through training and other forms of educational endeavour, including research and practice development. More importantly, intellectual capital incorporates the insights and experiences of day-to-day interactions about which approaches work, in which particular contexts, and with whom. A significant amount of this type of knowledge can be made explicit, and embodied in guidelines, protocols, manuals and procedures. A great deal of knowledge, however, is tacit – in that, as mentioned above, it consists more of 'know how' than of 'know what'. Intellectual capital that is 'know-how' is best shared, explored and understood in groups, networks, and communities of practice.

COMMUNITIES OF PRACTICE

The concept of 'communities of practice' was the result of different approaches to learning theory by two academics from quite different academic traditions. Jean Lave, a social anthropologist and Etienne Wenger, an expert in artificial intelligence, came up with a model of 'situated learning'. This proposed that learning is not separated from our daily working lives and is not best experienced in the typical didactic pupil–teacher–classroom context, but rather, learning involves a process of engagement within a community of practice. Wenger and Lave argue that communities of practice are everywhere, and we are generally involved in a number of them as core members or on the boundaries. Wenger (1998) argues that a community of practice is defined by (1) its purpose – what it is about, how that is understood and redefined through its membership, (2) how it functions – how the membership engage with each other into a socially cohesive group and (3) what capability it produces – for example, the shared repertoire of communal resources (routines, products, documents, language, events, approaches) that members have developed over time. A community of practice needs to involve, therefore, a great deal of interaction, debate and practice. Wenger (1998) argues that the interactions involved, and the ability to undertake complex challenges, projects and activities, requires co-operation that brings practitioners together, and which facilitates, in turn, relationships and trust. Ultimately, through the concept of communities of practice, Lave and Wenger (1998) position learning as something that is done, and knowledge acquired, through relationships with others.

THE NOTTINGHAMSHIRE INNOVATION NETWORK MODEL

At Nottinghamshire Healthcare NHS Trust, the R&D department is responsible for undertaking and supporting high-quality, relevant, mental health orientated research. With the inception of clinical and research governance, and the emphasis that the Commission for Health Inspection and Audit place on the management of evidence-based practice, R&D offices are critical in ensuring that best practice and high-quality research evidence is disseminated and implemented, where possible, in practice. In Nottingham, the R&D office is responsible for seeking out areas where the organisation is pursuing, or might pursue, opportunities for the development and application of new evidence from research programmes and feed these into the service planning process. The R&D office has developed an Innovations Unit that will have two key functions – one is the diffusion of evidence to practitioners, and the other is the development of innovation networks based around care groups and specific clinical themes. The Innovation Unit is, in effect, a virtual unit, consisting of R&D staff and associates to support the two functions mentioned. The Innovation Unit will provide support and a hub for the purposes of knowledge management and strategy development to a range of 'innovation networks'. The innovation networks are responsible for creating, sharing and diffusing knowledge, expertise, ideas and service innovations, that in themselves lead to new researchable ideas and the development of proposals for research funding or service development. The R&D office is running three pathfinder innovation networks: primary mental health care, arts and mental health and a practice-based evidence network. These pathfinder networks are in the process of developing their strategies, and were launched in early 2004. A proposal to recycle R&D funding to invest in up to twenty such innovation networks has been approved by the Trust Board and these will be launched in 2004. The pathfinder networks are developing their strategies for the marketing, PR and communication of the networks, alongside their strategies and business plans.

A strategy for the marketing, PR and communication of the Innovation Unit and networks needs to be developed alongside the delivery plan.

The Trust has agreed to fund these innovation networks on the basis of a number of expected features or critical success factors. These are listed below.

Features of a funded innovation network

1. Leadership
    i. Intellectual (academic) lead
    ii. Clinical lead
    iii. Network co-ordinator
2. Membership
    i. Academic
    ii. Clinical – multi-disciplinary

   iii. Service users

   iv. Carers

   v. Other interested parties

3. Funding (£5K pump-priming)
4. A strategy, including aims, objectives, vision
5. A work plan
   i. Collaborative projects
   ii. EBP – sharing best practice
   iii. Research proposals (external funding)
   iv. Seminar series or planned events
6. Communication strategy (internal, external, PR and 'scientific')
7. Performance management
   i. Annual Report
   ii. Regular briefings to Research Executive Team
   iii. R&D Annual Report
   iv. Research and Clinical Governance Reports.

Critical success factors

Ability to provide evidence of

1. Impact and influence on clinical services within the network field
2. Impact and influence on clinical governance
3. Publication profile
4. Research and other grant income profile
5. Membership profile (research-based qualifications, grants, publications).

CONCLUSION

The emphasis of these networks has been on the generation of innovations, the sharing of good practice and the building of a research culture through shared understanding and knowledge. Although there is a focus on clinical and research governance, our intention is to develop communities of practice that are not stifled by the imperatives of governance and 'the must dos' but to allow individuals the necessary 'head-space' to explore and make sense of their working environments and lives in a way that allows innovative approaches and responses to research and practice. Wenger (1998) describes communities of practice as having a range of developmental stages. He describes these as (1) potential – where people face similar situations without the benefit of a shared practice or exploring commonalities; (2) coalescing – where members come together and recognise their potential, and explore connections and define their common goals; (3) active – where members engage in developing a practice – joint activities, creating products and artefacts and influencing practice; (4) dispersed – where members no longer engage intensely but the community is very much an active entity where members contact each other for advice; and finally, (5) memorable – where the community is no longer central but people still refer to it and tell stories about 'its work' and refer to its products.

Wenger (1998) also describes how communities of practice may have different types of relationships to the official organisation and corporate structure and strategy. He describes these as unrecognised (or invisible to the organisation), 'boot-legged' (only visible informally to the circle of people in the know), legitimised (officially sanctioned as a valuable entity), strategic (widely recognised as central to the organisation's success) and transformative (capable of redefining the organisation as a whole).

Beyond the unrecognised and boot-legged communities of practice, the innovation networks within the Trust may operate in different relationships to the organisation – so all of them may be legitimised, some may be strategic, while perhaps a few may evolve into networks that have transformative potential. Interestingly, by offering the unrecognised and boot-legged networks some legitimacy through funding and organisational support, we may have the potential to leverage some very powerful innovations as their work becomes more readily available to the whole organisation.

The challenge for the organisation, R&D and the innovation networks is to ensure that they do not become stifled by elitism through the establishment of cliques rather than networks, or by short-term organisational pressures, management demands, bureaucracy or political pressures. At the same time, it is vital that they are sufficiently porous as to ensure that new ideas are absorbed and considered, and that interests, stakeholders and approaches are accepted and considered within the networks. The insights and ideas developed from the fields of innovation diffusion, sociology, and networking, coupled with the emerging insights from practitioners of social and intellectual capital have a powerful role to play in contributing to robust and influential innovation networks.

Finally, the work of Wenger and Lave in developing the concept of communities of practice is a significant contribution to the debate around the research–practice gap, and the development of true praxis through innovation networks in mental health care and other settings.

References

Amabile, T. (1988). A model of creativity and innovation in organizations. *Research in organizational behavior*, **10**, 123–67.

Bero, L.A., Grilli, R., Grimshaw, J.M., Harvey, E., Oxman, A.D. and Thomson, M.A. (1998). Closing the gap between research and practice: an overview of systematic reviews of interventions to promote the implementation of research findings. *British Medical Journal*, **317**, 465–8.

Cross, R. and Prusak, L. (2002). The people who make organisations go– or stop, *Harvard Business Review*, **80**(6), 105–12.

Department of Health. (1990). *National service framework for mental health.* HMSO.

Department of Health. (2000). *The NHS plan.* HMSO. DoH Website, Accessed February 2004: http://www.dh.gov.uk/PolicyAndGuidance/ResearchAndDevelopment/ ResearchAndDevelopmentAZ/NationalNHSRDFunding/fs/en).

Downs, G.W. and Mohr, L.B. (1976). Conceptual issues in the study of innovation. *Administrative Science Quarterly*, **21**, 700–14.

Expert Advisory Group on Cancer to the Chief Medical Officers of England and Wales. (1995). *A policy framework for commissioning cancer services. (The Calman-Hine Report).* Department of Health, London.

Ferlie, E. and Pettigrew, A.M. (1996). Managing through internal networks: some issues and implications for the NHS. *British Journal of Management*, **7**, Special Issue: S81–99.

Granovetter, Mark. (1973). The strength of weak ties. *American Journal of Sociology*, **78**, 1360–80.

Haines, A. and Donald, A. (1998). Making better use of research findings. *British Medical Journal*, **317**, 72–5.

Haines, A. and Jones, R. (1994). Implementing findings of research. *British Medical Journal*, **308**, 1488–92.

Halliday, T. (1985). Knowledge mandates: collective influence by scientific, normative and syncretic professions. *British Journal of Sociology*, **36**, 421–47.

Harrison, A. and New, B. (2001). The finance of R&D in healthcare. *Healthcare UK: the King's Fund review of health policy*, pp. 26–44.

Haynes, R.B. (1990). Loose connections between peer-reviewed clinical journals and clinical practice. *Annals of Internal Medicine*, **113**, 724–8.

House of Lords Select Committee on Science and Technology. (1988). *Priorities in medical research.* HMSO, London.

Kitson, A., Harvey, G. and McCormack, B. (1998). Enabling the implementation of evidence based practice: a conceptual framework. *Quality in Health Care*, **7**, 149–58.

Lave, J. and Wenge, E. (1991). *Situated learning legitimate peripheral participation.* Cambridge University Press.

Lazarsfeld, P. and Merton, R. (1964). Friendship as a social process: a substantive and methodological analysis. In *Freedom and control in modern society* (eds Berger, M. *et al.*). Octagon, New York.

Menzel, H. and Katz, E. (1955). Social relations and innovations in the medical profession: the epidemiology of a new drug. *Public Opinion Quarterly*, 19, 337–52.

NHS Executive South-East Regional Office. (2000). *Managed clinical networks.* NHS Executive, South East Regional Office, London.

Rogers, E.M. (1983). *Diffusion of innovations.* New York Free Press.

Stewart, T.A. (1997). *Intellectual capital: the new wealth of organizations.* Doubleday, New York.

Strategic Reviews of Research and Development – Mental Health, DoH, 2002 – available at: http://www.dh.gov.uk/assetRoot/04/06/87/03/04068703.pdf. Accessed March 2004.

The Scottish Office. (1998). *Acute services review report.* The Stationery Office.

The Scottish Office. (1999). Introduction of managed clinical networks within the NHS in Scotland. MEL (1999) 10. The Scottish Office.

Tarde, G. (1903). *The laws of imitation.* (Translated by Porson, E.C.). Holt, New York.

Wenger, E. (1998). *Communities of practice.* Cambridge University Press.

Wenger, E. (1998). Communities of practice. Learning as a social system, Systems Thinker, http://www.co-i-l.com/coil/knowledge-garden/cop/lss.shtml. Accessed January, 2004.

17

Prison mental health

David Sallah and Alistair McIntyre

INTRODUCTION

The modernisation agenda for health care in the Prison Service has been given a greater impetus by the establishment of the Prison Health Task Force in 1999. The enormity of the task to be resolved as far as health needs are concerned, however, seems to be endless. For example, about 90% of all prisoners have a diagnosable mental health or substance misuse problem or both. It is also estimated that 5,000 prisoners are seriously mentally ill and the rate of suicide in prisons is sixteen times that of the general population. Furthermore, 10% of female prisoners and 7% of male prisoners have a history of self-harm, and 20% of prisoners who misuse illicit drugs by injection (and there are about 16,000 prisoners) are infected with hepatitis B and 30% with hepatitis C, about 13% of the prison population has a diagnosis of asthma and 80% of all prisoners are smokers.

Given these figures, the need to identify, treat and manage prisoners (particularly those with mental health problems) and promote positive mental health practice has been identified as a crucial health-promoting activity by the European region of the World Health Organisation (WHO) Health in Prisons Project (WHO 2000a). The potential harm that imprisonment can have on the mental health of prisoners is described by WHO as important for everyone and not only for those who have been diagnosed as suffering from mental disorders, because it underpins all health and well-being in the prison setting. This theme is further strengthened in the *NHS plan* (DoH 2000), which earmarked resources to employ 300 additional staff to enable the necessary changes to happen.

While it is appropriate that prison regimes are necessarily structured around the need for containment and control, it is true that this focus of emphasis tends to create tension between security and therapeutic ethos of any secure institution. This dilemma is a clear reality for practitioners who care for prisoners with health care needs, particularly of those with mental health problems.

The focus of current policy development is that the NHS should have direct accountability for the health care needs of prisoners; this change in approach is known as the 'principle of equivalence'. In this chapter, we chart some of the key milestones in providing care to prisoners. Furthermore, we develop our thinking by outlining some of the consequential aspects of this so called 'principle of equivalence' and discuss what we believe should be done to improve the mental health needs of prisoners.

HISTORICAL CONTEXT

Society in the middle ages controlled its 'least desirable or unacceptable elements' (for example, those with contagious diseases e.g. leprosy) through excluding them from society, cities (and other communities) and 'locking them outside the gates'. In the sixteenth century, with the eradication of leprosy from Western cities, society faced a challenge to its social order. Its response was to maintain a social structure by demoting citizens they perceived as having the lowest social standing to fill the vacant role of 'underclass'. This new 'underclass' became the new societal outcasts. By the middle of the seventeenth century, exclusion from the cities had become an inadequate means of control and with the opening of the 'Hospital General' in Paris, in 1656, this was the first time confinement had been used as a form of control for the anti-social and unsocial elements of Western society. However, people with mental illness remained, for the most part, living in the community assimilated within a larger group comprising the morally disreputable, the poor, vagrants and minor criminals (Foucault 1974).

Over the next three hundred and fifty years, advances in knowledge and understanding and their application to the 'care and treatment' of people with mental health problems has gradually, but steadily, changed. Notably societal attitude, acceptance of diversity and government policy contributed to engineering the gradual development of society which is becoming increasingly tolerant (knowledgeable and supportive) towards those experiencing mental health distress. This apparent cultural maturation and 'civilisation' of Western society was a witness to a marked transformation in attitudes to those suffering with mental illness.

In the middle ages, the pervasive doctrine of the day (predominantly Christian) had dominated the care and treatment of those suffering mental distress with an out-of-sight-out-of-mind policy (Scull 1979). It was not until the work of Franz Joseph Gall on the 'new science' of phrenology, in the early-nineteenth century that an increasingly scientific view was brought to bear in this context. Gall had claimed that psychological phenomena were at last able to be studied through scientific means – through observation and not speculation (Gall 1807). A challenge to the domination of the religious order and its rights to administration over the 'insane' was made by the medical professions and the role of religion in the care and treatment of the mentally ill was to diminish (mirroring it's weakening in society at large). It was not until the late-twentieth century that any real challenge of note to the established paradigm of confinement and treatment was to emerge. This despite reported successes of more homely care and treatment such as the Geel Community in Belgium, which still exists (Goldstein J.L. and Godemont 2001) and its Quaker-led 'clone' at The Retreat in York, England (Scull 1979).

In the UK, early asylums and the like had been established as business enterprises, but the Poor Law Act of 1927 and the Local Government Act of 1930 signalled an end to the era of the workhouse. With this growing interest amongst physicians in the care and treatment of the mentally ill, and the National Health Service Act of 1946, a system of care and treatment developed (see also Webb, Sydney and Beatrice 1910).

The Mental Health Act of 1950 (and its revision in 1983) established a framework of rights that sought both to protect individuals in society, and establish rights for the individual experiencing distress. This legislation helped to prepare society for the acceptance of subsequent government policy on community care and further development of the rights of the individual, as in the Human Rights Act 1998. Like other clinical areas of health care in England, the pace of change (modernisation) in the NHS has been swiftest during the last decades of the twentieth century. In the 1990s, challenges to the models of care that had existed previously saw the beginnings of the 'community care' movement with policy changes heralding the closure of the 'old' long-stay institutions to be replaced by new and smaller units attached to general hospitals (HMSO 1990). However, a subsequent twenty-year gap in the development of government policy to support new models of service and the lack of any earmarked funding helped to sustain a service development vacuum. Consequently, progress on developing models of community support was to be most notable elsewhere. The very services that had been most inspired by the progress made in the UK were themselves to become international leaders and inspire a new generation. These services had viewed the closure of asylum care as a direction of travel and not a destination; they had asked questions about the care system such as: If the asylum closes, what next? What if the model of care and support is different? How would this affect an outcome for the client/patient? What do citizens value and how can we develop services to support that?

SERVICE DEVELOPMENT

A small number of services began to try out alternative models of care. For example, the Mental Health Center of Dane County in Madison Wisconsin (USA) had worked to provide support and maintenance for people outside of the traditional hospital setting and clients reported better outcomes, confirming some of the earlier successes from the communities at Geel and York. The acceptance of these new models of care and treatment for people with severe and enduring mental illness has been slow. In the twenty years since action was first taken a ground swell of opinion has grown, steadily championing the cause of the patient (service user) with an accompanying grudging acceptance (by some custodians of treatment) that treatment for people with mental illness in the community could deliver improved results for the service user.

Of course, there have also been advances in the development of more effective psychotropic and psychological treatments and these have contributed to a reduction in the number of care beds and the gradual demise of long-term institutional (asylum) care. A return to community was heralded as the new doctrine with services in Vermont and also in Keene, New Hampshire, rated as the best mental health services in all of the 50 States of the USA. In these services, a holistic approach was taken, including provision and support for housing, for access to leisure and support for employment. In the 1990s, reported success of these services began to stimulate interest in other countries leading to the beginnings of a much-needed paradigm shift in policy development and direction in the UK.

The UK Government's mental health strategy *Modernising mental health services* (DoH 1998) set out a new direction for the Government in its mental health policy. This shift in policy direction was quickly followed by the *National service framework mental health* (DoH 1999), which was designed to focus activity and the *NHS plan* (DoH 2000), which set out the strategic deliverables for the NHS. These mental health policies of the late 1990s have been broadly welcomed as they reflect a trend across the Western world of increasing access and choice. The mental health services responded by developing a strong consumer focus, and this in turn contributed to the creation of a growing divide between the choice and standards of care and treatment for those outside, and those inside, prison. It is time to redress this imbalance and to provide answers to the questions we raised earlier.

The conviction for a criminal offence is not a just cause for the removal of access to the same standards and quality of health care as is available to any member of the community. The Human Rights Act 1998 set out a set of basic human rights which the UK Government signed and adopted; albeit fifty years late. The Reed Report (1992), which examined the care and treatment of mentally disordered offenders was a milestone in the development of services for mentally disordered offenders. Over a decade after the publication of the Reed Report, it is clear that with the new paradigm for care and treatment outside of prison together with the modernisation programme for the NHS, the current situation of differentiation of care and treatment between NHS patients and prisoners cannot remain unchanged.

CURRENT STATE OF PRISON MENTAL HEALTH SERVICES

In 2003, the Prison Service reported that over 200,000 people entered or left prison on a daily basis. Of this number, the Office for National Statistics reported that the prison population in England and Wales increased by 20% between 1997 and 2003. This means that at the end of July 1997 there were 61,944 detainees in prisons in England and Wales but by December 2003 this number had risen to 74,084 prisoners; an increase of 12,140 prisoners and rising. There is also a corresponding rise in prison establishments from 131 prisons in 1997 to 140 prisons in 2003. These figures include considerable numbers of prisoners with significant mental and physical health problems. Some were receiving treatment before entering prison, but others have serious undiagnosed conditions. In a recent survey by the prison service, it found that 90% of those entering prison had a mental health or substance misuse problem (*Prison health handbook* 2003). Surveys conducted by the Office for National Statistics in 1997 indicated that nine out of every ten prisoners have at least one of the five disorders considered in the survey (neurosis, psychosis, personality disorder, alcohol abuse or drug dependence); while between 12% and 15% of female prisoners have four of the five disorders (see also Tables 17.1 and 17.2 below). The picture is even worse among young offenders (under 21 years of age), since 95% of them have a diagnosis of mental illness, or substance abuse problem, or both, and many also have personality disorders (*Changing the outlook* 2001). Clearly, imprisonment provides invaluable opportunities to address some of these health issues.

HEALTH CARE IN PRISONS

It has always been the aim to ensure that prisoners get health care to standards equivalent to those in the NHS, a concept commonly referred to as 'the principle of equivalence'. But it is generally recognised that this aim is not met in many prisons and in some places the gap between NHS standards of care and prisoner care is obvious. Health care in prisons should promote the health of prisoners i.e. identify prisoners with health problems; assess their needs and deliver treatment or refer to other specialist services as appropriate. It should also continue any care started in the community.

Because prisons vary in size, type and prisoner need, the aim according to the prison service must be to provide mental health services that respond to individual prisoners' needs (*Changing the outlook* 2001). However, it is somewhat curious that prison health services have been the responsibility of the Home Office while health services for the general population have been with the Department of Health. This has led to a less than equal service for prisoners, especially mentally disordered prisoners. This is why, in an effort to secure higher standards of health care in prisons, the establishment of a formal partnership between the Prison Service and the NHS was agreed in 1999. The partnership was originally led by two national joint units, a Policy Unit and a Task Force Unit, which came into being on 1st April 2000. In order to strengthen the work of these policy changes, the Government announced the transfer of funding for prison health care from the Prison

Service to the Department of Health and the re-organisation of the Policy Unit and Task Force Unit into a central unit. These changes set the stage to enable and sustain change in all prisons across the country to take place. This partnership for providing appropriate services and delivering appropriate care was therefore accepted as the bedrock for change in the prison service (*Prison health handbook* 2003).

The important thing is to understand that effective health care delivered to a good standard while in custody, even for a short period, can make a significant contribution to the health of individuals. As 80% of those people in prison are there for only six months or less, it is essential that continuity in care provision is assured, so as to equip prisoners with the skills and confidence they need to return to, and make a positive contribution to, their local communities. Tackling the mental health problems of prisoners can contribute to reducing crime and re-offending rates, as well as helping to respond to the problems caused by social exclusion. The prison service should be seen to be providing treatment to offenders in prisons as a contribution towards the Government's wider goals of reducing crime and social exclusion.

INCIDENCE OF MENTAL ILL HEALTH AMONGST PRISONERS

The most comprehensive study of the prevalence of mental illness in the prison population in England and Wales was carried out in 2000 by the Office for National Statistics (ONS). Tables 17.1 and 17.2 below summarise both the sample size against the category of prisoner and the corresponding numbers of prisoners by category of detention at the time of the survey in 1997.

In total, 3,142 prisoners completed the survey. Table 17.2 shows the percentage of those prisoners who were interviewed, by the main

Table 17.1 Sample size		
Prison population July 1997	Prisoner category	Sample size
46,872	Male sentenced prisoners	1,250
12,302	Male remand prisoners	1,121
2,770	Female prisoners	771

Table 17.2 ICD10 categories			
Diagnostic category	Male remand	Male sentenced	Female
Personality disorder	78	64	50
Psychotic disorder	10	7	14
Neurotic disorder	59	40	76
Suicidal thoughts (lifetime)	46	37	59
Alcohol misuse	58	63	39
Drug dependence	51	43	41

classification of mental disorders (using the International Classification of Disease −10).

Figure 17.2 shows that personality disorder was prevalent most amongst male remand and sentenced prisoners. These prisoners tended to be young, unmarried, from a white ethnic group and had been detained for acquisitive offences (robbery, burglary or theft), or violent behaviour.

Female prisoners had a higher prevalence of psychotic and neurotic disorders, and also had a higher prevalence for self-harming behaviour and were the group who had thought about or attempted deliberate self-harm most during their lifetime. They were found to be more likely to report experiencing neurotic disorders than their male counterparts. This was across all sub-categories, apart from obsessions and compulsive disorders. Furthermore, hazardous drinking and illicit drug misuse were reported as higher in male prisoners and the characteristics of this group were similar to the characteristics of the group with personality disorders – reflecting a high level of co-morbidity of these disorders. Furthermore, the survey revealed that the median 'quick test' scores of intellectual functioning were lower than would be expected in the general population.

CO-OCCURRENCE OF MENTAL DISORDERS

A large proportion of prisoners interviewed were identified as having several mental disorders. Fewer than one in ten showed no evidence of any of the five disorders considered (personality disorder, psychosis, neurosis, alcohol misuse and drug dependence) and no more than two out of ten in any sample group had only one disorder. Generally speaking, it is a fair assumption that at any one time 80–90% of prisoners have a mental illness. Gunn *et al.* (1991) reported that of the 5% of the prison population in significant distress, 2% are psychotic and 3% requiring transfer to an NHS facility. The Office of National Statistics (White 1997) found that 7% of male prisoners and 14% of female prisoners were experiencing significant mental distress. Overall, it was found that this distress was more than just the psychological reaction to imprisonment.

Another aspect of note is the impact of imprisonment on people from ethnic minorities. Three million people in Britain, 6% of the population, do not classify themselves as white and are assumed to belong to minority ethnic groups (ONS 2000). A further 1.5% of the British population are born in Ireland, with the total number of people of Irish descent (first and second generation) reaching as much as 1.7 to 1.95 million people or 3.5% of the population. In inner city areas, up to 45% of the population are from the black and minority ethnic groups, showing a predominance of cultural and ethnic groups that were traditionally considered to be in the minority, and are still considered as immigrants, despite significant levels of integration and acculturation.

The influence of culture on the expression of distress, on its recognition during consultations, and on illness behaviour, offer challenges to the prison service. Reviews of the mental health care of black and minority ethnic people in the USA and the UK show a similar picture of over-representation among forensic populations, different rates of treatment with medication and variations in access to care. NACRO, the crime reduction charity, asserts that the inmate population of prisons in England and Wales contains five times the number of black people found in the population at large. It further revealed that black people found guilty of offences are sentenced to custody sooner and for longer periods than white people (Nacro 2003). The ethnic representation in the prison population in 2000 was 18% of all male and 24% of all female prisoners, which is significantly higher than in the general population.

Such findings have prompted special concerns about discrimination, inequity in care provision and the need for policy response to organise changes in practice which lead to systematic improvements in the quality of care offered to minorities. The higher rates of detention in in-patient services from the black community, and the greater likelihood that black patients will be detained during their treatment, raise special concerns about the use of coercion where there is a cultural gap in communication. This view is espoused variously that such systematic differences in outcome may be the outcome of institutionalised discrimination enshrined in routine mental health care practice. This presents greater challenges to mental health services to be both culturally and racially sensitive to provide the necessary range of different skills and attitudes required to provide effective care and treatment to prisoners from black and ethnic minority backgrounds who also have significant mental health needs. Clearly, the case for change in the care of prisoners is overwhelming.

THE POLICY CONTEXT

That the prison environment may not be good for physical or mental health is hardly a new revelation; for example in 1992, the Reed Review indicated that the care and treatment of mentally disordered offenders was poor. Seven years later, in 1999, Her Majesty's Chief Inspectors of Prisons described the prison service as overcrowded with poor quality of prisoner care, shortage of resources and inactivity. Marshall and colleagues, in developing a toolkit for prison health needs assessment, argued that prisons can act as breeding grounds for many communicable diseases, introduce prisoners to new unhealthy practices and consequently seriously worsen their mental health (Marshall 2000). Furthermore, the current state of mental health service provision in prisons has been highlighted as a growing concern as it is now recognised that the incidence of mental health disorder amongst prisoners is increasing (DoH 1999 and 1998a; Home Office 1996).

The English mental health strategy (DoH 1998b) set out Government policy and started a sea change in the direction of mental health policy and practice. The mental health policies of the late 1990s have been broadly welcomed and this has greatly increased access and treatment to services. These services have also responded by developing a strong consumer focus, and this in turn has created a greater divide between the standards and care of treatment for those both outside and inside prison.

The modernisation agenda for health care in the Prison Service has been given a greater impetus by the establishment of the Prison Health Task Force. We have outlined the enormity of the task to be resolved and it seems to be endless. Consequently, the need to identify, treat and manage prisoners with mental health problems and promote positive mental health practice has been identified as a crucial health-promoting activity even by the European region of the *World Health Organisation health in prisons project* (WHO 2000a). The potential harm that imprisonment can have on the mental health of prisoners is described by the project as important for everyone and not only for those who have been diagnosed as suffering from mental disorders, because it underpins all health and well-being in the prison setting. Clearly, the task ahead covers a vast range of issues; from basic awareness of maintaining positive mental health to the identification and intervention of severe mental illness. This theme is further strengthened by the *NHS plan* (2000) which earmarked resources to employ 300 additional staff to enable the necessary changes to happen. In order to manage the problems in prison health care, the Prison Service and the NHS have agreed to work together to achieve an effective service (*Prison health handbook* 2003).

The Prison NHS Partnership, launched in 1999, set out to open up access to comprehensive health care with the same standards as are available to people in the wider community. To provide a strong link to the central strategy teams, regional health authorities and their local prison area managers set up prison health task forces to support local prisons in conducting health needs assessments and the provision of action plans to modernise health care, deliver services which met the needs identified in the assessment process and ultimately to oversee the transition of prison health care to the NHS.

EMERGENCE AND ROLE OF PRIMARY CARE TRUSTS

Shifting the balance of power (DoH 2002) has, the government would have us believe, moved decision making and accountability to a more local level than any previous arrangement. Replacing 90 commissioning bodies (health authorities) there are now 260 Primary Care Trusts that receive funding directly from the Department of Health. Of these Primary Care Trusts, approximately half have a prison within their boundary and will become the commissioner responsible for prison health care services for the population during 2004 to 2006 (there is a phased transition with health care in approximately twenty prisons due to transfer from April 2004). This proliferation in commissioning responsibility has indeed taken decision making to a more local level. It has also created a significant number of commissioners eager to develop skills and experience in this area – this is a huge challenge both to the

NHS and to prison health care. Health care commissioners now have performance targets, which ensure appropriate provision of services to meet the needs of prisoners returning from prison to live in their areas.

NEW DEVELOPMENTS

In the light of this policy pronouncement few initiatives are in train to improve the quality of care to prisoners. Mental Health In-Reach is the service for the improvement of mental health services for prisoners in line with the objectives of the *NHS plan* (DoH 2000). The NHS funds the establishment of multi-professional teams (in-reach teams), offering to prisoners the same sort of specialised care as they would have if they were in the community. It is likely that all prisoners with mental health needs will benefit to some degree from the in-reach services, but the early focus is on those with severe and enduring mental illness. In-reach staff have the advantage of working in local prisons while being employed by the NHS, and are therefore able to develop and maintain links between both areas. In-reach is essentially wing-based, with the relevant staff providing counselling services and mental health promotion for prisoners and support for prison staff. They also ensure prisoners have equal access to the services to which they are entitled.

The first phase of in-reach schemes started in April 2001 in 12 prisons in England and 4 in Wales. A further 6 prisons came on-stream in November 2001 with another 40 prisons during 2002 to 2003, and ultimately, the 60–70 prisons considered to have the greatest mental health need during 2003 to 2004. The in-reach project is supported through the 'collaborative' approach, where the learning and experience can be shared among those involved. However, those prisons in which it is established should not assume that in-reach by itself will solve all the mental health problems of their population. These teams come together at regular intervals to consider their work and options identifying what has worked well and what has been less successful. The collaborative is supported by a central co-ordinator. They have to complete a detailed review of mental health needs, based on their existing health needs assessment work, to identify gaps in provision between what was available and to develop action plans to implement the changes needed to fill these gaps.

As part of this partnership, there are already 150 new NHS mental health staff and this number will double by the end of 2004. This will ensure that 5,000 prisoners at any one time will receive more comprehensive mental health services, reaching in to prisons and treating people on the wings. The intention is that every mentally ill prisoner would have a care plan on release and a care co-ordinator to help him/her engage with services once back in the community. In order to measure the effectiveness of the strategy as a whole there are some clear performance indicators, such as a reduction in the number of prisoners located in prison health care centres. Other performance indicators are a reduction in the average length of time mentally ill prisoners spend in the health centres and a more appropriate skill mix among those providing mental health care. This is so that prisoners have access to the right range of services at NHS standards and have quicker and more effective arrangements for transferring the most seriously ill prisoners to appropriate NHS facilities, and receiving them back to continue their sentence, where appropriate. The Care Programme Approach (CPA) is one of the key elements of mental health care policy and is now extended to prisoners. Prisoners who were on CPA before entry to prison now have their treatment programmes set out for them and continued as far as possible within the prison setting. Another model of enhancing the quality of care for prisoners is through day care services, an arrangement that offers the benefit of access to more specialised services. The aim of this new service is to provide a non-threatening therapeutic environment, which helps individuals to identify specific problems and receive appropriate interventions for them. The establishment of day care within prisons is particularly beneficial to prisoners who receive care with minimum disruption to them and to prison staff, who will be able to focus on the provision of care without the added problems of supervision.

SUICIDE PREVENTION

Suicide prevention is a major goal of the Prison Service since 9% of all suicides in prison occur during the first 24 hours in custody, 27% during the first week and 43% during the first month (*Changing the outlook* 2001). Recently, five women killed themselves in a Manchester prison, making the issue of self-harm and an attempted suicide in Britain's jails a major theme. It has been suggested that a way to prevent this would be if courts stopped sending people with serious mental health problems to prison (Bright 2003). The picture in the NHS is somewhat different. The reform and modernisation agenda is beginning to deliver real change and benefit to patients. Waiting lists and times are shorter and mental health has reported that the suicide rate is continuing to fall.

The first annual report outlining progress with the implementation of England's national suicide prevention strategy (see DoH 2001) is showing a sustained fall in the number of suicides. Although the overall rate of suicide is falling, there are still around 4,500 deaths from suicide in England each year. The prison service's experience on the other hand is showing very little improvement.

WORKFORCE IMPLICATIONS

The challenges of the NHS in modernising its mental health services pail into insignificance when the paradigm shift that is required to bring the prison mental health services to the NHS current standards is considered. Here, we will concentrate on the workforce issues that need to be identified and met for the change in philosophy and approach to be delivered. We discussed some of these problem areas earlier, particularly from the perspectives of the health needs of prisoners and the policy shift necessary to meet those needs. Given the rapidly changing nature of the prison population and the gravity of health problems that need to be managed, continuous training and development of all prison staff is a very necessary undertaking. Continuous development as both a philosophy and as a process activity should be built on the new culture of lifelong, self-directed, problem-based learning. Concentration on basic mental health training and awareness should not be seen as adequate to meeting the changing needs of prison staff. Charlton (2001) provided the underlying philosophy to this viewpoint by maintaining that in promoting continuous development of staff, training should not be seen as an end point but just an attainment of a standard. In a survey in one of the larger local prisons in the West Midlands health region, researchers from the University of Wolverhampton compared data from the general population were compared with the proportions obtained from prison staff. In order to do this the data were transformed into binary groups using a cut-off point derived from the national study. Table 17.3 below shows the results; significant differences are highlighted. It should be noted that because several tests have been done there would be an increased risk of the possibility of type one errors occurring.

The null hypothesis for each test was that there would be no difference in the proportions agreeing or disagreeing between the prison staff and the general population. Significant differences were found with the following items. 'One of the main causes of mental illness is a lack of self-discipline and will-power' ($p < 0.001$) with 84% of the prison staff sample disagreeing with the statement compared to 66% in the general population. When asked should 'less emphasis be placed on protecting the public from people with mental illness' (16%) of the prison staff agreed compared to 34% of the general population ($p < 0.001$). Seventy-four per cent disagreed with the statement 'people with mental illness should not be given any responsibility', compared with 86% of the general population ($p < 0.001$). The probability was less than 0.001 when 65% of the prison staff agreed with the statement 'people with mental illness are far less of a danger than most people suppose', 34% of the national sample were in agreement with this item. Forty-four per cent of the national sample compared with 31% of the prison sample strongly agreed with the statement 'as far as possible mental health services should be provided through community based facilities' ($p < 0.001$). When asked how far they agreed with the statement 'residents have nothing to fear from people coming into their neighbourhood to obtain medical health services', 53% of the prison sample stated that they agreed, whilst 33% of the national sample did ($p < 0.001$). The probability equalled 0.001 for the question 'as soon as a person shows signs of mental illness he/she should be hospitalised' with 58% of the prison sample strongly disagreeing compared with 42% of the general population.

The probability was less than 0.05 for the following question 'mental hospitals are an outdated means of treating people with mental illness'; 30% of prison staff agreed with this statement compared with 40% in the general population sample. The item 'virtually anyone can become mentally ill' was agreed to by 97% of the prison population and 92% of the general population. Nationally, 19% agreed with the statement 'most women who were once in a mental hospital can be trusted as babysitters' compared to 26% of the prison sample.' Finally, 44% of the general population strongly agreed with the statement 'as far as possible mental health services should be provided through community based facilities' as opposed to 31% in the prison sample.

Another revealing aspect of this study was that training to equip prison staff with the required knowledge, skills and attitudes was said to be less of a priority to the prison hierarchy. It is important here to

Table 17.3 Four binomial tests comparing percentage of agreement/disagreement on attitudes to mental illness scale items between prison staff and the general population

Question	Agree/disagree	n	% Prison staff	% General population	Significance
One of the main causes of mental illness is a lack of self discipline and will power	*Disagree*	92	84	66	.000
There is something about people with mental illness that makes it easy to tell them from normal people	Disagree	78	71	64	.079
As soon as a person shows signs of mental disturbance, he/she should be hospitalised	Strongly Disagree	64	58	42	.001
Mental illness is an illness like any other	Agree	74	67	76	.021
Less emphasis should be placed on protecting the public from people with mental illness	Agree	18	16	34	.000
Mental hospitals are an outdated means of treating people with mental illness	Agree	33	30	40	.017
Virtually anyone can become mentally ill	Agree	108	97	92	.030
People with mental illness have for too long been the subject of ridicule	Agree	98	88	85	.201
We need to adopt a far more tolerant attitude towards people with mental illness	Agree	97	87	88	.479

Table 17.3	Continued				
Question	Agree/ disagree	*n*	% Prison staff	% General population	Significance
We have a responsibility to provide the best possible care for people with mental illness	Agree	103	93	94	.369
People with mental illness don't deserve our sympathy	Disagree	101	91	88	.205
People with mental illness are a burden to society	Disagree	87	76	83	.121
Increased spending on mental health services is a waste of money	Disagree	101	90	90	.425
People with mental illness should not be given any responsibility	Disagree	82	74	86	.000
A woman would be foolish to marry a man who has suffered from mental illness, even though he seems fully recovered	Disagree	52	47	42	.174
I would not want to live next door to someone who has been mentally ill	Disagree	49	44	49	.177
Anyone with a history of mental problems should be excluded from taking public office	Disagree	92	83	76	.056
No one has the right to exclude people with mental illness from their neighbourhood	Agree	71	64	71	.063

Table 17.3   Continued

Question	Agree/ disagree	n	% Prison staff	% General population	Significance
People with mental illness are far less of a danger than most people suppose	Agree	71	65	34	.000
Most women who were once in a mental hospital can be trusted as babysitters	Agree	29	26	19	.037
The best therapy for many people with mental illness is to be part of a normal community	Strongly Agree	40	36	43	.083
As far as possible, mental health services should be provided through community based facilities	Strongly Agree	34	31	44	.003
Residents have nothing to fear from people coming into their neighbourhood to obtain mental health services	Agree	59	53	33	.000
It is frightening to think of people with mental health problems living in residential neighbourhoods	Disagree/ Don't Know	96	87	81	.060
Locating mental health facilities in a residential area downgrades the neighbourhood	Disagree/ Don't Know	79	71	76	.140

remember that a large proportion of prisoners have a mental health or substance misuse problem. When prison staff were asked when they last received any training, 24 out of 111 completing a questionnaire (22%) had either never received training or none had been offered. Others had missed training that had been arranged for them because of staff shortages on the wing resulting in training being cancelled.

The study discussed above has implications for policy makers, prison governors and the NHS in developing and implementing the 'principle of equivalence' of care provision to its successful conclusion, which is to provide appropriate and effective treatment and care to people with mental health problems in prisons. Given the prevalence of mental health problems in the prison population and the key issues highlighted in this study, the need to prepare prison staff to meet these problems effectively is a Herculean task. The views expressed in Table 17.3 above by prison officers should demonstrate a higher level of understanding in all aspects examined in this study compared with that held by the general population.

THE FUTURE PERSPECTIVES

The problems discussed so far require considerable change in structure, people and quality of treatment and care in order to meet the complex health needs of prisoners effectively. During the latter half of the 1900s, the high security hospital system had existed as a system within, but outside, of the mainstream NHS. Until the 1990s, the three high security hospitals had been funded directly by the Treasury and accounted separately from the rest of the NHS through a Special Health Authority to the Secretary of State for Health. As a reaction to the Fallon Inquiry (1999), the growing number of calls that a third of the high security psychiatric estate was redundant based on the needs of patients and the inevitable consequences of reform in the NHS, change reached the high security hospital system. The three high security hospitals were merged into the mainstream of the NHS to become part of local mental health NHS Trusts.

Working together with new regional commissioners the three hospitals developed a set of key performance indicators including forensic case management to support the emerging local NHS specialist commissioning arrangements in their task of managing the necessary movement of individuals to more appropriate placements and to deliver on targets set out in *NHS plan*.

The West Midlands health region's *Strategy for forensic mental health services 2001–2006* focuses on the levels of security offered in mental health services and attempts to identify key aspects of service provision and delivery based on the PDSA (Plan Do Study and Act Cycle) methodology (Berwick 1998) adopted by the prison service nationally to drive service change. This approach is being developed in collaboration with general mental health services and within the substance misuse field. Within this model, local NHS teams of clinicians, service users, carers and other stakeholders together map out a service by identifying the time taken at each stage and between each stage in the identified process as it actually works at the time. The team then agrees on the way to improve the process focusing on the following key principles:

- The Care Programme Approach (CPA) is established in prisons
- The mental health promotion element of the health promotion strategy is implemented in prisons
- Transfers between prisons and other NHS facilities are improved
- Training needs arising from the collaborative process are identified and provision made.

The move to integrate prison health care with local NHS services is a strong and much-needed change. However, much effort will be needed to ensure that beyond the transfer of financial responsibility the partnerships forged over the last two years remain strong and healthy and based on assuring an effective structure, governance and accountability. This should then be the foundation upon which improvements relating to access to, and choice of, services underpinned by a greater sense of promoting race and cultural sensitivity should be made. Integration brings new opportunities for the prison workforce to be developed and trained and commissioners of services to acquire and strengthen new skills.

The future development of health care for prisoners has to go beyond promoting healthier living. The strength of local partnerships must be greater than simply having the human resource to produce more glossy reports describing local issues and needs. The focus of change and for research and development has to be the sharing of effective evidence-based interventions and other supports that are linked to informed and competent commissioning. There needs to be clear evidence that commissioners do more than tinker with last years investment and activity and that the total financial envelope is reviewed and utilised to underpin service modernisation. Put simply, it is about developing and sharing knowledge; what works, as well as working to integrate the cultures of custody and punishment with that of access to high-quality health care, which is delivered by culturally well-informed and responsive staff. In addition to this, there are issues relating to the medicines management concordance and choice that has been agreed by the prison service and the NHS. This concordance should not be viewed from the cost control perspective alone, but also to foster a more open dialogue with the prisoner with mental health problems, to allow and support the development of consistency in prescribing regimes and monitoring of (self-managed) medication to reduce drug dependence. Importantly, in this approach to managing drug dependency, there is a need to explore ways in which information about medication and its benefits and side-effects can be balanced with the experiences of the same by the prisoner.

We started from the basis that it is a major goal of policy makers to ensure that prisoners receive the same quality of care as in the NHS. This aspiration would not be achieved unless those with obvious or diagnosable mental health problems received appropriate treatment and care while those with less obvious levels of mental illness are identified and treated. Prison officers should be aware and play a key role here, as they are in a position to observe prisoners' behaviour daily on the wings, as it is known that not all cases of mental ill health could be spotted at reception. As we outlined, there is a need for staff to be appropriately trained so as to recognise these problems, something that is not the case so far. For instance, as we reported in the University of Wolverhampton study, we found that prison officers had received little or no training in mental health care, and exhibited the same misconceptions as the general population (see also Armitage *et al.* 2003).

CONCLUSION

The Chief Inspector of Prisons reported that there is a clear gap between treatment and conditions in which sentenced and unsentenced prisoners were held; the balance of advantage lying invariably with sentenced prisoners (Her Majesty's Chief Inspector of Prisons 2000). He concluded that as a result of this, many mentally disordered individuals enter prison as remand prisoners without any prior assessment by mental health staff. In much stronger terms, the Chief Inspector of Prisons described the culture in most prisons as being plagued with the apparent cynical way prison officers viewed the introduction of new programmes and changing work practices. He explained further that this cynicism, which is clearly noticeable amongst older staff, is affecting new recruits who begin with enthusiasm but are ground down by domination and intimidation, which he described as a pernicious way of influencing colleagues (Her Majesty's Chief Inspector of Prisons 2000). Prison regimes are necessarily structured around the need for containment and control. This focus of emphasis tends to create tensions between security and the therapeutic ethos of any secure institution. This dilemma is a clear reality for practitioners who care for prisoners with health care needs, particularly those with mental health problems. Clearly, the prison environment is not the best place to care for mentally ill and vulnerable people. The task ahead for the care of mentally disordered offenders is therefore formidable without evidence, which is grounded in the experiences of the key stakeholders. We are certain that we have provided a picture of how things are currently and have outlined the key steps that needs to be in place in order to make a success of current initiatives designed to improve the care needs of prisoners.

References

Berwick, D.M. (1998). Developing and testing changes in delivery of care. *Annals of Internal Medicine*, **128**(8), 651–6.

Bhopal, R.S. (1998). The spectre of racism in health and health care: lessons from history and the USA. *British Medical Journal*, **316**, 1970–3.

Department of Health and Home Office. (1992). Departmental review of services for mentally disordered offenders. *The prisons group report (Reed Review)*. The Stationary Office.

Department of Health. (1998a). *Psychiatric morbidity among prisoners in England and Wales*. The Stationery Office.

Department of Health (1998b). *Modernising mental health services: safe, sound and supportive*. The Stationery Office, London.

Department of Health. (1999). Joint Prison Service and National Health Service Executive Working Group. *The future organisation of prison health care*. The Stationery Office.

Department of Health. (2000). *The NHS plan: a plan for investment a plan for reform*. The Stationery Office, London.

Department of Health (2001a). *Safety first: five-year report of the national confidential inquiry into suicide and homicide by people with mental illness*. Department of Health Publications (Ref 23425), London.

Department of Health. (2001b). *Shifting the balance of power*. The Stationery Office, London.

Department of Health. (2002). *Shifting the balance of power: the next steps*. The Stationery Office, London.

Fallon, P., Bluglass, R., Edwards, B. and Daniels, G. (1999). The Report of the Committee of Inquiry into the Personality Disorder Unit, Ashworth Special Hospital. The Stationery Office, London.

Foulcault, M. (1974). *Madness and civilisation.* Vintage, 4 Chambliss, W. New York.

Gall, F.J. (1807). Gall first declares that insanity due to brain illness or defect. Doktor Gall über Irrenanstalten. *Allgemeine Zeitung,* 21, Supplement, 81–3.

Changing the outlook. (2001). *Changing the outlook: a strategy for developing and modernising mental health services in prisons.* Prison Service.

Goldstein, J.L. and Godemont, M.L. (2001). *A community mental health care legend. Whatever happened to Geel?* A discussion at 129th meeting of APHA, Atlanta GA.

Gunn, J., Maden, A. and Swinton, M. (1991). *Mentally disordered prisoners.* Home Office, London.

Her Majesty's Chief Inspector of Prisons. (2000). Report of a full announced inspection of HM Prison Birmingham. Home Office, London.

Home Office. (2002). Prison Mental Health Collaborative Launch Document.

Home Office. (1996). *Patient or prisoner? A new strategy for health care in prison.* HM Inspectorate of Prisons, London.

Home Office. (1999). *Changing the outlook: a strategy for developing and modernising mental health services in prisons.*

Home Office. (1999). *Her Majesty's Chief Inspector of Prisons Annual Report.* Stationery Office.

HSC. 1999/223. *National Service Framework for Mental Health. Modern standards and service models for mental health.* Department of Health.

Johnson, B. (2003). *Audit of arrangements for mentally disordered offenders.* NIMHE. West Midlands.

Marshall, T., Simson, S. and Sterens, A. (2000). *Toolkit for health care needs assessment in prisons.* University of Birmingham.

McIntyre, A. (2001). West Midlands Forensic Mental Health Strategy 2001–2006. NHS Executive West Midlands.

Nacro. (2003). http://www.nacro.org.uk/publications/index.htm

Prison Health Handbook. (2003). www.prisonshandbook.co.uk/info.html

Prison Service. (1999). The Future Organization of Prison Health Care: Report by the Joint Prison Service and National Health Service Executive Working Group: Prison Service/NHS Executive – (Free).

Reed, J. (1992). *Review of mental health and social services for mentally disordered offenders and others requiring similar services: Vol. 1: Final summary report.* (Cm. 2088). HMSO, London.

Scull, A. (1979). *Museums of madness: the social organization of insanity in nineteenth-century England.* Allen Lane, London.

Singelton, N., Meltzer, H., Gatward, R., Coid, J. and Deasy, D. (1997). *Psychiatric morbidity among prisoners.* Office for National Statistics.

Webb, Sydney and Beatrice. (1910). *English poor law history.* Longmans Green and Co. London.

White, P. (1997). *The prisonpopulation in 1997: a statistical review.* Home Office Research and Statistics Directorate Research Findings no. 76. ISSN 1364-6540, London.

WHO. (2000a). *WHO health in prisons project.* http://www.hipp-europe.org/resources/

WHO. (2000b). *WHO guide to mental health in primary care.* Royal Society of Medicare Press and www.mentalneurologicalprimarycare.com.

Conclusions

David Sallah and Michael Clark

This book is written to fill the gap that exists for a credible source book addressing the key issues of research and development in mental health particularly as the work of the National Institute for Mental Health in England (NIMHE) evolves. Combining research with development is a crucial aspect of closing the gap that exists between research and practice. We are confident that mental health practitioners and those preparing to enter the research field will find the issues addressed in the chapters of this book both useful and informative.

There is often a complex, convoluted and usually lengthy process of conducting research and of getting research into development and then identifying further research needs. The Department of Health has recognised this and has taken some steps to address some of the problems across its whole NHS R&D strategy, for example, the research governance framework. Where the focus of research was once determined by the sometimes idiosyncratic interests of the individual health professional – usually a doctor – now it is more coordinated by central government and interested groups and reflects the areas that the government considers central to its programme of NHS modernisation. Recent policy statements indicate that research should be undertaken close to where clients and patients are being cared for rather than by academics in academic settings, research that often takes a generation or longer to get into practice. The illustration of this theory/practice divide is presented in the case of Thomas Arnold who was Superintendent of the Leicester Asylum in the mid-nineteenth century and who formulated three principles of mental health care. As is shown in Chapter 4, this could be achieved through early detection of illness, preparing appropriate interventions and developing good social support once the patient was discharged.

In mental health, the creation of the Mental Health Research Network in readiness for a co-ordinated approach to identifying what works and what should be done to implement these findings is a step in the right direction. Hopefully, this approach will improve the organisation, delivery and implementation of research and its findings in mental health. Perhaps the Health Research System model in Chapter 1 will eventually help to develop better theory driven strategy and allow comparison with, and learning from, other countries. In Chapter 9, the authors have dealt with this issue by highlighting how the Department of Health is now more systematically trying to develop a research and development strategy across the mental health portfolio. It is worth pointing out here that this effort on the part of the Department of Health is largely in terms of a more coherent research strategy that is aligned with development needs defined nationally, with a better infrastructure to deliver larger scale projects through the Research Networks. While there are strengths and weaknesses in such an approach (overall a very positive approach), the question is: does the approach provide a better strategy for research and development to ensure research is actually taken up into development? There is some progress on this but the jury is out.

There are challenges to the world of research and the methodologies employed within mental health. For example, as shown in Chapter 2, much of the challenge in mental health research has been the development of discrete and valid outcomes measures and verification that these are clinically relevant. Another element of work is to elucidate, specify and evaluate complex interventions, which are the mainstay in mental health care. The emphasis on quantitative research has been checked recently by demands for more meaningful research into the values found in mental health settings, user-focused research and research into the therapeutic value of relationships. This call for a different form of mental health research seems over-determined where it seeks to render quantitative research methods meaningless, or remote from the concerns of the public and of patients. The authors of Chapter 2 have asserted that complementarity between diverse research traditions has rarely been achieved, but active debate at the 'edges' of specific research paradigms is promising. In Chapter 3 the author developed the case for qualitative approaches. The author in making a case for qualitative approaches, maintained that while all research is important to the development of knowledge within and across disciplines, there are arguments that support the idea that research ought to show its value to the wider community. However, no one single research paradigm can provide all the different knowledge that is required for a discipline, neither can it meet all the knowledge needs of the community. What qualitative research does, then, is to attempt to understand, describe, explain and make sense of the social world. It is, therefore, a valuable means of creating an understanding of a phenomenon. Accordingly, qualitative research is necessary for the knowledge, practice, education and policy related goals of some mental health professionals and the formal area of mental health care. In Chapters 2 and 3 we set out the place of both quantitative and qualitative research within mental health settings and mental health care. The key message emanating from the various contributions on methodologies is inclusivity, partnership building and managing diversity. Clearly, this message is resonating with the policy responses detailed in Chapters 9 and 10. The role of networks in delivering a sustainable research and development programme is an interesting one in terms of linking research and development as shown in Chapter 16. The successes of the national Mental Health Research Network will in part depend on learning the lessons of other, local networks such as those as described in Chapters 16 and 12. The achievements of Dementia Plus, as discussed in Chapter 12, show a successful different approach which is focused on developing a network that sits astride a number of worlds – different organisations, localities and professions – and can link across them but which also provides a link between research and development by taking research to organisations in the form of training, consultancy and innovation. While involving localities and communities directly in research is clearly a positive approach, another problem to address is making research and evaluation directly relevant to practice through local partnerships.

We have outlined and discussed various areas for research in the future in this book; for example, in the areas of race and mental health and women and mental health. In the case of race, ethnicity and mental illness/health there is a growing body of knowledge helping to deconstruct the complexity and contradictions for research therein. Subjectively these topics evoke a variety of emotional responses that could range from fear to denial and prejudice. Utilising these constructs in research therefore brings us to one of the most contentious spheres of knowledge construction as well as to policy and service development in mental health. Concentrating on what works is a better approach to managing these contradictions. Much of the published research on women's mental health has used methodologies such as anecdotal, qualitative and narrative approaches, which are less powerful in terms of scientific replicability or predictability. Qualitative approaches nonetheless are extremely valuable in defining the 'right questions' and in grounding future theories and hypotheses. There are some powerful and consistent messages, which come from women's individual testimonies. However, qualitative approaches are not seen as 'powerful' in terms of bidding for service development resources. Qualitative approaches lack replicability, and if their conclusions are overstated, may perpetuate ineffective interventions. Better-funded 'mainstream' research and audits do not analyse powerful data sets by gender or by ethnicity routinely and thus there is insufficient attention to these differences in response to various therapies and interventions. Gender differences in presentation and response to interventions should be evaluated more systematically and should receive an appropriate share of the 'research revenues' leading to more cost-effective delivery of a range of services. Another area where personal accounts of individuals should inform mental health research and development is that of building resilience and ownership in managing one's own problems or illness. The concept of recovery is relatively new within the field of psychiatry and mental health services with much of the current research emanating from the field of psychosocial rehabilitation and focusing on evidence-based treatments such as family psycho-education, employment and assertive community treatment. In Chapter 15, the author has shown that previous efforts on behalf of mental health service users have focused on finding ways of coping with, and managing, perceived pathological experience rather than focusing on issues of resilience and recovery. While it is true that very little rigorous evidence is available to support the value that recovery has made to mental health service users' health, this evidence must be found.

The specific problems posed by mental health in the prison service have been dealt with (Chapter 17). It is clear there is a need to have access to and to engage fully with prisoners and prison staff in developing a credible research and development plan. The full integration of the service within the NHS in terms of health care provision presents a great opportunity for this to happen.

We set out in this book to explore theoretical, methodological policy and practical issues relating to developing evidence that underpins the evolving modernisation agenda in the mental health field. In order to deal with the key issues of capacity and capability adequately, the contribution that higher education can make should not be overlooked. Higher education institutions will also need to work closely with the NHS in identifying its clinical and effectiveness needs in order that a programme of research that meets the needs of all can be developed. It is here that the development programme meets the research agenda. The NHS policy framework is geared towards increasing the numbers of existing staff studying for higher degrees as the need for knowledge and evidence base for mental health increases. Consequently, most academic institutions are revising their curricula to increase access, particularly on part-time bases. Additionally, current NHS policy for R&D is to develop a greater strategic alignment with NHS priorities, of which mental health is one. Hence, there is a significant amount of effort underway at national and local levels to develop more and higher quality research programmes in mental health that have relevance to service development needs. This pool of new learners needs a concise, authoritative and accessible source book to refer to. We are confident that we have achieved this.

Index

U.W.E.L. LEARNING RESOURCES